PSYCHOTIC DEPRESSION

Psychotic depression is a distinct and acute clinical condition along the spectrum of depressive disorders. It can manifest itself in many ways and be mistaken for schizophrenia. It often induces physical deterioration, mortally dangerous acts toward self or others, or completed suicide. This book aims to help clinical practitioners and trainees describe their observations of psychotic depression, formulate treatment, and express expectations of recovery from illness. It focuses on all facets of the disorder, from clinical history to coverage of the current state-of-the-art diagnostic and treatment protocols. Medical readers of this book will come away able to diagnose and readily treat psychotic depression and thus will be able to serve their patients better. Non-physician readers will come away with the message that this is a terrible illness, but there is hope. This book fills an important gap in the realm of psychiatric literature.

Dr. Conrad M. Swartz is a board-certified psychiatry professor who has written and lectured extensively on depression, anxiety, and the use of electroconvulsive therapy for severe depression.

Edward Shorter is a historian of psychiatry who has written three books on the history of psychiatry and psychosomatic illness.

Also by Edward Shorter

A History of Psychiatry (1997)

Historical Dictionary of Psychiatry (2005)

Psychotic Depression

Conrad M. Swartz
Southern Illinois University School of Medicine

Edward Shorter
University of Toronto

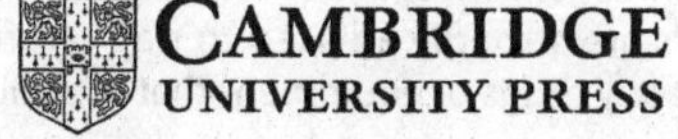

CAMBRIDGE
UNIVERSITY PRESS

32 Avenue of the Americas, New York NY 10013-2473, USA

Cambridge University Press is part of the University of Cambridge.

It furthers the University's mission by disseminating knowledge in the pursuit of education, learning and research at the highest international levels of excellence.

www.cambridge.org
Information on this title: www.cambridge.org/9780521878227

First published 2007
First paperback edition 2012

A catalogue record for this publication is available from the British Library

Library of Congress Cataloguing in Publication data

Swartz, Conard.
Psychotic depression / Conrad M. Swartz, Edward Shorter.
p. cm.
The practitioner's guide to patient-centered psychiatric treatment; v. 1
Includes bibliographical references and index.
ISBN 978-0-521-87822-7 (hardback : alk. paper)
1. Psychotic depression. I. Shorter, Edward. II. Title. III. Series.
DNLM: 1. Affective Disorders, Psychotic – therapy. 2. Affective Disorders, Psychotic – diagnosis. 3. Depressive Disorder – diagnosis. 4. Depressive Disorder – therapy. WM 207 S973P 2007
RC537.S895 2007
616.85′270651–dc22
2007002288

ISBN 978-0-521-87822-7 Hardback
ISBN 978-1-107-40629-2 Paperback

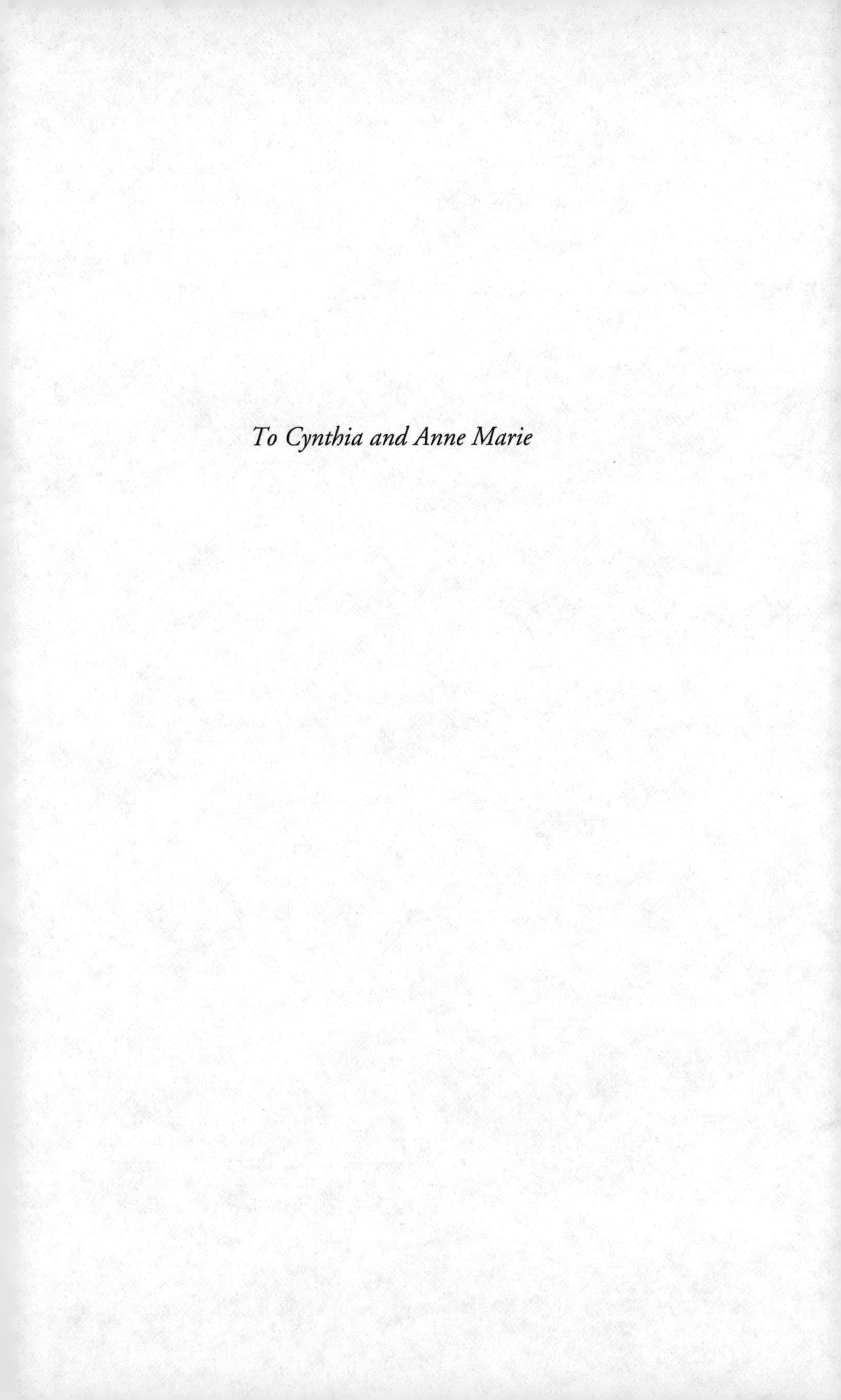

To Cynthia and Anne Marie

Contents

Preface

PSYCHOTIC DEPRESSION is an alloy of psychosis and depression that is not separable into psychosis and depression. Psychosis is a symptom that thought and behavior have become unrelated to reality. It is, in other words, a symptom of madness just as biological as delirium. Psychologists and psychodynamicists often understand illnesses as psychological conditions, caused by psychological conflicts and blamed on unconscious psychological mechanisms. Saying "illness" does not denote "biological" to them. We should like readers to perceive the old-time biological meaning of madness, not through the psychology of the unconscious. Depression is an illness that includes, among other symptoms, the loss of ability to think things through. Patients with psychotic depression have an illness with symptoms of disordered thought, behavior, and mood. They are both delusional and suffer a mood disorder. They are truly physically ill, and their illness represents a terrible suffering for patients and their families, worse so because they cannot describe it. This book aims to help health care professionals find the words to describe their observations of psychotic depression, to work together with their patients to formulate treatment, and to express expectations of recovery from illness. The following pages contain the past, the present, and the future of patient-centered concerns about conventional, and some not entirely conventional, ideas concerning its diagnosis and treatment.

We are trying to reach mainly physicians here, because it is upon their shoulders that responsibility for diagnosis and treatment rests. But we have tried not to make the book so forbiddingly "medical" as to be inaccessible to those outside of medicine such as the patients themselves, their friends and families, and all others interested in or curious about psychiatric illness. It's hard to write both for doctors and patients, for obvious reasons. The pharmaceutical armamentarium so familiar to physicians is a jumble of unfamiliar terms to everyone else. Physicians are accustomed to thinking cooly about diagnoses that patients experience as the horrors of hell and to rationally considering treatments that everyone else deeply fears. The whole alphabet soup of instruments and procedures that doctors take in with the mother's milk of medical school is usually entirely unfamiliar to patients, except terms such as "EEG" that they have encountered in their own experience.

Thus, patients may not consume avidly every last line of the diagnosis chapter because they are mainly interested in the one illness that they have, not in the entire range of phenomena that they could conceivably have but don't. And physicians may smile indulgently at the chapter on subjective aspects of psychotic depression – psychotic depression as the patients experience it. But they should not. Knowing your patients' experience of illness, and being able to succor and advise them appropriately, is part of the practice of medicine. At some level doctors realize they do not feel what their patients experience until they go through the same condition themselves or with a close relative. Of course, this awareness is easily overlooked in the everyday demands of clinical practice. Doctors, please do not imagine that you know all that your patients go through, because you cannot.

Medical readers of this book will come away able to diagnose and readily treat psychotic depression, and thus be able to serve their patients better. Nonmedical readers will come away with the message that this is indeed a terrible illness, but that there is hope. This can be a precious message.

Conrad Swartz is a practicing psychiatrist and an academic scholar who has published on many subjects, and a specialist in medical treatment, electroconvulsive therapy, and psychopharmacology. Much of his research reflects his engineering PhD along with his MD. Edward Shorter specializes in the history of psychiatry and psychopharmacology, and is a PhD. Shorter comes to the story via the trail of age-old suffering; Swartz has spent a lifetime treating patients. Both perspectives are useful and offer a comprehensive picture of what one is up against in this disease called psychotic depression.

Conrad M. Swartz
Edward Shorter

Acknowledgments

SUSAN BÉLANGER, Heather Dichter, and Ellen Tulchinsky in the History of Medicine Program of the University of Toronto have been of great help in various aspects of the preparation of this book. We should especially like to acknowledge the sage advice and practical experience of Marc Strauss of Cambridge University Press and our copy editor Anula Lydia.

1

Introduction

On JUNE 20, 2001, Andrea Yates of Houston, Texas, drowned her five children one by one in the bathtub in her home. She was clearly seriously ill and had been treated with the drugs sertraline (Zoloft), olanzapine (Zyprexa), haloperidol, and lorazepam among other remedies. Her attending psychiatrist had rejected electroconvulsive therapy (ECT) for her on the grounds that it was "for far more serious disorders" (Denno, 2003). She was said to have committed this terrible act in the grips of major depression. But that cannot be right. "Major depression" is not a specific illness. She had psychotic depression. She was improperly diagnosed, evaluated, and certainly inadequately treated. Her illness gave her an overwhelming compulsion or she would not have pushed the heads of her children underwater in the delusive belief that she was saving them from Hell.

Andrea Yates herself was caught in the jaws of Hell. An editorial in the British medical weekly *Lancet* in 1940 called depression "perhaps the most unpleasant illness that can fall to the lot of man"

(*Lancet*, 1940), and in the midst of a psychotic depression, Yates had opportunity to experience this. Psychiatry could have rescued her, but confusion about her diagnosis and her treatment interfered.

The Andrea Yates story had one more chapter, in which the reality of her illness from psychotic depression was finally understood. An appeals court overturned her original conviction because of inaccurate evidence from Park Dietz, a forensic psychiatrist who had testified for the prosecution. In July 2006, Yates again went before a jury, which found her not guilty. "The jury looked past what happened and looked at why it had happened," said her former husband. "Yes, she was psychotic. That's the whole truth." This time Yates was sentenced to an indefinite term in a maximum security hospital (Associated Press, 2006). Thus the story had an end that lifted slightly the flap of public ignorance about this disorder.

What happened to Andrea Yates between her 2002 and 2006 courtroom trials is also noteworthy. In 2002 she was physically fit. In 2006 she was hardly recognizable, flabby and overweight. In television views of her in prison before the 2006 trial she was unkempt and poorly groomed. Under psychiatric treatment her appearance strikingly deteriorated. What types of psychiatric treatments cause such deterioration, and what do not? People avoid psychiatrists because they are afraid of being stigmatized or controlled by psychiatric treatment. Success in treatment includes avoiding stigmatization and behavioral deterioration from the treatment.

Marc Cherry was the producer and scriptwriter of the TV series *Desperate Housewives*. He said that, like Andrea Yates, his mother was at the cusp of a similar experience. He and his mother had been watching the news coverage of the Yates trial one evening and she grunted, "I was once almost there myself." Cherry was so surprised that he said to himself, "If my own mother was once so desperate, then every woman has probably felt the same thing" (Kreye, 2005).

But no! Andrea Yates killed her children in the grips of a delusional depression. However stressed, every woman does not have a psychotic depression, any more that every woman has a pancreatic tumor or a spinal infection. Psychotic depression is as much a medical illness as tuberculosis. It is not a blip on the stress continuum. Mrs Cherry, at one point, as her son said, set to throw her children out the car window, may or may not have had a psychotic depression. But it is a disease, not a normal response.

What is psychotic depression?

There is a classical psychiatric tradition of dividing depression into two types.[1] As Michael Shepherd, the dean of British psychopharmacology, pointed out in 1959, there were hospital depressions and then there were "large groups of loosely termed 'neurotic,' 'reactive,' or 'exogenous' depression often admixed with the clinical manifestations of anxiety. Many of them run a chronic, fluctuating course." They were certainly not suitable for admission to hospital. Most of these patients "do not come to medical attention at all but rely rather on the advice of the chemist [pharmacist] or on self-medication" (Shepherd, 1959).

In one type of depression – Shepherd's hospital depression – brain biology takes over. The depression happens out of the blue. The patients

1 Aaron T. Beck seems to prefer, among possible polar depression types, the "distinction between endogenous and reactive depressions." A. T. Beck. 1967. *Depression: Clinical, experimental, and theoretical aspects*. New York: Hoeber/Harper & Row, p. 66. For his discussion of the difference between "neurotic" and "psychotic" depressions, see pp. 75–86. See also David Goldberg and Peter Huxley. 1980. *Mental illness in the community: The pathway to psychiatric care*. London: Tavistock. The authors argue that there may be a continuum in depressive illness. Yet "... [s]omewhere on this continuum the line must be drawn between those whose mood disorder is impairing their social and psychological functioning, and those in whom normal homeostatic mechanisms may be expected to operate." (p. 15) See, e.g., P[er] Bech. 1988. A review of the antidepressant properties of serotonin reuptake inhibitors. *Adv Biol Psychiatry* 17: 58–69; "We will analyze the depressive inpatients and the depressive outpatients as two different diagnostic entities" (p. 60).

are very sick and may have delusions and hallucinations or sink into stupor. In 1920 German psychiatrist Kurt Schneider, then in Cologne, proposed a term for this kind of depression in which the patients were terribly slowed. He called it endogenous depression,[2] borrowing from the great German nosologist Emil Kraepelin the term "endogenous," by which Kraepelin meant biological, indwelling in the brain, and dominating the body. Schneider contrasted endogenous depression with a second type, which he called "reactive" depression, usually seen outside of hospital settings. Reactive depression has almost nothing in common with psychotic depression except maybe sadness. Yet reactive depression can also be quite serious, the patients hovering on the brink of suicide. But reactive patients are not psychotic nor do they experience the same kind of "psychomotor retardation," to use the technical term for thought and action being slowed. There are two different illnesses here, one involving a terrible, pathological slowing among other symptoms and the other dependent on external events.

Whether there are two depressions or one – and, if two, whether they may be divided into endogenous and reactive – has long been controversial.[3] We step into a snake pit here. But the massive evidence of the history of psychiatric illness does indeed suggest that there are two. For the sake of convenience we call them here endogenous and reactive-neurotic, fully aware that future generations may find these

2 K. Schneider. 1920. Die schichtung des emotionalen lebens und der aufbau der depressionszustaende. *Zeitschrift fur die gesamte Neurol Psychiatr* 59: 281–6. "Bei der betrachtung der depressionszustaende gehen wir von den beiden, in ihren extremen auspraegungen wohl characterisierten typen aus, der reinen motivlosen 'endogen' und der rein reaktiven depression" (In considering the types of depression, we use as a basis the two forms that have been best characterized in their extreme forms, the purely motiveless "endogenous" and the purely reactive depression; p. 283.)

3 Joe Mendels and Carl Cochrane (1968) began the revival of the endogenous-reactive split: The nosology of depression: The endogenous-reactive concept. *Am J Psychiatry* 124 (Suppl): 1–11. Another important early contribution was I. Pilowsky et al. 1969. The classification of depression by numerical taxonomy. *Br J Psychiatry* 115: 937–45. See also the work of Michael Feinberg and Bernard J. Carroll. 1983. Separation of subtypes of depression using discriminant analysis. *J Affect Disord* 5: 129–39.

terms inadequate. Yet the present state of science does not permit us to go beyond them, and whatever one chooses to call them the fundamental reality is that two classes of depressive illness exist, as unalike as chalk and cheese. Most practitioners will probably agree with this, even though they are forced into the procrustean one-depression bed by the official diagnostic schema – the *Diagnostic and Statistical Manual (DSM)* of the American Psychiatric Association – that is now current.

One distinguished believer in the two-depression concept is Joe Schildkraut at Harvard. In 1965 Schildkraut devised one of the most influential ever biological theories in psychiatry. He said that affective disorders (depression and mania) result from disturbances in the metabolism of the neurotransmitter norepinephrine. Chemically, norepinephrine belongs to the "catecholamine" class of neurotransmitters, and Schildkraut's ideas became famous as the "catecholamine hypothesis of affective disorders."[4] Schildkraut, as other observers, saw that there were two kinds of depression. Later, he characterized the endogenous disorders as "running out of gas depressions" and the reactive as "chronic characterological depressions." (He actually did not use the term reactive but rather "depressions with much more in the way of . . . self-pity and histrionics." Yet it means the same thing: a chronic character meets a distressing environmental event.) Schildkraut called the endogenous concept "more a European notion, a notion that might be called by some vital depressions, because you didn't have to have a depressed mood. It was based on having a loss of vitality, anergia, anhedonia and psychic retardation." He said that such depressions, unlike the reactive, "did not readily change with ongoing interpersonal interactions or environmental events. It was a kind of fixed-stuck disorder."[5]

4 Joseph J. Schildkraut, interview. 2000. The catecholamine hypothesis. In David Healy (ed.) *The Psychopharmacologists*, vol. 3. London: Arnold, pp. 111–34, at p. 131.

5 See note 4.

A tradition exists of calling endogenous depression melancholia. Psychiatrists once resisted the term melancholia because it harked back to the days when deep depression was associated with humoral theories of "black bile" and the melancholy constitution. Yet the term melancholia has such historical heft that many prefer it to the rather jargonish-sounding "endogenous." Bernard Carroll affirmed emphatically in 1982, after discovering that a biological test (the dexamethasone suppression test) was relatively specific for melancholia, "Our results give unequivocal support to the view that melancholia is a categorically distinct entity from non-endogenous depression" (Carroll, 1982). In 2006 Michael Alan Taylor and Max Fink re-endorsed in a comprehensive overview the existence of melancholia as a separate diagnosis (Taylor and Fink, 2006). In our view, melancholia is one type of endogenous depression, but when speaking generalistically the two terms are interchangeable.

There are various types of endogenous depression. In catatonic depression, the extreme form of which is stupor, movement and speech are slowed. In melancholic depression, the patient has a sickly persona, and movement and speech may also be "retarded." In this book, we are interested in the type of endogenous depression called "psychotic," characterized by delusions and hallucinations. As Chapter 3 explains, there are various forms of psychotic depression that are really more or less independent illness entities in their own right. Psychotic depression is not actually a disease of its own but a collective term for a number of illnesses having the common properties of depression and psychosis. Of hospitalized patients with endogenous depression, about half are psychotic.[6]

Psychotic depression is highly dangerous. The patients' thinking becomes so delusive that, having lost contact with reality, they

6 Of 225 patients with primary unipolar affective disorders admitted to the Iowa University Psychiatric Hospital between 1935 and 1940 (part of the "Iowa 500 Study"), 52% revealed delusions. See William Coryell and Ming T. Tsuang. 1982. Primary unipolar depression and the prognostic importance of delusions. *Arch Gen Psychiatry* 39: 1181–4.

contemplate suicidal behavior, taking poison perhaps to kill off the hallucinated bug infestation (although it kills them). As London psychiatrist Thomas A. Munro, a psychiatrist at Guy's Hospital in London, pointed out in 1949, "The treatment of depression is always a great responsibility. The patient's life is at stake" (Munro, 1949).

Psychotic depressions can also be risky for others. As with Andrea Yates, periodically there are terrible stories of psychotically depressed parents who murder their children to save them from the fires of Hell or the doom the parents know lies ahead. Thus, the English *Drug and Therapeutics Bulletin* advised in May 1965 as follows: "Another reason for admitting severely depressed patients to hospital is that on occasion they murder relatives or friends in an attempt to spare them imagined pain."[7]

In psychotic depressive illness we are therefore discussing a variety of endogenous depression, depressions that may end up in hospital. Reactive depressions, on the other hand, come on slowly, under stress, and are filled with anxiety, anger, or dissatisfaction. The symptoms of reactive depressions tend to be vague, formless, and primarily subjective. In today's psychiatry, reactive distress tends to be called by a range of terms that are really all over the map, from adjustment reaction, major depression, depression "not otherwise specified," or dysthymia, to the whole anxiety spectrum, such as generalized anxiety disorder or some other anxiety diagnosis, to personality disorders such as borderline personality, or even dissociative disorder. The term neurosis formerly applied in many cases. The psychoanalysts once considered these patients, perhaps not incorrectly, as having a character disorder. A number of additional conditions doubtless huddle under the shelter of reactive distress, including chronic fatigue syndrome (formerly neurasthenia), weltschmerz, and the emotional consequences of poverty, pain, and threatening medical illness.

7 See May 28, 1965, Antidepressant therapy, *Drug and Therapeutics Bulletin* 3(11): pp. 41–3, at p. 42.

In the vast mass of "depression" diagnoses that are handed out today, many patients will have such a reactive depression: the depression comes on in response to bad news rather than out of the blue. The patients' thought and movement are not abnormally slowed as in endogenous depression. Unlike psychotic depression, which answers readily to ECT, reactive depressions do not respond so well to ECT. The phrase "reactive depression," by the way, was abolished in 1980 in American psychiatry with the advent of a new recipe-based classification manual called *DSM-III*. Yet, the term reactive depression delineates a basin of distressed patients with a mixture of sadness, weariness, and anxiety that is difficult to circumscribe well, and there is no reason why it should not soldier on.[8]

Endogenous depression is an entirely different beast. The patients are not necessarily sad but slowed in thought and deed, sometimes to the point of stupor. The patients complain that their minds move slowly and their movements are laborious and painful. In the psychotic variety of endogenous depression the patients are not always slowed, and may have a hint of mania, exhibiting such features of agitation as pacing and repeating "It's my fault, it's my fault." Yet the main point is that the patients are tormented by delusions of various kinds; in an earlier era their delusive thoughts often involved their irremediable sinfulness; today, hypochondriac delusions about one's organs turning to concrete and the like come to the fore. Endogenous illness does not have the same favorable promise of remission that is lent to reactive depression, although after about 8 months most untreated endogenous patients get over it (for the time being). Patients with endogenous depression are often inclined to seek oblivion, so that suicide is always to be feared, as

8 It is true that reactive depression has not been without its critics. As Swiss psychiatrist H. J. Bein put it, "It must, of course, be borne in mind that . . . in all the so-called reactive depressions, the qualifier 'reactive' is only a reflection of the investigator's empathy for a given situation." H. J. Bein. 1978. Prejudices in pharmacology and pharmacotherapy: Reserpine as a model for experimental research in depression. *Pharmakopsychiatrie Neuropsychopharmakologie* 11: 289–93, at p. 291.

actually happens in perhaps one in seven of the untreated cases. (But in nonendogenous depression too the patients may attempt suicide, and the psych emergency wards are very familiar with them.)

"Endogenous depression should be looked upon as an acute disease, like appendicitis; it cannot wait," one Swedish psychiatrist told a Scandinavian symposium from the floor in 1960. He remembered a patient from his practice in Linköping, referred with the following information, "The patient is recommended for examination at a psychiatric clinic." There was nothing more. "We phoned the doctor but he was not in, and then we wrote – as we usually do – requesting details of the case. Three days passed before we got any news and the same day the patient committed suicide, taking with him a daughter of five years."[9]

Finally, endogenous depression is "autonomous"; it does not get better with good news.[10] Your lover has just moved back in? Guess what, your psychotic depression has not improved. As psychopharmacologist Donald Klein once told Robert Spitzer, the mastermind of *DSM*-III, in a moment of irritation, "I think that the distinction between the relatively autonomous depression and the relatively reactive depression is a strikingly important one that should be present in this edition [the forthcoming *DSM*-III-R in 1987]. That also speaks for the utility of a mood-reactive depressive disorder."[11]

DSM-IV in 1994, no longer under Spitzer's control, did incorporate the notion of mood reactivity, but made it a characteristic of major depression with "atypical features," meaning what is often called "atypical depression." Yet the disease designers included alongside "mood reactivity," "interpersonal rejection sensitivity," which means basically

9 Gerdt Wretmark, in discussion. In Erik S. Kristiansen (ed.) 1961. *Depression: Proceedings of the Scandinavian Symposium on Depression, 26–28 October 1960.* Copenhagen: Munksgaard, pp. 138–9.

10 Pioneering the distinction between "autonomous" and "reactive" depressions was English psychiatrist R[obert] D[ick] Gillespie. 1929. The clinical differentiation of types of depression. *Guy's Hospital Reports* 79: 306–44.

11 Klein to Spitzer, March 19, 1986; American Psychiatric Association, Williams Papers, *DSM-III-R*, box 2.

thin skin (American Psychiatric Association, 1994). The disease designers had in effect asserted that thin skin is the autonomous dimension of major depression.

The basic problem with *DSM*, though, is that it fails to recognize endogenous depression. The manual styled itself as "atheoretical," meaning making no assumptions about causation. But by dismissing causality, *DSM* is more agnostic than diagnostic. In all other fields of medicine, causality is crucial in diagnosis and intimately tied to evidence and scientific observation. Psychiatrists must not be so totally agnostic (if they want to be effective or to practice on the basis of modern science).

After Kraepelin lumped mania and depression together in 1899 as a single illness,[12] "manic-depressive psychosis," for about the next half century endogenous depression often was referred to as manic-depressive illness. Yet the majority of patients had no evidence of mania, and many patients with mania had no history of depression. Today, authors distinguish between genuine manic-depressive illness, also called "bipolar-1" disorder, and unipolar disorder (depression without mania). This book is mainly about unipolar disorder and about psychosis in the depressive phase of bipolar illness. But, to be frank, some clinicians think that sooner or later many of the depressed hospitalized patients will develop an episode of mania, and that on a lifetime basis the distinction between unipolar endogenous depression and bipolar disorder is meaningless.[13]

To recap, this basic distinction between endogenous and reactive depression has today almost been lost sight of. Since Kurt Schneider, the classification of depression has become rather a parlor game for insiders, with countless varieties being proposed. In particular, the all-encompassing amorphous label of major depression and a pseudospecific

12 Emil Kraepelin. 1899. *Psychiatrie: Ein Lehrbuch für Studirende und Aerzte*, vol. 2, 6th edn. Leipzig: Barth, pp. 359–425.

13 See, e.g., Heinz E. Lehmann. 1971. Epidemiology of depressive disorders. In Ronald R. Fieve (ed.) *Depression in the 1970's*. Amsterdam: Excerpta Medica, pp. 21–30; proceedings of a conference held in 1970.

subtype called atypical depression enjoy popularity at the moment. Yet there are not countless varieties. There are really only two master illness entities here. Schneider's distinction between endogenous and reactive has a solidity that has withstood the test of time. This book is about psychotic depression in its varieties because it is threatening, yet repairable.

There are commonalities between the two depressions. They may have sadness in common or a diminished sense of self-worth and overarching distress. Both may be triggered by stress, but endogenous depression must also have a biological trigger, not just a psychological one. Jet lag, high cortisol, insomnia, starvation, and stimulant drug abuse may all serve as behavioral disturbances that provoke the physical brain changes of endogenous depression. As L. G. Kiloh and R. F. Garside at the University of Durham observed in 1963 in a classic article, "It is often correctly pointed out that many attacks of endogenous depression are precipitated by adverse circumstances and are therefore in this sense reactive, but this does not necessarily indicate that the precipitants play an important causal role" (Kiloh and Garside, 1963).

And sin! While psychotically depressed patients are covered in it, patients with community depression feel they deserve to be treated better. They do not dread punishment for having sinned unforgivably in the eyes of God, or fear that they are dead.

Thus, two diseases. It is just as tuberculosis and pneumonia are two different diseases, although they may have fever and coughing up phlegm in common. Lumping the diseases of endogenous and reactive depression together as "depression" makes about as much sense as lumping tuberculosis and pneumonia together: They have different prognoses, entirely different responses to treatment, and presumably different biochemistry and genetics. That means we are talking about utterly different diseases, not variations on a theme.

In this book we look at the whole question of the diagnosis and treatment of psychotic depression afresh, without the preconceptions of industry-marketed psychopharmacology and *DSM*-nonspecific nosology that have made psychiatry today a field that needs upstanding principles instead of accommodating every viewpoint. It is not as though we had a huge conventional wisdom about psychotic depression to overturn, because in the past 30 years psychiatry has not paid much attention to the condition (nor has psychiatry bothered much about the other kinds of endogenous depressions either). But psychiatry has paid inordinate attention to the public marketing of what is officially called "major depression," which is a mixture of melancholia and dissatisfaction, or of psychotic depression and reactive depression if one will. A single class of drugs – the selective serotonin reuptake inhibitors (SSRIs) – has been offered by industry as the treatment of choice of major depression, although the drugs are not effective for serious depressions.[14]

So there is a conventional wisdom out there: the SSRIs as the ideal treatment for major depression. And the conventional wisdom is wrong. There is no specific thing as major depression, and the SSRIs are poor antidepressants, although they have efficacy in treating other types of mood changes, such as worry. The enormous success of the SSRIs as the treatment of choice for major depression – a nontreatment for a non-illness – has left many clinicians frustrated as their patients fail to recover until their illnesses have run their natural cycle. It has also left the patients chasing futilely one ineffective treatment after another rather than receiving accurate diagnoses and therapies that might make them genuinely better.

14 In an unguarded moment, Robert Temple, head of the Office of Drug Evaluation I of the Food and Drug Administration (FDA), admitted in front of a microphone at a meeting of an advisory committee, "[We need] to find out whether the [SSRI-style] drugs actually provide some benefit, even in people who seem to be doing well on them . . . I mean, as Tom [Laughren] has pointed out repeatedly, the failure of most of the drugs to show effectiveness doesn't mean they don't work. On the other hand, we don't have evidence that they do work, and that is not irrelevant either." FDA Archives, Joint Meeting of the CDER Psychopharmacologic Drugs Advisory Committee and the FDA Pediatric Advisory Committee, September 14, 2004, transcript p. 55. Although the meeting was given over to pediatric suicide with antidepressants, Temple made this comment in the context of the treatment of adults. Laughren was head of the psychopharmacology evaluation unit of the FDA.

As we said above, the ideal treatment for psychotic depression is ECT. Yet the view has squirmed into today's psychiatry that the way to go is a combination of antipsychotics and antidepressants.

As one warning flag among many: At the University of Iowa, Paul Penningroth collected a series of four patients with psychosis and depression treated with antipsychotics who suicided (at ages 21, 23, 24, and 38), despite seeming to have responded.[15] Antipsychotics do not remove all the thought disorder, and that is the problem. Moreover, they cause substantial impairment. So the combo of antipsychotics and antidepressants is clearly not the first choice. The first choice is ECT. The second choice is a tricyclic antidepressant (TCA) or a drug Glaxo SmithKline markets called generically bupropion (Wellbutrin), to which about a third of psychotic depressives respond. Then comes a miscellany, for example, drugs that inhibit the enzyme monoamine oxidase, called MAOIs, such as phenelzine (Parke-Davis's Nardil); in the miscellany is lithium plus TCAs. In the last place, and not win, place, or show in the horse race, is the combo of TCAs plus antipsychotics.

Patients

The year is 1889. We are in the closed wing of the Holloway Sanatorium for the Insane, in Virginia Water outside of London, a private nervous clinic for the middle classes. Constance, D., 35, is brought in for "acute melancholia." She had given birth about 2 months ago, and 3 weeks after the delivery, as one of the medical certificates stated, she had taken on "a terrified expression, [is] nervous and wrings her hands, is afraid she is going to be boiled alive, and asks for a knife with which to end her life." Before the onset of the present

15 R. Paul Penningroth, "Schizophrenia, depression, and suicide." Psychiatry Grand Rounds, University of Iowa Hospitals and Clinics, November 16, 1976.

illness she was said to have been "strong, active, healthy and temperate, very fond of music." Then after the baby's arrival she started to lose her appetite and was sleepless (a nanny apparently looked after the child). She began to dread impoverishment although there was no objective reason for doing so. As noted in her chart, "She said she was miserable enough for suicide but lacked the necessary courage. She appeared to take no interest in her child." She came into the care of Dr George Savage, a prominent London psychiatrist who also once had Virginia Woolf as a patient, and Savage arranged for her committal to "Holloway House," as it was called.

At Holloway House, the clinicians noted that she had a scar on her left hand, where she had attempted to open a vein. Mentally she is suffering from "melancholia agitata," with delusions that she is about to undergo some horrible torture. She clutches her hair, wrings her hands, looking the very picture of abject misery, begging that she shall be removed to some dark room and just locked up where no nurse can reach her, as they are on the point of taking her into the bath and boiling her alive." Every time the doctor visited her she would say, "This is the last time, all is pretence and sham, that they are now preparing the boiling pitch for her."

That was in March. By May she was well enough to play tennis on the clinic's "airing court," yet filched a nurse's keys and plunged down the embankment in order to launch herself into the Thames. She continued to pick her face into open wounds, "continues the nervous habit of blowing on her hands whilst talking, and adheres to the same absurd statement that this is her last day as she is about to be put into the 'boiling bath.'"

In August, Savage had her discharged to her home in the hope that familiar surroundings might make a difference. (Apparently there were servants enough to keep an eye on her.) By October Savage informed the clinic doctors that Constance D. was indeed much improved, washing and dressing the baby and being mistress of the house at the head of the table. "The only suspicious feature respecting her cure being that she still says, 'she ought never to have been sent away from home,' and 'that her husband is a fool.' "[16]

This was a psychotic depression, brought on by the birth of a child. Constance D. had been ill for about 10 months, which was fairly standard. In 1889 they had no specific treatment for depression, only weak sedatives such as the foul-smelling paraldehyde for patients who were highly agitated, and her doctors and family just waited the illness out.

Fifty years later, psychiatrist Eliot Slater recalled the typical delusional melancholic patient in the early 1930s at the Maudsley Hospital on Denmark Hill in South London: The chronic melancholic "would be a thin, elderly man or woman, inert, with the head lifted up off the pillow. There were some sort of Parkinsonian-like qualities, mask-like face sunk deep in misery, and speaking in a retarded way. If you could get them to say anything, it would be something about how hopeless things were, how they were wicked, doomed to disease, death, and a terrible afterlife, if there was one." Could these patients be helped? "There wasn't anything you could do," said Slater, "except to try to make them sleep, try to get them to take some food, tube-feed them if they were refusing food, which happened frequently." It was when they started to revive from this kind of stupor that suicide was to be feared, said Slater.[17]

At this point psychotic depression, as well as the other endogenous depressions, suddenly became among the most treatable of all psychiatric disorders. In 1935 Budapest psychiatrist Ladislaus von Meduna originated the first of the convulsive therapies, using the convulsive drug pentylenetetrazol, sold in Europe under the trade name Cardiazol, in the United States under Metrazol, to trigger the seizure. Although Meduna intended to treat schizophrenia with Metrazol, it soon became apparent that depression responded even better to the new treatment, including

16 Holloway Sanatorium, patient files, at Wellcome Library for the History of Medicine, London. MS 5157, case no. 404.

17 Eliot Slater. 1993. Interview. In Greg Wilkinson (ed.) *Talking about psychiatry*. London: Gaskell, p. 4.

psychotic depression.[18] Three years later, in 1938, Rome psychiatrist Ugo Cerletti determined an even better way of inducing convulsions, with electricity; ECT was born.[19] ECT was thought to be superior to Metrazol convulsive therapy because it caused the patients less anxiety in the stage of waiting for the fits to begin – with ECT unconsciousness is immediate; also, Metrazol was plagued by the problem of partial seizures. ECT remains today the preferred treatment for psychotic depression.

Questions

These momentous developments left several questions unanswered, and they remain question marks even today.

First, why has the frequency of psychotic depression declined considerably over the years? Today, it is certainly not an uncommon ailment, and 15–30 percent of endogenous depressions are said to have a delusional component. But in mental hospital admissions in the past the figure was much higher. At the Royal Hospital in Edinburgh, a psychiatric hospital, among female patients the number of delusional depressions per 100 depressions admitted dropped from 75 percent in 1892 to 39 percent in 1942–3, to 30 percent in 1981–2. The decrease is statistically significant (the decrease in male patients, though parallel to that of females, is not statistically significant; Eagles, 1983). Of course it is possible that the hospital decided to admit more delusional depressives at one point than another: were the quieter cases kept more at home in the earlier period? Or perhaps later generations of family

18 L. C. Cook and W. Ogden. 1938. Cardiazol convulsion therapy in non-schizophrenic reaction states. *Lancet* 235: 885–7. Four of five patients with "psychotic depression" responded well to Cardiazol.

19 For details on these developments, see Edward Shorter and David Healy. In press. *Shock Therapy: The History of Electroconvulsive Treatment in Mental Illness*, forthcoming from Rutgers University Press, September, 2007.

doctors, intent upon treating their patients' (now treatable) bodily woes, simply missed the delusions in their depressed patients and did not recommend them for admission. It is also possible that "schizophrenia" has increasingly replaced the diagnosis of psychotic depression, given that the presence of psychosis in depression, if chronic, could easily be considered schizophrenia. Thus, in various ways the finding could be an artifact, but it is probably not because several other series confirm it.

In Scotland at the Crichton Royal Hospital (formed out of two nineteenth-century institutions), the percentage of depressed patients with delusions declined in women from 77 percent in 1880–9 to 19 percent in 1970–9; in men from 78 percent to 31 percent. On an epidemiological basis, per 100,000 population at risk, the declines were of a similar magnitude, so it is not just a question of possible changes in the patient mix. Meanwhile in Scotland, the percentage of delusions in patients with schizophrenia was relatively unchanging (and per 100,000 population actually rose).[20]

Finally, in Finland at the Helsinki University Psychiatric Clinic, among patients with severe depression (called "depressive psychosis" but not necessarily delusional), the percentage of patients experiencing "strong manifest guilt," a surrogate for delusions, declined from 30 percent in 1900–9 to 9 percent in 1930–9, to 5 percent in 1960–9. The trend for "religious symptoms in abundance" was similar.[21]

Because the trend in all three of these studies is sharply down, it is unlikely that we are dealing with some kind of artifact of registration; a genuine epidemiological change seems to have occurred, lessening the frequency of psychotic depression. Because big changes over time in

20 A. D. T. Robinson. 1988. A century of delusions in South West Scotland. *Br J Psychiatry* 153: 163–7. For a not entirely convincing critique of this study, see M. J. S. Morton, letter, 1988. *Br J Psychiatry* 153: 710–11.

21 P. Niskanen and K. A. Achté. 1972. Disease pictures of depressive psychoses in the decades 1880–89, 1900–09, 1930–39 and 1960–69. *Psychiatria Fennica* 95–100; delusions increased somewhat between the 1880s and the 1890s.

illnesses with a significant genetic component, such as delusional depression, are not to be anticipated, we may be dealing with some external factor activating or deactivating an underlying predisposition. The puzzle is exactly similar to that surrounding a possible increase in the incidence of schizophrenia during the nineteenth century.[22] Some external circumstances seem to make these brain illnesses more or less common, and getting at it would help cast a light upon etiology.

Second, what kind of a brain disease are we dealing with here? We know that in elderly patients, for example, the new onset of psychotic depression can literally be a mixture of endogenous depression and such coarse brain diseases as Parkinson's, stroke, or prodromal dementia. Analogously, in younger patients is psychotic depression a mixture of endogenous depression and a separate psychotic process? It is clear that endogenous depression, psychotic included, differs from reactive depression, and is an illness sui generis in that sense. But what is the link between psychotic depression and schizophreniform illness (once called "acute schizophrenia")? Since mania and depression can occur together, might the opposing changes in affect that each causes cancel out and leave the otherwise secondary psychotic features predominant? This would make for an illness that looks like schizophrenia but is not. When schizophreniform illness is not interrupted by treatment, can the brain pattern of illness harden into chronic psychosis? That is, can chronic schizophrenia result from withholding effective early treatment? This seems to have been what happened to the Russian ballet genius Vaslav Nijinsky. Nijinsky did not have true childhood-onset core schizophrenia; he had an acute illness that hardened in the absence of proper biological treatment. (He was started in Switzerland on a course of insulin coma therapy, got better, wanted to continue it with specialists in New York, and then had to abandon it because the U.S. consulate would not grant him a visa!)

22 See Edward Shorter. 1997. *A history of psychiatry from the era of the asylum to the age of Prozac*. New York: John Wiley, pp. 60–4.

There is a whole concept of major psychiatric illness as a single disease process, suggesting that schizophrenia might be the chronic untreated form of psychotic depression and of psychotic mixed manic-depressive states. The notion that depressive psychosis and "madness" were somehow related was launched in German psychiatry in the nineteenth century under the banner Einheitspsychose, or unitary psychosis (Shorter, 2005). It is indeed possible that there exists no separate entity of "schizophrenia," and that the chronic psychotic state we call schizophrenia is initially the same disease as psychotic depression. Perhaps the mild form is affective disorder, the severe acute form is psychotic depression, and the extreme persistent form is schizophrenia. As early as 1922 August Hoch, the former director of the New York State Psychiatric Institute, and John T. MacCurdy wrote, "It may be possible to differentiate between the benign and malignant melancholias, relating the former to manic-depressive insanity and the latter to dementia praecox [schizophrenia]" (Hoch and MacCurdy, 1922). Could psychotic depression be among the malignant melancholias?

Recent research has been heading in this direction, seeing psychotic depression as closer to schizophrenia than to nonpsychotic depression. In 2004, S. Christian Hill and colleagues at the University of Illinois at Chicago and at the University of Pittsburgh studied "neuropsychological dysfunction" – meaning defects in memory, attention, executive function, and the like – in a group of patients experiencing their first episode of unipolar psychotic depression. They found that, for example, the deficit in motor skills and executive function of these patients differed "dramatically" from that of patients with nonpsychotic depression and resembled that of schizophrenics. They concluded that "psychosis appears to be associated with a common profile of diffuse neurocognitive dysfunction, regardless of whether it occurs in . . . schizophrenia or depression" (Hill, 2004).

The following year, in 2005, a group at the Institute of Psychiatry in London found that white matter deficits in schizophrenia and in psychotic forms of manic-depressive illness tended to occur in the same areas of the brain, the frontal and parietal lobes. The same was not true of gray matter, where there were extensive deficits in schizophrenia and virtually none in psychotic depression. The white matter is responsible for carrying the nerve impulses across the brain, and the authors thought their findings were "in accordance with the hypothesis that both major types of psychosis represent a disorder of anatomical connectivity between components of large-scale neurocognitive networks" (McDonald et al., 2005). (A historian cannot help remarking that these findings are an unwitting throwback to one of the first biological theories of psychosis, German psychiatrist Carl Wernicke's "sejunction theory" in 1900, which claimed "paranoid states" as being a disorder of the "association fibers" of the brain; Wernicke, 1900.)

These findings are all of interest because they suggest a common underlying biological basis to the two great illnesses, psychotic depression and schizophrenia.

The bottom line: in psychotic depression there are answers and questions. The answers concern how to make patients better, for effective treatments are at hand. The questions concern the nature of the psychotic, endogenous beast, and what we may learn of it that might apply to other mysteries of psychiatry.

2

History of Psychotic Depression

IN PSYCHIATRY, the past can be a storehouse of wisdom. Very often the older diagnoses and remedies are superior to the newer patent-protected drugs and industry-promoted diagnoses. It is for that reason that some understanding of the history and diagnosis of psychotic depression is useful.

We know historically that psychotic depression seems to have a specific response to treatment and a specific prognosis. That matters today. If you as a physician did not have a distinctive treatment to offer, it would not matter so much whether psychotic depression differs from other illnesses, just an academic exercise, really. But here therapeutic choices exist. Also, there are different kinds of psychotic depression, with different responses to treatment (see Chapter 8). Finally, you can tell a troubled family what they can expect in the future. So these diagnostic hairsplittings are not academic.

Psychiatry has long yearned for such choices. As Robert Gaupp, professor of psychiatry in Tübingen, said in 1926:

What we want and need as physicians are diagnoses and classifications that don't let us down when we're in front of a living human being, a human being who stands ill before us and whose apprehensive family wants to know what's going to happen, recovery or chronic suffering, return to normality or death after years or decades of decline. *What's going to happen? What should we do?*"(Gaupp, 1926; emphasis in the original)

So chiseling psychotic depression from the mass of undifferentiated depressive illness is quite a practical exercise.

Some forms of melancholia involve madness, some do not. Awareness of this is really as old as medicine itself. Any disease with a heavy genetic component will have been familiar to physicians across the ages, and psychotic depression is no exception. So it is probably as pointless to ask who penned its "first" description as to ask who first described tuberculosis or sore throat. In 1621 Oxford cleric Robert Burton, a melancholia scholar, looked back upon a thousand years of medical writing on the subject, together with describing his own experiences as a melancholic:

Fear of Devils, death, that they shall be sick of some such or such disease, ready to tremble at every object, they shall die themselves forthwith . . . that they are all glass, and therefore they will suffer no man to come near them; that they are all cork, as light as feathers; others as heavy as lead; some afraid their heads will fall off their shoulders, that they have frogs in their bellies.[1]

Medical observations of psychotic melancholy go back a long way.

Of equally antique lineage is the historic inability of physicians to offer relief to these patients. Felix Platter, the city physician of Basel at the beginning of the seventeenth century, often had to deal with them. "The wife of a painter was by nature inclined to solitude, was industrious in domestic matters, pious, sad and melancholic." She was also inclined to jealousy because her husband once confided to her that he had loved another woman before he married her. Then in January 1600, the false

1 Robert Burton. 1948/1621. *The anatomy of melancholy.* New York: Tudor, p. 328; quote from the edition published in 1651.

news arrived that her absent son had been killed in a quarrel. This triggered a severe melancholy.

Now the old jealousy of her husband from the early days of her marriage flamed back into life. Even the son's return at the behest of her physicians did not suffice to distract her from this idea, and despite frequent bleedings and purgings, she complained of ever greater mental distress. She became so agitated that she ran from one side of the house to the other ceaselessly day and night. Now, she called ardently for death and asked friends to give her poison.

"Finally she despaired that God would never forgive her, that she was damned, and repeated that she had begun to feel the tortures of Hell. After this had gone on for four months, her delusions assumed such a degree that she completely persuaded herself that her husband and children wanted to administer poison and thus accomplish her death." All entreaties of friends proved vain and she persisted in the opinion that people wanted to poison her. She took no food, drink, or medication. When given nourishment by force, she spit it out, wiped her mouth, and maintained that she had to remove the last remaining bits of the poison. Even when friends demonstratively ate from the vessels in front of her to show the harmlessness of the food and drink, she claimed that it might not be poisonous for them but that it was for her. Even though she strictly abstained from taking anything offered her,

> she nonetheless lived on for ten days and as many nights, which was the more surprising as she was already emaciated and weakened from her illness over the past four months. Shortly before she died, she looked heavenward and said, "Upwards, upwards I shall be borne to Heaven." As she was no longer able to speak she folded her hands, as she was requested, as though for prayer, and breathed her last on April 4, 1600, at 4 o'clock in the morning.

Just imagine. Platter had to stand by and watch his patient expire of self-starvation because of the psychotic delusion that enveloped her.[2]

2 Felix Platter. 1963/1602. *Observationes: Krankheitsbeobachtungen.* Berne: Huber, pp. 75–7, case 71.

For Platter, this was a straightforward case of melancholia, in retrospect in its agitated psychotic form. When does psychotic depression start to be identified as a special form of melancholia? And when does awareness dawn that it has a prognosis and treatment of its own?

Differentiating melancholy

In the early days of psychiatric diagnosis, melancholy and mania were thought of as way stations on a long road that led from wellness to dementia: First the patient would develop melancholy, then progress to mania, then to dementia. Each way station was described correctly with the distinctive symptoms of that particular disorder. Yet, one way station led inevitably to another and thus to terminal dementia and death. This is not exactly the same concept as "unitary psychosis," which means there is only one underlying brain disease that produces the symptoms of depression or schizophrenia. But it is a concept of madness that goes back to the ancients. Late in the eighteenth century, with writers such as William Cullen, this single "unitary insanity" view began to give way to a proper nosology, seeing the separate psychiatric illnesses as different diseases.

So carving nature at the joints in psychiatric illness has a long tradition. In 1799 London physician James Sims subdivided the psychiatric diseases in terms that are quite familiar today. He described melancholics in the first stage of their illness: "Their speech is slow, sedate, solemn, measured, and argumentative; and they are mostly buried in sorrow." Then melancholics would become frankly delusional: "Their silence gives way, in some degree, and they complain of some action that they have done against some friend or relative, or some crime that they have committed, which can never be forgiven by God or man. This action is often totally imaginary." Paranoia soon sets in as "[t]hey become suspicious of all around them, and imagine they see conspiracies against them in the most trifling occurrences. They think all their friends are become enemies, which induces a taedium vitae, ending often in suicide." Still further on, "[t]hey lose all regard to the common civilities, or even decencies, of life." Sims thought poorly of writers who insisted that "melancholy was partial, and mania universal insanity," which was the traditional view. "I believe there is no universal insanity except in some cases of idiocy and delirium." (Sims concluded with an admonition quite apposite even today: "Everything in Nature is a continuing chain, without those breaks and intervals which even the accurate describer is obliged to make, in order to keep up due discrimination, and to render himself intelligible.") (Sims, 1799) In this manner, numerous authors – of whom Sims is merely a good example, and not necessarily the first – began to carve a distinctive picture of melancholy from the great block of madness.

Among the first to slice melancholy into distinct subgroups was Joseph Guislain, professor of psychiatry in Ghent in Belgium. In a widely quoted textbook in 1852 he described as "general melancholy" what was in fact the psychotic version:

> These melancholics accuse themselves. They should have done this, they say; they should have done that. They imagine that they have committed a deplorable, criminal action. One might say, I have offended God; another pretends to have signed away his fortune or the fortune of his children .... Another is prey to sinister premonitions: the police will raid his home; he will be imprisoned, he will offer the world the sight of a man punished for having grossly abused his position. (Guislain, 1852)

Then Guislain said there are the "special" forms, such as melancholy without madness, having a large mood component (the "without madness" [*sans délire*] part was borrowed from French psychiatrist Philippe Pinel, who wrote of "mania without madness," meaning without deterioration of the personality). There were also hypochondriacal melancholy and anxious melancholy. Guislain's focus was not strictly on affective disorders, sweeping in other kinds of symptoms as well. But it was quite a refined differentiation.[3]

The nineteenth century belonged mainly to the great German heavyweights, giving rise to the aphorism that if French was the language of diplomacy, German was that of psychiatry. The Germans soon began to draw a separate profile of psychotic melancholy.

The central figure in German psychiatry in the mid-nineteenth century was Wilhelm Griesinger, professor of psychiatry first in Zurich then in Berlin, before his premature death of appendicitis in 1868 at the age of 51. Griesinger is remembered for his dictum that psychiatric illness is a brain disease and for placing German psychiatry on a thoroughly organic footing. But he is recalled as well for his textbook, the influential second edition of which was published in 1861. Here he distinguished between psychotic and nonpsychotic melancholy, illnesses having different courses and treatments. As he wrote of the melancholic "deliria," "At the beginning, and in some cases throughout the entire duration of the melancholy, an actual psychosis [delirium] may be absent; the patients have good judgment of their situation and the surrounding world; they correctly analyze their feelings, and wish avidly to be rid of them but are incapable of doing so."

Griesinger continued:

> Among the cases of frank melancholia there is an important difference, whether the patients are in a deep dreamlike condition or whether their relations with the surrounding world are quite perceptive. The former cases usually arise more acutely, resemble the condition of "melancholy with stupor," and have in general a better prognosis than the second variety, which usually are of gradual onset and have a more chronic duration. The former tend to end quickly, as though in a sudden awakening, the latter never. (Griesinger, 1861/1964)

Thus, for Griesinger, psychotic melancholy had a sudden onset, dramatic symptom picture, and equally quick termination; the nonpsychotic

3 J[oseph] Guislain. 1852. *Lecons orales sur les phrenopathies, ou traité théorique et pratique des maladies mentales*. Ghent: Hebbelynck, pp. 105, 111, 119, 126. Guislain proposed still other forms of melancholy as well.

variety tended to be chronic.[4] (A bit of hairsplitting may be necessary here: Griesinger with his dream-like condition might also have been referring to catatonic depression, stupor or delirium being key features of a catatonic form of depressive illness that is closely related to psychotic depression but precedes it in diagnostic terms: If you are depressed, stuporous, and hallucinating, you have catatonic depression.)

After Griesinger came a virtual parade of contributions. The second of the big nineteenth-century German figures weighed in 2 years after Griesinger, in 1863. Some authorities believe that Karl Kahlbaum was among the greatest psychiatric writers of the nineteenth century because of his insistence on using the clinical method to study psychopathology. Kahlbaum also drew clear portraits of catatonia and "cyclothymia," a variety of manic-depressive illness (MDI) (the concept of circular illness was already well known) that did not end in dementia. In his system of nosology, written as a postdoctoral thesis while he was still a junior staffer in the East Prussian asylum at Allenberg, Kahlbaum distinguished between melancholia, a major form of madness (a Vesania) with a downhill course, and "dysthymia meläna," by which he meant non-deteriorating melancholia (meläna is one of the Greek black-bile terms for depression). Kahlbaum claimed to be proceeding in an entirely empirical way, throwing aside first principles and describing only what he had seen in Allenberg.

For Kahlbaum, melancholia was the first stage of a "typical psychiatric illness," an innocuous expression for a process that he meant in a very malignant sense: a major psychosis progressing to dementia. This became a template for Emil Kraepelin's dementia praecox three decades later. Dysthymia meläna, by contrast, a "Vecordia" rather than a "Vesania," meant a depressive temperament as well as a depressive syndrome with a fluctuating course. Vesaniae progressed to dementia

4 Wilhelm Griesinger. 1964/1861. *Die Pathologie und Therapie der psychischen Krankheiten,* 2nd edn. reprint Amsterdam: Bonset, p. 233. Griesinger believed in "madness" as a unitary process, beginning with melancholia, ending in dementia.

whereas Vecordiae did not. The symptoms of both the melancholia and the dysthymia involved psychosis (Kahlbaum, 1863). (A century and a quarter later, the APA in *DSM*-III in 1980 unwittingly resurrected Kahlbaum's dysthymia to mean minor chronic depression, formerly called "neurotic depression." The manual actually had difficulty differentiating it from chronic grumpiness and said, "When Dysthymic Disorder is of many years' duration, the mood disturbance may not be easily distinguished from the person's 'usual' functioning" (APA, 1994). It is a depression that is less than a depression.) Kahlbaum had obviously included in his vesanic melancholia a number of cases of schizophrenia. Yet in the Vecordia he did single out a nondeteriorating psychotic form of melancholia, his dysthymia.

In an era of upper middle-class patients who languished away months in "open" private nervous clinics (no bars or locks), a diagnosis such as "dysthymia" was pure gold because it meant good news for the patients: They were not going to become insane and die demented, in an era when so many men in particular died insane and demented of neurosyphilis. At the time, the cause of neurosyphilis was not known. It was not even called neurosyphilis but "general paresis of the insane" (GPI), which was thought to be the result of masturbation or overwork, and it scared the pants off everybody. So to have a diagnosis such as dysthymia, really just a spot of trouble rather than insanity, became a precious calling card in the hands of private practice neurologists and hydrotherapists, who did psychiatry for outpatients (psychiatrists proper worked in asylums or university hospitals). Therefore, it was a Russian psychiatrist with a considerable interest in the private sector – Theodor Tiling in St. Petersburg – who said, hey, guess what? Dysthymia can be nonpsychotic. Not only do patients with these diagnoses not deteriorate, but dysthymia also does not create the presumption of craziness because the patient is not clinically crazy.[5]

5 T[heodor] Tiling. 1879. Ueber Dysthymia und die offenen Curanstalten. *Jahrbuch für Psychiatrie* 3: 171–86; Tiling himself was an asylum psychiatrist but he had a strong interest, for unclear reasons, in "open" private clinics.

Thus, we have Kahlbaum's psychotic dysthymia and Tiling's nonpsychotic dysthymia, a rehearsal for the split between psychotic depression and nonpsychotic depression today.

Of course Tiling's dysthymia had a good prognosis and a favorable response to massage, mud baths, electricity, dietary therapy, and the rest of the armamentarium of physical therapy, or else patients would not be spending their money on these spalike open clinics, as unlike asylums as night is from day (Shorter, 1990). Just as chronic fatigue syndrome today, these were diagnoses in social demand.

Meanwhile, other German scholars were attentive to the differentiation of melancholia on the basis of physical signs. In 1878, Heinrich Schüle, director of the Illenau asylum, named the "Omega sign" the characteristic arching of the inner ends of the eyebrows in "silent melancholia," an arching of the muscles that Charles Darwin in 1872 had already nicknamed "the grief muscles." This was in contrast to "active melancholia" with its suicidality and loud lamentations, physically betrayed by a narrowing of the visual field.[6]

This was an era of anatomical pathology, attributing syndromes to brain lesions, and with the work of Theodor Meynert, professor of psychiatry in Vienna, the frontal lobes became incriminated, in an almost prescient way, in psychiatric illness. It was Meynert's student Johann Fritsch who claimed in 1882 that the seat of psychotic melancholia lay in the frontal lobes (Fritsch, 1882). (In recent years the "hypofrontality" thesis has boosted a resurgence of interest in the frontal lobes.)

Thus far we have examined a series of mostly now ill-remembered German investigators. Yet one important French contribution, now completely forgotten, must be mentioned. It was Georges Dumas, a student of Théodule-Armand Ribot in Paris, who in 1895 convincingly

6 Heinrich Schüle. 1878. *Handbuch der Geisteskrankheiten*. Leipzig: Vogel, p. 439. See Charles Darwin. 1965/1872. *The expression of the emotions in man and animals*. Chicago: University of Chicago Press, pp. 176–91.

described melancholia as an illness of the entire body, not just of mood or intellect. (For him, melancholia was mainly psychotic.) Dumas said melancholia can have two origins: one intellectual (loss, shock) and one somatic (a fever, anemia). Yet, both proceeded via seizing the entire body with slowing, not just slowing the mind. The blood pressure, all the "secretions," all bodily functions were down in melancholia. He noted Darwin's description of the oblique upturning of the eyebrows and downturning of the corners of the mouth. "Melancholia is thus truly an organic disease, and it is on the organism that the physical and psychological causes that produce it initially reverberate."[7] Dumas said that delusional thinking came in due course, in association with disturbed body function.

Whether German or French matters less. European psychiatry of those years has really become a kind of lost continent. Subsequent Anglo-Saxon writers have vaguely suspected its importance, yet the vast dimensions of European writing of those years still lie underwater. One will search in vain for Dumas in the standard guides. Kahlbaum is a name few have heard of, despite his enormous impact on his contemporaries. Tiling has vanished completely from the radar. Yet, Emil Kraepelin, by contrast, is a name on the tip of the tongue of anyone today knowledgeable about psychiatric diagnosis. The inspiration of *DSM*-III in 1980, a volume that made the American *DSM*-series the world bible of psychiatry, was said to have been "Kraepelinian."

Emil Kraepelin was professor of psychiatry at two prestigious German medical schools: Heidelberg in the 1890s and Munich before World War I. He is probably the central figure in modern psychiatry, at least with regard to diagnosis. Somewhat peculiarly for today's readers accustomed to gleaning medical progress from journal articles, Kraepelin communicated new knowledge in the form of successive

7 Georges Dumas. 1895. *Les états intellectuels dans la mélancholie*. Paris: Alcan, quote on p. 138. As Dumas qualified medically in 1894, this reflective work must have been a doctoral thesis. Dumas went on to become a professor of psychology at the Sorbonne.

editions of a textbook. His *Psychiatry: A textbook for students and physicians*, first appeared in 1883. But it was only in the editions published after he became professor of psychiatry in Heidelberg in 1891 that things started to get interesting. At the Heidelberg University Psychiatric Hospital, he began keeping precise notes on each of his patients and was able to put little one-sheet summaries of their clinical records into piles, on the basis of the patient's subsequent course. He noted that the patients in the downhill pile, those whose personalities deteriorated and who died demented, had a number of clinical features in common: Madness seemed to strike them early in life, and their illness withdrew them from social contact; young men and women with mask-like faces, whose illness left them unresponsive to human interaction save in moments of wild psychosis. In the 1893 edition of his textbook, Kraepelin decided to give these patients the diagnosis "dementia praecox," or "premature dementia" (in fact they were thought-disordered and psychotic but not demented).

A brief aside: In 1908 Zurich psychiatry professor Eugen Bleuler rebaptized these patients as having "schizophrenia" (he thought dementia praecox was awkward to use as an adjective; also, he focused on core symptoms other than psychosis and thought disorder; he believed that patients had a milder prognosis than did the gloomy Kraepelin). Bleuler's followers have not hesitated to call any and all serious mental illness schizophrenia, based on his teachings.

Then in the sixth edition of his textbook that appeared in 1899, Kraepelin pointed to another pile of slips and said that these patients seem to run a fluctuating course, sliding wave-like from psychosis to recovery and back again. Also, mood symptoms seemed more prominent in their courses than in the dementia praecox patients. Kraepelin decided to call these patients "manic-depressive" an illness that was totally different from dementia praecox. His textbook then went through two further editions, a final eighth edition completed in 1915. This final edition (the clinical volume of which appeared in 1913) represented Kraepelin's definitive views. After World War I, he died while at work on yet another edition and it was brought out by his assistant Johannes Lange.

As for the psychotic versus nonpsychotic distinctions of his predecessors, the patients in Kraepelin's two big diagnoses were almost all psychotic. Psychosis was strewn like grass-seed throughout his large category "manic-depressive illness." But he did make some differentiations within the large basin of MDI that are not without interest. In his 1913 volume he distinguished among clinical forms of depression within the overarching category MDI.[8]

First, there was simple depression: "The mildest forms of depressive conditions are characterized by the appearance of simple psychic retardation [Hemmung] without hallucinations and without well-defined delusional notions. The patient finds thinking difficult ... he cannot collect his thoughts, nor come to the point; it is as though the patients are paralyzed and cannot make headway" (Kraepelin, 1913).

Then came a series of fully psychotic depressive subtypes: depressions with all kinds of psychotic ideas. Kraepelin used the German term "Zwangsvorstellungen," which literally translates as "compulsive thoughts," but from the text he clearly means delusional thinking. In addition, he described a form of depression with mainly melancholic features; then there was another form where hallucinations predominate; there was also a stuporous group, the most serious; another "delirious" group of depressive illness also existed, meaning "a deep dreamlike disturbance of consciousness" (Kraepelin, 1913). These were, of course, not separate illness entities but just clinical variants of depression in MDI. They did not have different prognoses or responses to treatment. (In dementia praecox, Kraepelin (1913) also said there were depressive symptoms.)

Yet, Kraepelin did admit the existence of differential response to treatment. He felt that bromium or the synthetic hypnotics then coming

8 E. Kraepelin. 1913. *Psychiatrie: Ein Lehrbuch für Studierende und Ärzte*, 8th edn, vol. 3 (2). Leipzig: Barth, pp. 1183–395 on "das manisch-depressive Irresein."

on the market in Germany were the treatment of choice for general depression, but for depression with anxiety he recommended a combination of bromide salts and opium (Kraepelin, 1913). Likewise, he thought that different clinical forms had different prognoses. Although he had given up the term melancholy for depression by 1913, nonetheless in this volume he did reserve it for a special set of depressions: melancholic depression in the middle-aged and older (Kraepelin, 1913). Before 1913 he had seen these "involutional melancholias" as quite a separate illness; in 1913 melancholy in this population became assimilated to MDI. But he thought it entailed structural brain changes and that it had a worse prognosis than the others (Kraepelin, 1913).

Within this magisterial structure of MDI, a single entity that had a dramatic impact on the next 50 years of psychiatry, there was one outlier: "psychogenic" depression, not a part of MDI. It did not correspond to "simple depression" described above, the mild form of MDI. Rather, it was not autonomous; unlike MDI it did not come out of the blue; unlike MDI it was also responsive to changes in the patient's social situation. He wrote,

A number of patients have been referred to me whose deep sadness, paucity of speech and anxious tension might have suggested a circular depression; yet it came out subsequently that we were dealing with dysphorias [Verstimmungen] caused by serious mistakes [the patient had made] and by looming legal procedures. Because the milder depressions of manic-depressive illness, as much as we can tell, fully resemble the motivated dysphorias of healthy psychic life – with the essential difference that they occur without motivation – in cases of this kind [psychogenic depression] one will not be able to interpret the symptoms correctly without knowledge of the patient's history. (Kraepelin, 1913)

This, therefore, marks the beginning of the endogenous-reactive distinction in depression that today looms quite large.

One final comment about Kraepelin: Toward the end of his life, he rather took it all back. In an article in 1920 he admitted that it had been a mistake to erect a firewall between dementia praecox and MDI, that in fact the two largely overlapped. This admission was crucial, of course, in conceiving of psychotic depression, which really does seem a mixture of schizophreniform psychosis and mood disorder. To be sure, Kraepelin insisted that there were pure forms of both illnesses, in the one patients with disintegrating personalities, in the other patients who recover. Yet, he did say that "[t]he emotional and schizophrenic clinical forms of madness [Irresein] actually do not represent the expression of well defined disease processes, but rather point solely to the mental domains in which they occur."[9]

Thus, in his major body of work, Kraepelin had at least raised the possibility of different illness entities – brain-driven MDI and reactive psychogenic depression; he had allowed for differential responsiveness and prognosis; in his afterthought of 1920 he had opened the door to the two supposedly separate diseases of schizophrenia and affective illness overlapping. With Kraepelin we are, therefore, halfway along the road to psychotic depression as a separate entity.

In 1920, as Kraepelin in Munich was contemplating the destruction of his own lifetime architecture, a few hours' train trip across Bavaria and up the Rhine River sat the very much junior Kurt Schneider in Cologne. Schneider distinguished between "endogenous" and "reactive" depressions, though he coined neither term. (In 1913 psychopathologist Karl Jaspers had commented on the frequency of "reactive depressive states" in his work that was familiar to Schneider (Jaspers, 1913). Schneider borrowed the term "endogenous" from Kraepelin, who talked about "endogenous psychoses," meaning psychoses entrenched in the very parenchyma of the brain itself.) It was Schneider who juxtaposed the two concepts of endogenous and reactive as the main typology of depression.

Reactive depression for Schneider did not necessarily mean reactions to external events but to feelings. Reactive depressions were situated at the level of emotions and involved mainly sadness; by contrast

9 Emil Kraepelin. 1920. Die Erscheinungsformen des Irreseins. *Zeitschrift für die gesamte Neurologie und Psychiatrie* 62: 1–29, quote on p. 27: "sondern lediglich die Gebiete unserer Persönlichkeit anzeigen, in denen sich jene abspielen."

endogenous depressions somehow seized the entire body and dragged down the sensation of "vitality" rather than confining themselves to a lock on emotions. So for Schneider, the basic dichotomy was feelings versus loss of vitality as reflected in numerous autonomic symptoms. This concept of vitality was long familiar in German psychiatry,[10] and Schneider spoke rather romantically about "vital sensations" instead of using a technical concept such as "autonomic nervous system." Yet, in reality, vitality meant roughly autonomic functions: vital feelings were regulated by sleep, appetite, vascular tone, bowel functions, and similar bodily events partly under autonomic control.

"What is striking," wrote Schneider, "is the fact that in endogenous depression, disorders of feelings of vitality find a much greater role [than in reactive depression]. We know that here [vitality], disorders of body and bodily sensations often dominate the picture completely, and that these disorders can precede the sadness of mood as well as outlasting it" (Schneider, 1920). The devitalization of Schneider's endogenous depression would later be described as "psychomotor slowing," or slowing in "psychomotor disturbance." (Psychomotor disturbance can also be agitated.)

Schneider was not so interested in psychosis. Thus, his 1920 article had the function of shifting the entire discussion of depression from psychosis to the autonomic nervous system. This was a major development: For 50 years, psychiatry lost interest in psychotic depression.

Before we continue the story, we want to shift the spotlight very briefly from this parade of Germanic professors to one non-German figure, who directly contrasted "simple melancholia" with the psychotic version, only to see his contribution forgotten later in the enthusiasm over psychoanalysis. It was Henry Maudsley, a wealthy private-practice psychiatrist in London who endowed the institution named after him,

10 [Carl Friedrich] Flemming. 1844. Ueber Classification der Seelenstörungen. *Allgemeine Zeitschrift für Psychiatrie* 1: 97–130, at p. 100; "Vitalitäts-Energie," "Vitalitäts-Verletzungen."

the Maudsley Hospital, as the most prestigious center for training and research in the United Kingdom. In his 1867 textbook, *The physiology and pathology of the mind*, Maudsley spoke of "partial ideational insanity," characterized by "delusion accompanied by a sad and oppressive passion," or "ordinary melancholia." "The feeling of oppression of self becomes condensed into a painful delusion of being overpowered by some external agency, demonic or human, or of salvation lost through individual sins." This clearly delusional depression was in contrast, Maudsley said, to "affective insanity," one variant of which was "melancholic depression without delusion. Simple melancholia" (Maudsley, 1867). It was a neat layout of psychotic depression versus nonpsychotic depression, later forgotten because Maudsley wrote so obscurely and in such an unsystematic manner.

Now we are in the 1920s. At this point a film of vaseline starts to be drawn over the lens of psychiatric diagnosis because of a complete disagreement between two competing schools about the cause and nature of depression. The Kraepelinians, as we have seen, believed MDI to be an endogenous psychosis: It came on unprompted, wrestled down the entire body, then went away again often without obvious cause. It was "autonomous." Freud, on the other hand, viewed depression as entirely reactive. As he explained in *Mourning and melancholia* in 1916, depression represented a response to the loss of a "love-object." Unresolved negative feelings became directed inward, resulting in a sense of worthlessness, despair, and thoughts of self-harm (Freud, 1946).

The Kraepelinians and Freudians were truly like two parallel universes. But the rising popularity of psychoanalysis, to the point that it literally took over American psychiatry after World War II, resulted in a loss of interest in "psychopathology," which meant observing patients' symptoms closely in order to determine what disease they really had. For the analysts there were no diseases, only intrapsychic conflicts with coping mechanisms of different varieties.

To be sure, the psychoanalysts differentiated between "neurotic" and "psychotic depression," but they had little interest in the latter. It was the former that was their bread and butter. As New York analyst Otto Fenichel wrote in 1945, "Neurotic depressions are desperate attempts to force an object to give the vitally necessary supplies [of self-esteem], whereas in the psychotic depressions the actual complete loss has really taken place and regulatory attempts are aimed exclusively at the superego" (Fenichel, 1945). One contrasts this with Kraepelinian and Schneiderian formulations about endogeneity and the like.

Swimming in and out of view

The history of psychotic depression as a concept from the 1920s to the present may be written as the story of swimming in and out of view, depending on the therapeutics of the day. When psychotic depression is seen as differentially diagnosable or treatable, it swims into view; when not, it swims out of sight.

In 1913 Karl Jaspers opined that melancholia was always psychotic (Jaspers, 1913). Thus, endogenous depression and melancholia were identical for him. The rather hesitant differentiation of psychotic depression from other forms of depression and melancholia began from this ground zero.

It begins in New York. In the twentieth century, outside of the German professors and their increasingly unfamiliar language, it was the Anglo-American tradition of psychopathological analysis that first caused psychotic depression to swim into view. The psychopathology was straightforward: sorting patients into categories on the basis of their symptoms. The initial attempt occurred in 1922 with two American psychiatrists August Hoch (who was actually of Swiss origin) and John T. MacCurdy, both New Yorkers. Hoch was the former director of the New York State Psychiatric Institute. They set out to differentiate what Kraepelin had called "involutional melancholia," or severe midlife depression that often got better, from the kind of chronic psychotic melancholia in the elderly that did not remit. Involutional melancholia in the middle aged recovered usually within 4 years and corresponded to psychotic depression; they associated it with "manic-depressive illness." Involutional melancholia in older people was often a deteriorating illness ending in dementia and more like schizophrenia. Younger people with psychotic depression, they said, were a good-prognosis group involving sadness, retardation, and thoughts of sinfulness; involutional melancholia in the elderly, by contrast was associated with "fearful delusions and marked anxiety, often with terrifying hallucinations; a strong tendency to hypochondria sometimes leading to fantastic delusions" (Hoch and MacCurdy, 1922). This marks an early twentieth-century attempt to separate a good-prognosis form of psychotic depression from the deteriorating brain diseases of the elderly.

In Britain in the 1920s and 1930s there was considerable interest in the question, one depression or two? Edward Mapother, the superintendent of the Maudsley Hospital, believed there was only one: Kraepelin's MDI. Yet, at a meeting where he presented his ideas, Thomas Arthur Ross of the Cassel Hospital in Penshurst spoke up and said that his own patients, labeled "neurasthenics," were in fact a mixture of psychoneurotics and psychotic depressives, for whom Ross also used the term "manic depressive." "While the psychotic-depressive on the whole tended to blame himself for his state, the psychoneurotic always blamed someone else." While the psychoneurotics responded greatly to psychotherapy, "[t]he manic-depressive psychosis was a disease which ran a course."[11]

This was the two-depressions school. British psychiatry began to think in terms of the difference between "autonomous depression," a term that neurologist Sir Farquhar Buzzard, then Regius Professor of Medicine at Oxford, proposed in 1931, and "the depression of the anxiety state." "The large majority of patients who sought advice for symptoms characteristic of nervous exhaustion," said Buzzard of his private practice

11 T[homas] A[rthur] Ross, discussion, Edward Mapother. 1926. Discussion on Manic-Depressive Psychosis. *BMJ* 2: 872–6; Ross's comment on pp. 877–8.

in Wimpole Street, "belonged to one of two categories: the anxiety-neurotic and the manic-depressive." The former were mixed cases of anxiety and mild depression, the latter psychotic. "The depression in the case of the psychotic was always at its worst in the morning; sleep might not be disturbed, but waking was horrible." "Cases of suicide were mainly cases of manic-depressive psychosis," said Buzzard.[12]

Yet, the soon-to-become major figure in British psychiatry was Aubrey Lewis, who trained at the Maudsley in the early 1930s under Mapother and who formally was identified with the one-depression school. Lewis, the outstanding clinician of his generation, was known for a 1934 paper he had written on depression, arguing that it could not be subdivided (Lewis, 1934). Yet, when Leslie Kiloh at the University of New South Wales and a co-worker did a cluster analysis in 1977 of the data on the sixty-one patients whom Lewis had treated at the Maudsley in the early 1930s, they discovered at least two clearly defined subtypes of depression: endogenous and neurotic. In the endogenous group, "ideas of influence" received the second heaviest weighting, meaning that the endogenous patients were largely psychotic (Kiloh and Garside, 1977). Later in life, Lewis himself said that he favored the subtyping of "psychotic," "reactive," and "neurotic" (Lewis, 1971).

Thus, the psychopathological tradition in the British Isles was the first in the twentieth century to profile the concept of psychotic depression, as opposed to other varieties.

Then psychotic depression swam out of view again. So many serious depressions responded well to ECT that it seemed to be a panacea, and the subtyping of depression braked after ECT was introduced in 1938. Such subtyping virtually vanished when the TCAs, the first chemotherapy for serious depression, were introduced in 1957. It was believed at the time, although this was later seen as not true, that all

12 E. Farquhar Buzzard. 1931. Treatment of nervous exhaustion. *BMJ* 2: 753–4. It is unclear whether Buzzard's patients were formally deluded, and he may have used the term "psychosis" as a synonym for seriously ill. Still, the link between "psychosis" and "depression" was clearly being made.

endogenous depressions yielded equally to imipramine. Given the general effectiveness of these new treatments, what need was there to retain psychotic depression as a separate diagnosis?

Events unfolded as follows: ECT was introduced by Ugo Cerletti in the university psychiatric clinic in Rome in 1938, and within 2 years had spread to almost every major center in the Western world. After his arrival in New York in 1940, German psychiatrist Lothar Kalinowsky, who had worked in Cerletti's clinic in the late 1930s, became the principal advocate of ECT in the United States. Kalinowsky believed ECT to be equally effective in all forms of depression, save the neurotic intermixed with anxiety. "We get the best results in shock therapy in patients with dramatic symptoms," he said in 1944. "Patients with neurotic symptoms superimposed on a psychosis and patients with borderline conditions in which the personality is preserved show the poorest response to treatment." All the severe depressions did equally well, in other words.[13] Kalinowsky, in his many writings, never singled out the psychotic form of depression as a special treatment target.

Max Hamilton in Leeds, the originator in 1960 of the famous depression scale named after him, was a big fan of ECT. He had little patience for the typologies of depression such as "psychotic vs. neurotic" or "endogenous vs. reactive." He called them all "pseudo categories." All these types could be equally severe, he said; there was no correlation between the various categories and the results of ECT.[14]

The introduction of the first TCA, imipramine, in Switzerland in 1957, in the United States in 1959, further erased the lines among endogenous depressive illness, melancholic illness, and psychotic illness. In 1959, at a big conference on imipramine at McGill University in Montreal – sponsored by Geigy (now Novartis) – a series of speakers

13 Lothar B. Kalinowsky, in discussion, in Kalinowsky et al. 1944. Electric convulsive therapy of the psychoneuroses. *Arch Neurol Psychiatry* 52: 498–504, quote on p. 504.

14 See, e.g., Max Hamilton. 1974. Prediction of response to E.C.T. in depressive illness. In J[ules] Angst (ed.) *Classification and prediction of outcome of depression (1973 symposium).* Stuttgart: Schattauer, pp. 273–9, discussion comments on p. 286.

stood up to say that, basically, one size fits all. Fritz Freyhan, at Delaware State Hospital in Farnhurst, said that whether it was manic depression, involutional depression, or psychotic depression, the patients responded about the same, 50–60 percent getting somewhat better (Freyhan, 1959). Hans Hoff of Vienna found imipramine effective for most of his patients with "true endogenous" depression: of fifty treated, thirty-three were much improved (Hoff, 1959). Further differentiation of "endogenous" was not necessary. (As we see in Chapter 7, the TCAs today would not be the first choice of treatment.)

Thus, in mainline psychiatry, psychotic depression swam out of view in the 1960s. The several English factor analyses in the 1960s that clearly differentiated endogenous from neurotic depression made almost no reference to psychosis.[15] In *DSM*-II, published in 1968, "psychosis" really served as a synonym for "severe" and did not entail loss of reality. What the manual called affective psychosis was really, as Don Klein observed, "simply a severe endogenous mood disorder" (Klein, 1976).

The St. Louis school associated with Washington University, then the premier advocates of biological thinking in American psychiatry, was also uninterested in psychotic forms of depression. Sam Guze, Eli Robins, and George Winokur, the school's leaders, were pushing "primary" versus "secondary" typologies of depression and scorned the qualifier "psychotic" as having been inconsistently used in the past. In a clinical study, Guze found that depressed patients with psychosis had no

15 See L. G. Kiloh and R. F. Garside. 1963. The independence of neurotic depression and endogenous depression. *Br J Psychiatry* 109: 451–63; M. W. P. Carney, M. Roth, and R. F. Garside. 1965. The diagnosis of depressive syndromes and the prediction of E.C.T. response. *Br J Psychiatry* 111: 659–74; these latter authors did, however, look specifically at psychosis and found that it correlated positively with endogenous depression. On the basis of a positive (abnormal) response to the dexamethasone suppression test (DST), in 1980 Bernard J. Carroll and co-workers at the University of Michigan reaffirmed the existence of endogenous depression as an independent diagnostic entity distinct from nonendogenous depression. Carroll et al. 1980. Diagnosis of endogenous depression: Comparison of clinical, research and neuroendocrine criteria. *J Affect Disord* 2: 177–94.

particular profile: "The results failed to support the validity of a classification of affective disorders based on the presence or absence of psychotic features" (Guze, 1975).

One of the pupils of the St. Louis school was Ming Tsuang, later an architect of the "Iowa 500" study, in which case records of patients admitted to the Iowa Psychopathic Hospital between 1935 and 1944 were retrospectively analyzed and the patients' destinies traced. Tsuang was puzzled by eighty-five cases of "atypical schizophrenia," where, although the diagnosis "psychotic depression" practically screamed in his face, he did not use it and instead expressed bewilderment at so curious a mix of psychosis and depression (Tsuang et al., 1976).

Another pupil of the St. Louis school was John Feighner, chief author of a famous paper that appeared in 1972 on the classification of psychiatric illness based on "operational criteria" (lists of possible symptoms) rather than clinical impressions; in Feighner's nosology, psychotic depression virtually disappeared. (The criteria were the work of many hands at St. Louis; Feighner was just finishing his residency, but Robins and Guze generously let him be first author.) In the "Feighner" (or "Robins-Guze") criteria, three big symptom groups were needed to make the diagnosis of "primary affective disorders." Under the middle group, which required five of eight possible criteria for the diagnosis of "definite" depression, psychotic was just smuggled in as criterion number 6: "Feelings of self-reproach or guilt (either may be delusional)" (Feighner et al., 1972). So, psychosis vanished from diagnosis of depression in St. Louis.

Psychotic depression also disappeared from therapeutics. For Leo Hollister and John Overall, among the pioneers of psychopharmacology in the 1960s, there was, to be sure, differential responsiveness in depression: imipramine was indicated for retarded depression, thioridazine for the anxious variety; psychosis as such was not one of their subtypes (Hollister and Overall, 1965; Overall et al., 1966). In a large study of antidepressant drugs that Gerry Klerman and Gene Paykel were undertaking in New Haven, Connecticut, in the early 1970s, the authors found no significant difference in response to TCAs in any of the depression groups, one of which was "psychotic depression."[16]

As the studies piled up, it looked as though psychotic depression was doomed.

The *DSM* series: psychotic depression as a subclass of "major depression"

The 1970s also saw the drafting of the dramatic new third edition of the APA's diagnostic guide, published in 1980 as "*DSM*-III." The guide basically buried psychotic depression, even though interest in the subject was rising among clinicians. How did this happen?

The story goes back to a big collaborative program in the "psychobiology of depression" that National Institute of Mental Health (NIMH) decided to fund in the 1960s. Marty Katz, the program director at NIMH, agreed in 1969 to fund a big conference in Williamsburg, Virginia, to kick off the program.[17] Gerry Klerman, then at Yale, was the program's chief investigator. Klerman, impressed by Guze's and Robins's thinking on "how to validate a diagnosis," invited them to Williamsburg, and Klerman and Robins (Guze did not come), together with several other investigators, agreed to rework the diagnosis of depression until then mired in psychoanalytic jargon.[18]

16 G. L. Klerman, E. S. Paykel, and B. Prusoff. 1973. Antidepressant drugs and clinical psychopathology. In Jonathan Cole et al. (eds) *Psychopathology and psychopharmacology.* Baltimore: Johns Hopkins, conference in 1972, pp. 177–93, see p. 186.

17 T. A. Williams, M. M. Katz, J. A. Shield Jr. (eds) 1972. *Recent advances in the psychobiology of depressive illness: Proceedings of a workshop sponsored by the Clinical Research Branch, Division of Extramural Research Programs, National Institute of Mental Health, hosted by the College of William and Mary in Virginia, Williamsburg, Virginia, April 30–May 2, 1969.* Washington, DC: GPO; DHEW Pub. No. [HSM] 70–9053.

18 On Spitzer's trip to St. Louis, see Samuel Guze, interview. 2000. The neo-Kraepelinian revolution. In David Healy (ed.) *The psychopharmacologists*, vol. 3. London: Arnold, pp. 395–414, especially p. 404. The Robins-Guze paper on

Klerman thought the classification of depression should be based on evidence.[19]

David Healy backgrounds this Williamsburg meeting:

> The NIMH collaborative program aimed at testing Joe Schildkraut's catecholamine hypothesis of depression [that depression was caused by a shortage of the catecholamine neurotransmitter norepinephrine]. The catecholamine hypothesis on one level seemed a simple matter to test. But the meeting at Williamsburg recognised that in order for any biological tests to make sense, relatively homogenous groups of patients had to be collected. This required researchers to speak a common language, which called for a second arm to the program – one that would look at diagnostic criteria. (D. Healy, personal communication, 2005)

In 1973 Klerman summarized the group's thinking on the diagnosis of depression. He invoked the "unipolar-bipolar" dichotomy, an outgrowth of Kraepelin's MDI, that Karl Leonhard was studying at the Charité Hospital in East Berlin and Carlo Perris in Sweden. Klerman mentioned the British debate about one depression versus two. "The current trend," Klerman said, "is to regard the depressions as a heterogeneous group."[20]

Bob Spitzer at the New York State Psychiatric Institute had been invited down to St. Louis to give a talk. He had a background in psychometrics and psychoanalysis, and until then had paid relatively little attention to depression. Yet, meeting with Robins and Guze hooked his curiosity, and the three of them agreed to move forward on the diagnostic side of the collaborative program. Spitzer was unhappy with the Feighner criteria of 1972 and thought that depression could be much more sensibly subdivided. They decided to take on other diseases as well in a study of the Research Diagnostic Criteria (RDC) of psychiatry.

---

diagnosis appeared in 1970 as Establishment of diagnostic validity in psychiatric illness: Its application to schizophrenia. *Am J Psychiatry* 126: 983–7.

19 See Myrna Weissman, interview. 1998. Gerald Klerman and psychopharmacology. In David Healy (ed.) *The psychopharmacologists*, vol. 2. London: Altman, pp. 521–42, especially pp. 528–31.

20 See note 16.

In 1975 Spitzer and Robins published a preliminary version of their RDC, dividing "major depressive disorder" into ten subtypes, such as "agitated" and "endogenous." One of the subtypes was "psychotic," meaning just that: psychosis. The authors did not see it as a measure of severity (unlike *DSM*-II) and they did not see it as the other end of a teeter-totter with "neurotic" (Spitzer et al., 1975). They also included such refined categories as "minor depression" and "schizo-affective disorder, depressed type." In terms of the typology of depression, this was something of a *coup de main*, making the crude *DSM* categories that came along in 1980 almost a scientific embarrassment. A definitive version of the RDC was published in 1978 (Spitzer et al., 1978). (As well, RDC reduced the required duration of illness in major depression from a month in Feighner to 2 weeks, a difference that was the universe in practical terms.)

Meanwhile, an entirely different powder train was being lit. Quite independently of Williamsburg and the Washington University of St. Louis school, the leadership in Washington of the APA was feeling the same ferment in psychiatry as Klerman, Spitzer, and Robins. A new nosology, or diagnostic schema, was needed that relied less heavily on psychoanalytic concepts, as in *DSM*-II, and that made some effort to identify treatment-specific subgroups, given the avalanche of new psychopharmaceuticals then sweeping across the pharmacies' shelves. In March 1973, Walter Barton, the medical director of the APA, decided to initiate this reassessment, not really appreciating what he was getting into, and in 1974 Melvin Sabshin and Theodore Millon, "Young Turks" within the APA, as two historians of these events put it, decided to ask Spitzer to head a task force to revise *DSM*-II (Kirk and Kutchins, 1992). (They identified Spitzer because his campaign in 1973 to delist homosexuality as a psychiatric illness had caught the eye of the leadership.[21])

21 See, on these events, Robert Spitzer, interview. 1973. A manual for diagnosis and statistics. In David Healy (ed.) *The Psychopharmacologists*, vol. 3. London: Arnold, pp. 415–30.

Throughout the late 1970s this task force, quite separate from the RDC people, struggled with the intellectual and political task of wresting psychiatric diagnosis from the hands of the psychoanalysts.

In the work of this task force, "melancholia" and "psychotic depression" were relegated to "fifth-digit" qualifiers of major depression. (In the discussions of the task force, in correspondence preserved in the archives of the American Psychiatric Association, the term "psychotic depression" is virtually never mentioned.) Endogenous depression was abolished. Depression as a whole was reduced from the rich typology of RDC to a single disorder, major-depressive episode; "dysthymia" was tacked on just before the publication of *DSM*-III as an afterthought to piece off the analysts. (The manual did include bipolar disorder and adjustment disorder as well.) So the one-depression crowd had triumphed at *DSM*! This savaging of the RDC might have been partly related to a rift between Robins and Spitzer, and Robins's virtual withdrawal from the *DSM* process, which he later scorned.

Early on, the task force had made the decision to ditch "psychosis," "neurosis," and the distinction between them. (According to Myrna Weissman, Gerry Klerman's widow, the disease designers were influenced by Gerry's and Gene Paykel's notion, published in 1970, that in depression there was a smooth continuum from mild outpatient depression to the severe inpatient variety, with no demarcation points along the way.[22]) At a meeting of the task force in September 1974, in New York, Spitzer summed up what really were his own views, which he represented as the consensus of the task force:

22 See Myrna Weissman, interview. 1998. Gerry Klerman and Psychopharmacology. In David Healy (ed.) *The Psychopharmacologists*, vol. 2, pp. 521–42, at pp. 522–3. Klerman died in 1992. For the first articulation of the Klerman-Paykel theory about a single "gradient from outpatient to inpatient facilities," in terms of "patient characteristics, particularly severity, and chronicity of illness," see E. S. Paykel, G. L. Klerman, and B. Prusoff. 1970. Treatment setting and clinical depression. *Arch Gen Psychiatry* 22: 11–21.

> It was . . . agreed that "psychosis" and "neurosis" are useful possibly as adjectives, but not as classificatory principles. The term psychosis has become vague in usage, and the conditions formerly described as psychoses may be found in people who are not at the time of observation, psychotic. Neurosis, a theoretical etiologic term [in psychoanalysis], suggests a more or less steady state, which does not adequately categorize what we now see as primarily episodic or transient behaviors.

Spitzer also said that "what has been known as depressive neurosis should be included among the affective disorders," thus wiping out the single most cherished diagnosis in psychoanalysis.[23]

The *DSM*-III types were plagued by an inability to decide what to do with depressive neurosis, and after flirting with such phrases as "minor depression," they decided, as noted above, to call it "dysthymia." The analysts were furious about these changes because (a) the "neuroses" were abolished and (b) the affective disorders were all presumably treatable with psychopharmacology, not exactly the analytic stock in trade.

Within the task force, the decisions to abolish "endogenous" and "psychotic" produced a good deal of unwill. Spitzer's colleague Arthur Rifkin at the Psychiatric Institute proposed a bit of tinkering with some of the terminology, then added, "Of course, all this is not preferable to the truth (endogenomorphic, chronic dysphoric, and disappointment reaction) but I assume you want mild surgery not major."[24] There were numerous comments of this nature, as veteran psychiatrists instinctively reached back to concepts such as endogenous that they recognized from years of practice, alarmed at the homogenizing of the complex depression picture involved in the all-devouring term, "major depression."

In February 1979, as the manual lay almost ready for approval, Barney Carroll at the University of Michigan fired a final warning shot

23 [Summary]. 1974. Task force on nomenclature and statistics, meeting of September 4, 5, 1974 in New York, APA Archives, Professional Affairs, box 17, folder 188, p. 5.
24 Arthur Rifkin to Robert Spitzer, March 30, 1978, APA Archives.

across Spitzer's bow: the "major depression" category sounded rather "endogenous" (people were using the term to mean mood autonomy). Yet, you let in, Carroll told Spitzer, "a sizeable number of patients with non-endogenomorphic depressions. Endogenous also meant psychotic, according to Carroll, "true pathological guilt (not simply demoralized self-reproach)." Yet, plenty of nonpsychotic patients would qualify for *DSM*'s major depression. Carroll closed with a prescient note, "I am sincerely suggesting these changes to you with the greatest possible sense of urgency. I honestly believe that you will be buying yourself (and the rest of us) a lot of grief if you allow the unitary category of major depressive disorder to remain. I have no doubt that there *are* [emphasis in the original] two distinct types of 'depression' and that it is essential for clinicians to make the distinctions both for clinical practice and for research."[25] (Carroll later returned to this subject in print: "If we do not differentiate among types of depression, then whatever we can say about psychopathology or genetics or biological mechanisms sounds as though it applies to all of them. Once that attitude gets abroad the stage is set for chaos in therapeutics and clinical pharmacology"; Carroll, 1981.)

In 1980, *DSM*-III was published, the two historic depressions of psychiatry scrunched into one sole category: major depression. "Psychotic features" became a qualifier of major depression, alongside melancholia. This classification was to remain in the *DSM* system right through to *DSM*-IV of 1994.[26] As Gordon Parker put it later, Barney Carroll was right: "In reality, 'major depression' is a pseudo-category, effectively homogenizing multiple expressions of depression, and with each likely to be associated with quite variable response rates to different interventions" (Parker, 2004).

25 Bernard J. Carroll to Robert Spitzer, February 19, 1979, APA Archives, Williams Papers, *DSM*-III-R, *DSM*-III files, box 1. Major depressive disorder.

26 *DSM*-IV also added catatonic features as a qualifier for major depression (p. 376).

Psychotic depression as an independent disease

The return of psychotic depression as a disease of its own began with the discovery of a new biological measure of depression: the dexamethasone suppression test (DST), advocated by Barney Carroll from 1972 on.[27] Dexamethasone is an artificial steroid. The cortex, or outer layer of the adrenal gland, produces a natural steroid, cortisol. If you give someone an injection of dexamethasone, the artificial steroid will tell the hypothalamus in the brain to signal the pituitary gland that the body has enough steroid on board, and the pituitary gland will signal the adrenal cortex to stop producing the natural steroid cortisol. Cortisol levels will drop in a normal person. They are "suppressed." In someone with severe depression, by contrast, an injection of dexamethasone fails to shut off the hypothalamus-pituitary-adrenal axis. Cortisol levels remain high, being "nonsuppressed." A measure of serious depression, said Carroll, was dexamethasone nonsuppression of cortisol. The DST test became widely used in psychiatry during the 1980s (and some observers feel that its subsequent loss of popularity was a serious mistake).

Patients with psychotic depression suppress dexamethasone very poorly, their cortisol levels remaining high; patients with nonpsychotic melancholia suppress dexamethasone very variably; and patients with nonmelancholic depression suppress dexamethasone quite readily and tend to have normal levels of cortisol soon after dexamethasone. A number of well-conducted research studies established this. In 1987 Dwight Evans

27 See B. J. Carroll. 1972. Control of plasma cortisol levels in depression: Studies with the dexamethasone suppression test. In Brian Davies et al. (eds) *Depressive illness: Some research studies*. Springfield, IL: Thomas, pp. 87–148; see also Carroll and George C. Curtis. 1976. Neuroendocrine identification of depressed patients. *Aust NZ J Psychiatry* 10: 13–21; B. J. Carroll, G. C. Curtis, and J. Mendels. 1976. Neuroendocrine regulation in depression. *Arch Gen Psychiatry* 33: 1039–57; Carroll. 1977. The hypothalamus-pituitary-adrenal axis in depression. In G. D. Burrows (ed.) *Handbook of studies on depression*. Amsterdam: Excerpta Medica, pp. 325–42; B. J. Carroll, M. Feinberg, J. F. Greden, and J. Tarika. 1981. A specific laboratory test for the diagnosis of melancholia. *Arch Gen Psychiatry* 38: 15–22.

and Charles Nemeroff at the University of North Carolina in Chapel Hill studied 166 consecutive inpatients who had depressive symptoms of some kind. One hundred and four of them had major depression, and of these

- sixty-two had major depression without melancholia
- twenty-three had major depression with melancholia
- nineteen had major depression with psychosis

The investigators administered 1 mg of dexamethasone orally at 11:00 PM, then took venous blood samples the following day at 4:00 PM to assay serum cortisol. They defined DST nonresponse as a blood concentration of cortisol greater than 5 μg/dl. Of these 104 patients with major depression, the following had high serum cortisol:

- 95 percent of those with psychosis
- 78 percent of those with nonpsychotic melancholia
- 48 percent of those without melancholia

Some of the 166 patients did not make it over the "major depression" threshold but merely had "depressive symptoms." Only 14 percent of them had high serum cortisol (Evans and Nemeroff, 1987).

There were several studies like this,[28] quite dramatic demonstrations that melancholic depression was a different animal from nonmelancholic, and that melancholia's psychotic variant was biologically distinct as well.

28 See, e.g., J. C. Nelson and J. M. Davis. 1997. DST studies in psychotic depression: A meta-analysis. *Am J Psychiatry* 154: 1497–503, who found, in an analysis of nineteen studies, that nonsuppression occurred in 64% of patients with psychotic depression, as opposed to 41% of nonpsychotic patients. In melancholia, nonsuppression was only 36%, and among nonmelancholic outpatients with "major depression" – the heterogeneous DSM category – nonsuppression was only 12%.

There was also the recognition that psychotic depression had a different prognosis as well as a different response to treatment and a distinctive cortisol metabolism.

A debate occurred about whether delusionally depressed patients committed suicide more often than others. MDI, for example, was seen as an extremely dangerous affair. Could delusional depression be worse than that?

Yes, in a nutshell, and the definitive answer was delivered in 2002 by Jules Angst, a psychiatry professor in Zurich, together with co-workers. In an extraordinary research project Angst had followed over 400 patients admitted to the university psychiatry hospital between 1959 and 1963 for almost 40 years, up to 1997. By that time 76 percent of them were dead. Of these 305 deaths, at least 44 were from suicide. But the depressive illness would have contributed to many other deaths as well, such as those from accidents and heart disease. Their death rate as a whole was 61 percent higher than that of the general population. Angst did not keep track of how many of these patients were delusional; of the sample as a whole, 61 percent had psychotic episodes over their lifetime. So we are looking at a group heavily infiltrated with psychosis.[29]

Overall, these patients had a suicide rate eighteen times higher than that of the population as a whole, and since we are dealing largely with delusional depression here, the prognosis is not especially favorable. But within the depressives, the unipolars had a suicide rate more than twice as high as the bipolars, reversing the conventional wisdom about the relative lethality of the two illnesses. Moreover, all the depressives were continually at risk from the time of their discharge until observation ended in 1997: Every year a certain percentage would suicide regardless how much time had passed since their discharge. (The implications of this for maintenance therapy are startling: Depression is a life-long

29 F. Angst, H. H. Stassen, P. J. Clayton, and J. Angst. 2002. Mortality of patients with mood disorders: Follow-up over 34–38 years. *J Affect Disord* 68: 167–81. Correct as written is the repetition in the paragraph of "61."

illness for many, and constant vigilance is required.) "Naturally, many of these patients commit suicide," wrote one British psychiatrist. "They may not hope to get to heaven but they know they are leaving hell" (Price, 1978). The bottom line is that psychotic depression does seem to have a distinctive prognosis: If you have been hospitalized for depression, your chances of living to old age are much worse than those of your anxious and nervous neighbors.

Psychotic depression also started to be profiled after the 1960s because there were a number of severely depressed patients who did not respond to TCAs, the treatment of choice in those days. In a conference in Boston in 1965, Klerman said, "Using MAO inhibitors and imipramine, we do get results in about half of our patients, but the other half do not seem to respond very well to them."[30]

Particularly in psychotic depression the new drugs proved unpromising. In 1961 P.-B. Schneider, the head of outpatient psychiatry at the Lausanne University Hospital, and a colleague were doing a trial of Geigy's new antidepressant drug opipramol (Insidon) in depression. Some types of depression did well on the drug; 62 percent of the patients with endogenous depression were helped by it. Yet, of those with "depressive schizophrenia," or psychotic depression, only one in eight was helped (Schneider and Villa, 1961). In 1961 Fritz Freyhan noted that the "ideational syndrome" in depression, including guilt and delusions, responded much less well than melancholia or agitation to antidepressants (Freyhan, 1961). Said Charles Friedman of a trial of fifty depressed patients at Springfield Hospital in London, "Of 8 patients whose illnesses were characterized by the presence of frank delusions of guilt or unworthiness and who were clearly the most severely ill in our series, none showed any significant response to Tofranil [imipramine], while 5 of them subsequently responded to E.C.T."[31] Two years later

30 Gerald Klerman, discussion. 1966. In Philip Solomon (ed.) *Psychiatric drugs: Proceedings of a research conference held in Boston*. New York: Grune & Stratton p. 89.

31 C. Friedman, M. S. De Mowbray, and V. Hamilton. 1961. Imipramine (tofranil) in depressive states: A controlled trial with in-patients. *J Mental Sci* 107: 948–53, quote

Anthony Hordern, in another English trial comparing impraime versus amitriptyline, found the same thing: Imipramine had no impact on deluded depression and amitriptyline only little. "Depressed patients with unequivocal depressive delusions should be given ECT," Hordern said (Hordern et al., 1963).

These were important early results. They suggested that there was a distinctive syndrome out there on which the new drugs did not work but on which ECT did. This kind of differential responsiveness points toward an independent illness entity. It was this differential effect of ECT on psychotic depression, in the presence of medication failure, that turned on the red light: We are dealing with a disease *sui generis* here.

But these were the years of deepest stigmatization of ECT. Most clinicians were as inclined to prescribe ECT for their depressed patients as leeching. Only late in the 1970s, when the terrible stigma that had buried convulsive therapy for generations began to lift, did psychiatry become more open minded toward it, and just at that moment Sandy Glassman at the New York State Psychiatric Institute came along.

In 1975 Glassman, 41 years old, was interested in drug metabolism. A chemist at PI named Jim Burrell had developed a method for measuring the concentration of imipramine in the blood, and Glassman wanted to see whether fast metabolizers had a better clinical response to imipramine than slow metabolizers. (This kind of metabolism seemed under genetic control, and he wanted to get at that.) "The old tricyclics probably worked two-thirds of the time," Glassman said in an interview. "And the question was, much of the time that they didn't work was it because of this individual difference in how people metabolize them?"[32]

---

on p. 952. See also A. S. Friedman, S. Granick, H. W. Cohen, and B. Cowitz. 1966. Imipramine (tofranil) vs. placebo in hospitalized psychotic depressives. *J Psychiatr Res* 4: 13–36, who found that imipramine failed to beat placebo in hospitalized patients with psychotic depression. For both groups, about three-quarters got better.

32 This research was published as J. M. Perel, J. Mendlewicz, M. Shostak, S. J. Cantor, and A. H. Glassman. 1976. Plasma levels of imipramine in depression. *Neuropsychobiology* 2: 193–202; Alexander H. Glassman et al. 1977. Clinical implications of imipramine plasma levels for depressive illness. *Arch Gen Psychiatry* 34: 197–204.

Glassman collected his patients carefully, keen to keep out anybody at all schizophrenic, because antidepressant drugs were thought not effective in schizophrenia. "So if anybody was the least bit crazy, to be colloquial about it, if they had been psychotic without being depressed, I eliminated them."

Glassman knew about ECT, having become familiar with it as a resident at Albert Einstein Medical College, where he had also been indoctrinated about psychotherapy. "To be honest, it was like a blow to my ego. Here I worked so hard with psychotherapy to make somebody better, and the only people that really got better were the people who got ECT. The only thing I was sure of at the end of my first year of residency was that I could make patients worse."

So Glassman included delusions in his blood-level study, as long as the patients never had delusions when they were not depressed.

"At any rate, we sat on this ward, and we didn't know what the blood levels were, we were blind to that. All we knew was that these people were all really getting Tofranil, and nature was giving some of them high levels and some of them low blood levels. But the one thing that really struck me clinically was none of our delusional depressions were getting better." As Glassman reported in his subsequent article, "At the end of the four-week active medication period, only 3 of 13 delusional patients had responded to imprimine hydrochloride. In contrast, 14 of 21 nondelusional patients had responded to the drug. This difference is significant." Glassman then gave the psychotic nonresponders ECT and nine of the ten who had not responded to the drug got better. In the article he concluded that "to treat delusional depressive patients with tricyclic antidepressants may well prolong their suffering, lengthen the period at risk for suicide, and expose them unnecessarily to the toxicity of the tricyclic drugs. According to our experience, ECT is the treatment of choice for these patients" (Glassman et al., 1975).

Yet, what really set Sandy Glassman's mind to whirring was not the effectiveness of ECT in psychotic depression. That had been long known. It was whether, on the basis of treatment response, psychotic depression was a separate illness. He started investigating the delusional depressives systematically: Their plasma norepinephrine levels, for example, were much higher than those of nonpsychotic depressives. He sent the results to Joe Schildkraut in Boston. Schildkraut said, "You must have made a mistake, they're so high, they can't really be real." Glassman then asked Alan Schatzberg, then at Harvard, about the delusional depressives' high cortisol levels. The delusional patients turned out to have fewer previous episodes of illness, different biochemical profiles, and much more psychomotor retardation than the nondelusional depressives. In an article in the *Archives of General Psychiatry* in 1981, Sandy Glassman and Steve Roose said that, "Taken together, these observations constitute increasing evidence that the separation of delusional from nondelusional unipolar depressions is a meaningful distinction" (Glassman and Roose, 1981). This is a nice way of saying it was probably a different illness.

Two years later, Glassman and Shepard Kantor, who was also at PI, did say that delusional depression was an illness *sui generis*. Writing in the *British Journal of Psychiatry* in 1977, after a review of the effectiveness of ECT and drugs in delusional depression, they said, "The relative unresponsiveness of deluded depressed patients to tricyclic drugs would suggest that they are in some biological sense different from nondeluded depressed patients. . . . For these reasons deluded depressed patients should be excluded from populations considered otherwise homogeneous for primary depressive disorder" (Kantor and Glassman, 1977).

There was huge resistance to news of the effectiveness of ECT because a significant body of opinion wanted to believe in psychopharmacology as the route to go. In 1978, Fred Quitkin, Don Klein, and Arthur Rifkin, colleagues of Glassman at PI, doubted that Glassman had given his patients high enough doses of antidepressants and pooh-poohed ECT as the first-line therapy in psychotic depression (Quitkin et al., 1978). Glassman and his team replied that Quitkin's patients just had not been very psychotic, to which Quitkin replied that Glassman really had not used a high enough dose.[33]

Still, Glassman's delusional depression began to make its way abroad as a distinctive kind of disease. The scene now shifts from the Upper West Side of New York, where the PI is located, to Australia, where Gordon Parker ran a mood disorders unit at the Prince Henry Hospital in Sydney. Parker and co-workers had a strong interest in classifying depression, and in a study of 137 consecutive patients, they determined that psychotic melancholia was different from nonpsychotic melancholia. It responded poorly to antidepressants, well to combo therapies of antidepressants and antipsychotics, and well to ECT (this was known). Also, the psychotic depressions had started later in life; clinically, they were more slowed and had more sustained mood disorders than the nonpsychotic melancholics. Psychotic depression was, in other words, a terrible illness of relatively late onset in life. Finally they said – and this was news – that even in the absence of patients reporting formal delusions and hallucinations, they might be treated as psychotically depressed if they were sufficiently retarded, including up to the point of depressive stupor.[34]

By 1997, Parker and his group had worked out the view that psychotic depression was a subtype of melancholic depression, and that neither was a subtype of *DSM*'s artifactual category "major depression" (Parker et al., 1997). (The term artifactual is ours, not Parker's.) This is important because it emphasized that the treatments for melancholic depression of all kinds would differ from the treatments for "major depression": antidepressant-antipsychotic combos and ECT for the former, Prozac for the latter. It was intriguing that the psychotically depressed patients often conceived themselves as less ill than did their doctors, possibly because the psychosis caused them to minimize

33 See the exchange of letters in *Am J Psychiatry*, April 1979, 136: 462–3.

34 Parker G. 1991. Distinguishing psychotic and non-psychotic melancholia. *J Affect Disord* 22: 135–48; see also their Psychotic depression: A review and clinical experience. *Aust NZ J Psychiatry*, 1991, 25: 169–80.

their depression, or because they experienced their depression in other ways than sadness, such as numbness, apathy, or loss of vitality.

New in Parker's argument – yet firmly fixed in the older German literature that today is increasingly unknown – was the idea that melancholia differed from community depression mainly on the basis of retardation, often called "psychomotor disturbance." Parker was arguing that retardation defines the whole melancholia class, of which the psychotic version is a subtype.

By 2000, Parker had come up with an arresting reclassification of unipolar depression as a whole. There were basically two types: melancholic and nonmelancholic; psychotic was a subtype of melancholic (Parker, 2000). The defining characteristic of nonmelancholic depression was depressed mood state; the core of melancholic depression was "psychomotor disturbance," otherwise known as retardation; the core of psychotic depression was, by definition, psychotic features. Melancholic depression, including its psychotic subtype, corresponds to what we and others have been calling endogenous depression. Nonmelancholic depression is basically reactive, community depression. These are different illnesses, have different courses, and require different treatments. Parker, therefore, emerges as the Kurt Schneider of his day, at least in the analysis of depression.

In the meantime, Alan Schatzberg and Anthony Rothschild were beavering away at psychotic depression, first at Harvard, then Schatzberg at Stanford. One of the most influential figures in American psychopharmacology, Schatzberg had an academic interest in psychotic depression, wanting it inserted as a separate disease in the *DSM* series; he also had a practical interest, developing a drug for it to replace ECT. In 1992, Schatzberg and Rothschild argued in the *American Journal of Psychiatry* that there were major biochemical, clinical, and genetic differences between psychotic and nonpsychotic major depression. As well, the condition responded infrequently to placebo, poorly to TCAs and well to ECT, to combo therapies, and to amoxapine alone (in fact, amoxapine, a full-strength dopamine-receptor blocker marketed as an antidepressant, decreases the most obvious symptoms of psychotic depression without fully treating it, any more than an aspirin treats pneumonia). How curious, moreover, that young patients with psychotic depression often developed MDI, whereas older ones did not. The authors concluded, "The data reviewed in this article point to both the rationale and the need for designating psychotic major depression as a distinct syndrome in *DSM*-IV" (Schatzberg and Rothschild, 1992).

Schatzberg and Rothschild then began to explore a compound called mifepristone that had a worldwide reputation as a "morning-after pill" for birth control. But they wanted to try it in psychotic depression. In 2002, together with Joseph Belanoff, the physician-CEO of a company they had founded called Corcept Therapeutics that possessed the rights to the drug for this indication, they described encouraging reports of the drug's action in "open-label" (nonblinded) trials. (Belanoff et al., 2002). Subsequent results have been less heartening. But still the concept remains stunning: from Kraepelinian despair to a condition that is as readily treatable with a pill as an infected finger!

Einheitspsychose, endogenous depression, psychosis, melancholia, depressive neurosis, nerves ... What a tangled skein this has been historically! Anything but a straight line, in a field such as medicine where knowledge is supposed to be cumulative and progress steady. Bob Spitzer raises a pen, and a hundred years of psychopathological refinement is blotted out. Kraepelin has a bright idea and a thousand-year discourse about melancholia vanishes. If there ever was a field where knowledge has not been cumulative and traditions exist merely to be kicked away, it is psychiatry. Yet, this is the best we have to offer right now. Psychiatrists have to treat patients with these concepts, however inadequate they may be. In the following pages, we see how to do it.

3

Diagnosis in Psychotic Depression

How does one make the diagnosis of psychotic depression? How does one differentiate it from other conditions that may have similar symptoms?

Although psychotic depression is usually referred to as a single homogeneous entity, it has several different presentations. Each deserves a different treatment and thus constitutes a different type of psychotic depression. There are other conditions that only resemble psychotic depression and whose treatments differ still further again. Distinguishing among these types and conditions is the essence of proper diagnosis, and it is crucial to helping the patient and avoiding harm.

Problems with the *DSM* definition of psychotic depression

The first issue is how the diagnostic manual of the APA called *DSM* deals with psychotic depression. The *DSM* discusses this issue under the category "major depression." If a patient has a *DSM* major depression, the formalities of psychotic depression are brief, and simply the presence of hallucinations or delusions will qualify the patient for this diagnosis. The *DSM* stipulates nothing about the contents, form, severity, intrusiveness, or behavioral effects of any hallucinations or delusions.

So, according to the *DSM*, psychotic depression is a major depression accompanied by hallucinations or delusions. Its formal and only name is "Major Depressive Episode, Severe With Psychotic Features." It is classified as an episode that is symptomatic of an illness; the illness may be bipolar or unipolar, a single episode or recurrent. About a third of patients with psychotic depression experience only a single episode of depression from which they recover entirely, or at least have several decades between episodes. On the other hand, a further third of such patients experience episodes of both mania and depression. For these patients and their families, bipolar illness causes long-term distress. The remaining third have an intermediate course.

Patients with psychotic depression are typically severely behaviorally disturbed and ill. They might be unable to discuss or even mention depression. Some are incapable of expressing themselves accurately or coherently or even of saying anything at all. The death rate of patients with psychotic depression is high: 40 percent died within 15 years of admission to Yale University Hospital, compared to 20 percent of patients with severe nonpsychotic depression also admitted there (Vythilingam et al., 2003). The former averaged 63 years old, the latter 58 years, but the difference in death rate remained significant when age effects were compensated for.

By the *DSM* method, psychiatric diagnoses are assigned according to details of the patient's appearance and history, not by what might cause the condition. The cause is assumed to be unknown. If a definite and current medical cause for psychotic depression is found the diagnosis is no longer psychotic depression. Formally it becomes "depression due to (the named medical cause)" The *DSM* attaches no subtype identification such as psychotic depression to this lengthy name.

There are several fundamental problems in this agnosticism about cause. The *DSM* dismisses causation if it is not definite but merely apparent or possible. Background factors are dismissed. If there is a probable but unknown medical cause, the diagnosis remains psychotic depression. Causation by drugs or anything else is dismissed if the drug exposure occurred more than 3 months before the symptoms, even if symptoms began with the drug exposure and have continued unbroken since. The *DSM* dismisses this causation even though drugs such as LSD, PCP, and amphetamines are known to cause a persistent autonomous psychosis. In this way the *DSM* discourages the doctor who is assessing psychiatric illness from considering causes of psychotic depression. It makes biological causation seem strange, peculiar, and unnecessary. This approach differs from other medical specialties where identification of possible evidence is encouraged.

If hallucinations or delusions are present, the *DSM* always invokes the specifier of "severe with psychotic features." Unfortunately, the automatic application of the word "severe" unrealistically removes the possibility of variation in severity. Patients with a psychotic depression that has only mild to moderate depressive symptoms might well receive a different diagnosis, such as delusional disorder, obsessive-compulsive disorder, schizophreniform disorder, or psychosis not otherwise specified. (This is germane to those elderly patients with delusional parasitosis who continue to manage their self-care needs.)

The *DSM* lists two subtypes of psychotic depression: "mood congruent" if the "content is entirely consistent with the typical depressive themes" and "mood incongruent" if otherwise. Persecutory delusions and several so-called Schneiderian thought disorder symptoms (insertion, broadcasting, external control) are cited as examples of incongruency. (The term Schneiderian refers to the criteria that the German nosologist Kurt Schneider laid down for schizophrenia in the 1920s.) This *DSM* dichotomy between typicality and variance from it is obviously oversimplistic, a subjective matter of opinion, and unreliable. It is no surprise that researchers have found mood congruency or incongruency to be irrelevant (Abrams and Taylor, 1983; Anton and Burch, 1993).

An aside about the technical use of the terms depression and psychosis in psychiatry: In ordinary language these words describe personal dramas of frustration and conflict; they often include figures of speech, allegories, and imaginative images. But these are literary and theatrical usages. Diagnosis for therapeutic benefit demands clarity, specificity, and discipline in applying the terms psychosis and depression. It demands, in short, the science of psychopathology.

By depression, the *DSM* means major depressive disorder. This is a heterogeneous category; that is, it includes several different kinds of depression. If we are talking about the kind of serious depression once termed endogenous or melancholic, it is one sort of depression. Yet serious "major" depression is a disease that comes from within and strikes some people yet not others for no psychological reason. Surely there is a reason for this, but not a psychological one because the disorder is not primarily psychological. The most basic element of *DSM* depression is that either depressed mood or loss of interest or pleasure must be present. Yet both are subjective complaints, and *DSM* does not require any observable sadness or apathy, nor insist that either be long present. As an unfortunate consequence, major depression in *DSM* is only a pro forma classification, made in name only and without evidence or physiological concept.

A first problem with *DSM*'s major depression is its heterogeneity, by including several separate conditions that deserve distinctly different treatments. One condition identified as major depression is an emotionally charged psychological hyperreactivity about injustices caused by other people, and another major depression is a distinctly biological illness that looks like influenza in which the patient blames himself, even for things he did not do. Major depression can be formed of nothing but subjective complaints, or it can have abundant observable stigmata. Subjective symptoms are unreliable because they are by definition unverifiable by other people. Basing a diagnosis on subjective symptoms also conflicts with the modern standard of evidence-based medical practice. With such vagueness in its core definition, the *DSM* major depressive disorder has a disordered character. We will discuss the more verifiable components shortly.

A second problem with *DSM*-compliant major depression is the issue of anhedonia, once defined by Karl Jaspers (1913) as "the feeling of loss of feelings." The *DSM*'s notion of loss of interest or pleasure does not conform to the long-standing basic concept of anhedonia. Anhedonia is not merely loss of interest or pleasure but loss of the desire for these. Any workaholic can claim loss of pleasure because "have to do" tasks have displaced all else. Patients with generalized anxiety disorder (GAD) typically complain that they deserve a more pleasant life situation and are deprived of pleasure. This is not anhedonia because the patient desires pleasure or is capable of experiencing it. These distinctions are crucial yet *DSM*-IV does not bother with them. Anhedonic behavior is observable as absence of taking pleasure in conversation, in looking good, dressing well, eating tasty food, sleeping, reading, music, and the many things we do for entertainment. There are exceptions and even miserably depressed patients will say they enjoy the company of their children; still, they will not appear to be happy. We have seen severely depressed patients laugh at a joke for 10 seconds then return to statue-like apathy and immobility. An ocean with a small island is still an ocean.

The subjectivity involved in *DSM*'s depression criteria extends far beyond depressed mood and lost interest, and into its nine features of depression. These are the famous "operational criteria" that initially, back in 1980, were intended to distinguish the psychiatry that was newly aspiring to science from the previously unreliable swamp of psychoanalytic hypothesis.

Then there is the inconsistency problem of "atypical depression." Here is an example of these nine subjective depression criteria in action, within the *DSM* concept of major depression: the patient who is dissatisfied, worried, and challenged by adverse real-life events, and has been for at least 2 weeks. Poverty, threatening behavior by others, or medical illness are the usual causes, and a rigid personality amplifies their effects. This patient claims to be sad, tired, insomniac, observably fidgety, too upset to enjoy himself, unsure of what to do, feels he has failed, wishes he were dead, and overeats to soothe himself, or at least has most of these nine problems.

In *DSM* terms, this is "depression with atypical features." As the least specific depression – and so the path of least resistance – atypical depression applies in fact to most patients diagnosed with depression. The atypical feature set has become the tail that wags the dog that is major depression. It is another name for an unhappy anxiety disorder, and treatment is the same as for GAD (see Chapters 7 and 8). Just as anxiety disorders in *DSM* cannot be psychotic or melancholic, neither can depression be with atypical features. In *DSM*, conversion reactions with pseudohallucinations and dissociative phenomena such as flashbacks, personal identity changes, and time loss are not psychosis and cannot justify a diagnosis of psychotic depression.

We prefer a different approach. To diagnose depression on the basis of evidence, bona fide and specific observable pathology is needed. Impoverished initiation of thought, of expression, of motor activity, or of emotional expression represent good observable evidence of melancholic or catatonic depression, in the absence of a medical, neurological, or pharmaceutical cause. Of the nine *DSM* features of depression, the one that best predicts response to treatment is psychomotor agitation or retardation (Nelson and Charney, 1981). (Psychomotor refers to expressing thoughts and moving the body, while retarded signifies extremely slow and inhibited.) But one has to be careful how this is observed: Many psychiatrists are willing to accept patients' self-reports as sole and persuasive evidence of depression, a misleading path. Further, agitation is an ordinary feature of anxiety disorders, adjustment disorders, and virtually every other psychiatric condition. Purely agitated melancholia is rare but when it does occur, agitation occurs without provocation, unlike anxiety and adjustment disorders. Conversely, a depression without any observable psychomotor disturbance is presumably not a biological depression such as psychotic depression.

Diagnosis and treatment revolve around this point: psychotic depression is biological. Typically the depressed patient who reports psychotic thoughts shows psychotic behavior or observable signs of depression that objectify the diagnosis. Although *DSM*-IV does not require objective evidence to diagnose psychotic depression, insistence on evidence (i.e., observable signs) should provide a more reliable diagnosis.

Issues with the *ICD*-10 description of psychotic depression

The *International classification of diseases*, Tenth Edition (*ICD*-10) is to the *DSM*-IV as an orange is to an apple, but comparison is unavoidable. A basic difference is reflected by their names; while *DSM* claims to diagnose *ICD*-10 offers merely to classify. An illustration of this difference is specification of illness duration. While *DSM*-IV stipulates minimum durations for major depression and schizophrenia, *ICD*-10 mentions none. Another notable difference is that *ICD*-10 does not identify schizophrenia as a diagnosis of exclusion. *ICD*-10 does not describe any distinction between catatonic schizophrenia and other disorders that have catatonic features. Indeed, *DSM*-IV's description of catatonic features under mood disorders is inseparable from *ICD*-10 catatonic schizophrenia. With *ICD*-10 expertise in diagnosis resides in the clinician rather than the document.

Still, there are conflicts pertinent to psychotic depression. *ICD*-10 describes schizophrenia as having characteristic signs and Schneiderian symptoms, while *DSM*-IV avoids this overreaching claim. On the other hand *ICD*-10 schizoaffective disorder is a diagnosis of exclusion and is superseded when psychotic depression (or other psychotic mood disorder) can be diagnosed, even when psychotic symptoms are mood incongruent. Although *ICD*-10 psychotic depression ("severe depressive episode with psychotic features, code F32.3") can be pronounced by the presence of delusions or hallucinations with major depression it does not require either of these psychotic symptoms. Rather, this classification applies in the presence of psychomotor retardation or stupor that obstructs ordinary social activities. By *DSM*-IV these would be diagnosed as major depression with melancholic features, or with catatonic features, respectively.

Differences between *DSM*-IV and *ICD*-10 in the features of psychotic depression are somewhat moot. If a patient is stuporous or has severe poverty of thought or speech, how can you reliably determine that psychotic thought is not occurring? Catatonic depressed patients often first mention delusions or hallucinations after they have partially improved. Presumably some patients were too ill before treatment to coherently identify delusions or even have them. For other patients delusions or hallucinations might disappear before the patient is able to discuss them. Conversely, severe poverty of thoughts or stupor can produce incoherent speech that is easily mistaken for hallucinatory behavior or delusions.

The psychosis

Depressive psychosis usually consists of delusions and is often referred to as delusional depression rather than psychotic depression. Purely hallucinatory depressive psychosis is rare; patients with depressive hallucinations usually attach delusional interpretations to them, such as infestation, poisoning, or spying.

Delusional themes in psychotic depression are typically unpleasant (Parker et al., 1991a), meaning guilt, paranoia, sickness, worthlessness, or nihilism (he does not exist, he is now dead). In sickness delusions, the patient typically believes he is full of waste, poisoned, infested with parasites, or his body organs have quit working, especially the intestines.

Examples of less dramatic delusions are that the patient believes he is unwanted by family, deserves to be punished, or has committed a serious error that either was not committed or is not serious. (For more on the content of delusions, see Chapter 4.) Delusions can be rigid and systematized. Except in the catatonic type, the patient expresses emotions and concern about the delusions; there is no indifference. In the catatonic type, emotional expression can be diminished or absent (i.e., flat affect). A patient's belief that he deserves to be punished can incite him into dangerous and even assaultive behavior.

When the psychotic content consists solely of paranoid delusions, the response rate to ECT appears to be lower. In one small series, a mere 45 percent of twenty patients having only paranoid delusions in psychotic depression responded to ECT, but 100 percent of seven patients with nihilistic delusions responded (Solan et al., 1988). This suggests that about half of psychotic depression patients with solely paranoid delusions do not have a type of psychotic depression that responds well to ECT, such as tardive, psychotogenic drug-induced, or psychosis-dominant that is equivalent to anxiety disorder. These types are explained below.

Psychosis is generally tied to the presence of hallucinations or delusions, and *DSM* requires one of these for psychotic depression. Oddly, *DSM* allows the diagnosis of "psychotic disorders" to include schizophrenia, schizoaffective disorder, or schizophreniform disorder without hallucinations or delusions. This last diagnosis is permitted if the patient has other phenomena considered psychotic such as incoherent speech, catatonic behavior, or marked deficits in using logic, in emotional expression, or in motivation. Any of these can occur in depression, but when they do *DSM* does not classify them as psychotic. That is, symptoms that are psychotic in schizophrenia are not psychotic in depression, and this is internally inconsistent. This inconsistency can be resolved by considering that depressed patients with these symptoms have a depression that is equivalent to psychotic depression. Then calling it psychotic depression is only a formality.

Psychosis and evidence

Just as with depression, in *DSM* psychosis can be diagnosed according to evidence or subjective symptoms. Insofar as the evidence available is nonspecific and can be faked, it is unreliable. We are medical detectives, and as such we need to list and inventory our evidence and judge its quality, piece by piece. Conrad Swartz says: In a class I recently taught I saw a medical student act the role of a patient with paranoid schizophrenia. First, I admired her acuity, then I sincerely felt visceral terror that she was psychotic. I was relieved when my thanks terminated her performance, but I felt humbled in reflecting on the false quality of the evidence. Although I have seen obviously bogus emulations of catatonia by deceptive patients, purely subjective psychotic symptoms are easier to fake. We do not consider the exaggeration of sad mood or anhedonia a serious issue. Yet it is the basis of *DSM*-compliant major depression, so it is nice – if not essential – to possess hard evidence.

Psychosis is not a psychological attitude, an opinion, an implanted suggestion, or a reasoned conclusion. It cannot be changed by discussion, psychological training, logical reasoning, hypnotic suggestion, psychoanalysis, or other forms of tireless repetition. Attempts to do so will be met by the patient with anger, agitation, suspicion, or resentment, if not blunt assault and battery. When a patient with a psychosis asks for your opinion about delusions or hallucinations, rapport will be ruined by expressing doubts or judgments about the patient's perceptions. Patients appreciate hearing from us that we see they are suffering and have no doubt of it, and mentioning this has been a good start when I have replied to their challenges. So far I have not upset any patient or decreased rapport by saying that I have not been able to see or hear the voices or signs that are distressing them.

True psychosis seems like pregnancy, in that either you have it or you do not. It differs from mood, which can vary widely and in tiny gradations. In this regard, the image of a particular 89-year-old lady comes to mind. She had told us she is 525 years old. We started her on a low dose of the antipsychotic drug quetiapine because of periodic agitation. Several weeks later she told us she is 525 years old but that for our purposes we should consider her 89. Another partially improved patient said that the device that allowed her to hear the voices of people who were not present must have been turned off because she did not hear them any more. These patients offered acknowledgment but no compromise. Their world of psychosis was black and white; with improvement there was no fade through gray, just a distancing.

Still, there are observable behaviors associated with hallucinations and delusions, and a malingering patient who has not studied the pathology of psychosis is not likely to show them. So these observable behaviors comprise diagnostic evidence. The matter is easier with psychotic depression because it is improbable that a patient with a verifiable motor-retarded depression and poverty of thought would have the initiative to invent and assert factitious delusions. In this circumstance the depression validates the psychosis. If the content of the delusions is typical, it has some probative value as evidence. Emotional expression, motor behavior, speech pattern, and cognitive function are also basic kinds of psychiatric evidence. Accordingly, appropriateness of affect to delusional content, hallucinatory behavior, illogical speech, and disorientation are specific signs on which to base a diagnosis of psychotic depression.

The behaviors of psychotic depression

Besides delusions or, rarely, hallucinations, symptoms in common among the various types of psychotic depression include diminished ability to solve problems, understand new complex situations, manage social interactions, and pay attention well. These four problems are associated with prefrontal lobe function and occur with similar severity in mania, schizophrenia, and delirium (Jeste et al., 1996; Hill et al., 2004a); they are less severe in nonpsychotic depression (Schatzberg et al., 2000) and the nonpsychiatric elderly population (Lesser et al., 1991).

These prefrontal lobe symptoms do not call attention to themselves. More obvious symptoms of most types of psychotic depression include expressed low mood, withdrawal from pleasurable activities, viscous rather than flexible reasoning, slow speech, slow bodily movements, slow learning, and deficient spontaneous expressions of new thoughts, emotions, and physical activity. Although these symptoms are the archetype of melancholic depression, they are more severe in psychotic melancholic depression (Schatzberg and Rothschild, 1992; Parker et al., 1997). Psychosis-dominant type psychotic depression has obvious symptoms too, but they are different from these above. Because we expect all these symptoms to fade when the patient achieves remission, the use of antipsychotic drugs prevents full remission because they cause most of these same symptoms.

When not in an episode of psychotic depression (or some other mood disorder episode that is part of the same illness such as mania), the patient should enjoy normal function and psychological performance. Nothing abnormal should be observable. At followup after hospital treatment, patients who were treated for psychotic depression were similar to patients treated for nonpsychotic depression in global functioning, overall health, and social interactions (Jager et al., 2005). Both depression groups functioned markedly better than patients with schizophrenia.

Melancholic psychotic depression with age of onset over 60 years tends to include hypochondriacal or nihilistic delusions (Gournellis et al., 2001). In hospitalized patients about to start ECT, those with psychotic depression describe substantially more severe guilt feelings, hypochondriasis, and paranoia, and show more motor retardation than those with nonpsychotic depression (Petrides et al., 2001).

Suicidal behavior

Psychotic depression is highly associated with risks of suicide and self-injury. (See also Chapter 4 on this.) Some surveys report more suicide attempts in psychotic than nonpsychotic depression (Johnson et al., 1991). In patients about to start ECT treatment, suicidal thoughts, threats, and suicidal behaviors are less common in psychotic than nonpsychotic depression. Before ECT such suicidal expressions were present in 27 percent of 132 psychotically depressed patients and 53 percent of 181 nonpsychotic depressed patients (Kellner et al., 2005). However, actions speak louder than words, and risks of actual suicide appear much higher in psychotic depression. Specifically, in a series of twenty-two completed suicides of mood-disordered patients, 64 percent had psychotic unipolar depression but only 12 percent had nonpsychotic unipolar depression (Roose et al., 1983). Taking these results together, nonpsychotic depressives are more likely to emphasize dissatisfaction and to seek help by warning others, through acts and words, about their suicidality. In contrast, while psychotic depressives are less help seeking, less expressive, and more likely to behave in a hopeless manner, they commit seriously suicidal acts without warning other people first.

Suicide risks should be higher in patients with a concurrent or consequent anxiety disorder, which carries its own suicide morbidity (Sareen et al., 2005). Unfortunately, suicide risk does not stop with hospitalization. Rather, the first couple of weeks in the hospital carry a markedly increased suicide rate, as do the first 4 weeks after hospital discharge, especially the first week. These suicide risks apply regardless of treatment and imply need for supervision.

During the first month after hospital discharge, the patient should have no direct access to weapons or medication doses deadly in overdose. During the first 2 weeks in the hospital, or any time an inpatient is restless or agitated, supervised protection is important. Restless, depressed, or psychotic patients commonly blame their discomfort on hospital confinement and promise safe conduct during time away from ward supervision. However sincerely they may talk or feel, their restlessness signals distress and irrational motivation for impulsive dangerous behavior, as well as a need for relief from uncontrolled illness. This makes supervised confinement necessary.

Both psychiatrists and the hospital psychiatric nurses need to personally examine the patient for possible signs of self-injury, recent or past. Each missing body part, scar, burn, or wound deserves inquiry. Tattoos sometimes cover up injuries. If the patient injured himself before, he knows how to do it again.

Because suicidality can be related to many different aspects of psychotic depression, there is no reliable way to ascertain its disappearance in individual patients. Suicidality can be cold but insightless logic to escape the miserable tension, or delusional logic to escape fearful circumstances that are not real. It can derive from the depressive thought disorder that death or punishment is deserved, or from a specific delusion that the patient has committed some terrible deed. Self-destructive acts can follow command hallucinations or thoughts so confused they cannot be explained. They can result from an unconsidered tense impulse, even one without intended injury, such as the desire to flee.

Of course patients with present or past suicidal urgency, impulses, or behavior are at higher risk than patients who have always denied suicidality and who provide convincing explanations of why they would not suicide. Patients with suicide risk who are discharged on antipsychotic drugs remain at risk. This is because the use of an antipsychotic tranquilizer signals that the patient did not achieve remission with treatment, and remains ill. Remission stops the thought disorder of psychotic depression but antipsychotic tranquilizers do not.

Who gets psychotic depression and the risks

The reported prevalence of psychotic depression varies greatly according to clinical circumstance. Among patients admitted for depression to tertiary care hospitals, 15–30 percent are psychotic (Coryell et al., 1984; Spiker et al., 1985a; Kuhs, 1991). Among elderly patients with depression, the prevalence of psychotic depression is higher, 35–45 percent (Myers and Greenberg, 1986; Parker et al., 1991b). In the landmark

Epidemiologic Catchment Area study of past and present illness, 14 percent of major depression episodes were psychotic (Johnson et al., 1991). The point prevalence of psychotic depression in the population is less than 1 percent (Kivela and Pahkala, 1989). Psychotic features are more common in bipolar depression than in unipolar depression (Stephens and McHugh, 1991).

There is no psychological reason for a person to develop psychotic depression. Patients with psychotic depression and those with neurotic depression have similar premorbid stressful life events and difficulties (Brown et al., 1979). That study antedates current diagnostic terminology; its neurotic depression corresponds to atypical depression or anxiety disorders, which are essentially synonymous. There are biological reasons for psychotic depression, including genetic predisposition, bipolar disorder, childbirth, deteriorative brain disease, and jet lag. Other reasons include exposure to substances that cause psychosis or depression or whose discontinuation can do so. Such substances include hormones and drugs with hormonal effects, such as anabolic or androgenic steroids, high-potency corticosteroids such as prednisone and dexamethasone, and thyroid hormones. Street drugs such as amphetamines and phencyclidine can cause psychotic depression, sometimes reversible. Paradoxically, antipsychotic tranquilizers can eventually exacerbate or cause psychosis and depression. Of course, only a small minority of people with childbirth, jet lag, or steroid exposure develop psychotic depression; presumably there is an inherited fragility. This is analogous to smoking or high blood pressure risking coronary vascular disease and cerebrovascular disease. An illustration of genetic predisposition is the six-fold prevalence of bipolar illness among relatives of delusionally depressed patients, compared to relatives of other depressives and controls (Weissman et al., 1984).

As we have seen, melancholic psychotic depression is more common in the elderly (Parker et al., 1991b). Its incidence increases progressively past the age of 60 (Gournellis et al., 2001), perhaps further evidence of physical brain deterioration (e.g., cerebrovascular disease) as a cause of this kind of depression. Psychotic depression tends to strike people with worse physical health, more depression in the family, or atrophy in certain areas of the brain. These are the left frontotemporal region and the brainstem, particularly the reticular activating system and the diencephalon (Simpson et al., 1999). On magnetic resonance imaging (MRI) two-thirds of patients whose psychotic depression had started after age 45 and who had no clinical signs of neurological disease showed abnormalities, including lesions in the subcortical (deep) white matter and cortical atrophy (Lesser et al., 1991). Such abnormalities occurred in fewer than 10 percent of a comparison group of nonpsychiatric elderly people.

These constitute clear risk factors. Yet the suddenness and unpredictability of onset of psychotic depression can be disorienting for the clinician, and better warned is better armed. An 18 year old previously normal middle-class girl started a brief course of 50 mg/day of the potent corticosteroid drug prednisone for acute asthma. She lived with her parents, never abused drugs, and was a good student in high school. Her asthma remitted but 4 days later she became delusional, disoriented, and agitated. She appeared puzzled and confused. Her speech was brief and not clearly understandable. She was hospitalized and started on intramuscular haloperidol up to 30 mg/day, which made no useful improvement. After 5 days in the hospital she died in her bed. There was no evidence of suicide or foul play. Death was attributed to cardiac arrhythmia. Such sudden cardiac death occurs excessively in patients of any age with marked unremitted psychotic symptoms who have signs of catatonia or who take high doses of antipsychotics such as haloperidol. Psychotic depression can start up suddenly without any previous hints in people who are well adjusted and happy.

As adolescents and before the onset of psychiatric illness, patients who later developed psychotic depression showed deficits in social functioning. Presumably this diminished functioning derived from the same biological problems that eventually generated psychotic depression (Sands and Harrow, 1995).

Schizoaffective or psychotic depression?

Differentiating between psychotic depression and schizoaffective disorder depressed type is a serious issue because the prognoses are quite different. Schizoaffective disorder carries the dire prognosis of unending psychosis, but the expectation for patients with psychotic depression is more sanguine (Tsuang and Coryell, 1993). There is a distressing arrogance in diagnosing schizoaffective disorder or schizophrenia on the basis of merely a few months of observable illness – or just on subjective symptoms – and thereby consigning the patient to a bad long-term prognosis, lifetime stigmatization, dependence, loss of career, and tranquilization with drugs that cause impairment of performance, personality change, and physical deformity. One psychiatrist colleague complains about psychiatrists who diagnose schizophrenia in a hospital emergency room on an initial patient encounter.

Sadly, many people do have an inescapable chronic psychosis that does not respond to treatment and requires antipsychotic tranquilizers. We know that by giving these patients antipsychotic tranquilizers we are diminishing their suffering and distress from illness. Our hearts go out to these unfortunate people and their families. Still, we believe there are still more people given the diagnosis of schizoaffective disorder or schizophrenia who did not have a chronic unremitting psychosis before they received long-term antipsychotic drugs and who would have not posed a danger to themselves or others if they had been treated appropriately without such drugs. We believe it is likely that these people have psychotic depression or psychotic mania. Conrad Swartz says: Although I have placed or continued many patients on long-term antipsychotic drugs, I have rediagnosed many more patients as not having schizophrenia. I discontinued their antipsychotics and discharged them from the hospital free of psychosis and depression. At discharge virtually all these patients were taking lithium, valproate, another anticonvulsant, or an antimelancholic antidepressant.

Diagnosing young patients in a first episode of psychosis as having schizoaffective disorder or schizophrenia and placing them on long-term antipsychotic tranquilizers becomes a self-fulfilling prophesy of disability and chronic psychosis. Antipsychotic drugs are two-edged swords: at first swing they cut psychosis, but when taken in sufficient duration (2 years in young patients, 2 months in elderly) antipsychotic drugs cause psychosis or depression. Then the antipsychotic is continued to cut the symptoms it brought on.

The poor reliability and specificity of psychopathology simply do not permit us to diagnose schizoaffective or schizophrenia in the first year of psychotic illness in a patient-centered manner. First, schizophrenia and schizoaffective disorder are diagnoses of exclusion (Carpenter and Buchanan, 1994). This means that if the patient could have a different diagnosis, that is what he gets. Second, there are no symptoms or signs (or groups of symptoms and signs) that occur only in schizophrenia or schizoaffective disorder and never in other disorders. This applies as well to the duration of symptoms and signs. There is nothing specific or characteristic of schizo-disorders. Third, schizoaffective disorder is a diagnosis in search of something to represent. Its defining criteria changed vastly from *DSM*-III to the next edition *DSM*-III-R and again with *DSM*-IV because of lack of reliability and meaning. A representative study compared patients with schizoaffective disorder, psychotic unipolar depression, and psychotic bipolar depression, finding no difference in depressive delusions, other psychotic symptoms, or affective symptoms (Breslau and Meltzer, 1988).

Worse yet, the diagnosis of "schizoaffective disorder" is usually made on patients who have been treated with psychotropic drugs, particularly antipsychotics. Yet this diagnosis cannot be made in a clear manner while the patient is under the influence of these drugs. This is because psychotropic drugs change psychopathology a lot; of course that is why we use them. In patients with psychotic depression, antipsychotic drugs can achieve any of the following: diminishing psychosis but not depression, diminishing depression but not psychosis, diminishing both, or diminishing neither. In the diagnosis of schizoaffective disorder, mood symptoms can be present only intermittently and not continuously whereas psychotic symptoms must be continually present. If mood symptoms are always present when psychotic symptoms occur, the diagnosis is a psychotic mood disorder (such as psychotic depression). These diagnostic distinctions cannot be assessed while the patient is under the influence of a potent psychotropic drug. (If he might have a tardive psychosis, you should also hold off on a schizoaffective diagnosis.)

However, mood disorder is subjective; it depends on the patient's own self-assessment, accuracy, insight, and ability to express himself. These are all impaired in patients with psychosis and in those who take antipsychotic drugs. There is no reliable clinical distinction between schizoaffective disorder and psychotic depression, and indeed, studies of psychopathologic data find no clear boundary between schizophrenia-like conditions and psychotic depression (Brockington et al., 1991; Johnson et al., 1991). Unless there is a compelling and clear reason to diagnose schizoaffective disorder, the Hippocratic "do no harm" pledge demands that the diagnosis of psychotic depression be used instead.

Swartz says: At one time I had supposed that the combination of delusions, auditory hallucinations, unrelated affect and frequent "witzelsucht" was characteristic of disorganized schizophrenia. Witzelsucht is a silly, shallow, meaningless, inappropriate laughter. I saw these signs and symptoms disappear in a 19-year-old female after ECT, as she achieved remission from the first occurrence of psychosis that began 1 month before. Then as an outpatient the symptoms returned. Although delusions and hallucinations are subjective, the unrelated affect and witzelsucht were easy to see. Giving an outpatient ECT switched off these signs and returned her to normal affect and behavior just 30 minutes later. After three outpatient ECTs she was maintained on lithium, betaxolol, and a tiny 4 mg daily dose of perphenazine, which we stopped after 4 months. She continued well on followup 4 months later. On the basis of its response to ECT, this was psychotic depression. By its psychopathology it was an acute psychosis, and if she had not received ECT it probably would have lasted 6 months and become schizo-something.

The terms schizoaffective and schizophrenia are stigmatizing. There is a political imperative on the psychiatrist to administer antipsychotic drugs to the patient who carries either of these diagnoses. You cannot stop the antipsychotic drug unless you accurately understand the patient's history, but you cannot get an accurate history. You are trapped into trapping the patient in a neuroleptic box. Put yourself in the shoes of the psychiatrist who joins a health care agency and inherits a group of patients who have been diagnosed as schizoaffective. I wore those shoes when I was a psychiatry resident; the resident who rotated before me at a county hospital diagnosed about two dozen seriously ill inpatients schizoaffective. He placed them on a neuroleptic drug and either lithium or tricyclic. If he is reading this I want him to know that I took every last one of those patients off the neuroleptic. They all did fine – and a lot better – without it, and only the man with excited psychotic catatonia needed ECT. Next suppose that the psychiatrist who diagnosed those patients as schizoaffective is now your supervisor and you both work in a government health care agency. Every rediagnosis is your message to your supervisor that his diagnosis was not proper. This is a serious dilemma that psychiatrists commonly face in government-run medical centers.

Delusional disorder versus psychotic depression

If you believed you are infested, you would be depressed too. Would you have delusional disorder or psychotic depression? The key *DSM* distinction is that, to make the diagnosis of delusional disorder, there be no marked depression or impairment outside the implications of the delusions, while delusions may be of infestation, poisoning, or infection, among others. This distinction is superficial but its implications are profound. How could a person believe he is seriously infested, poisoned, or infected without showing generalized distress or distinctly decreased ability to enjoy life? If you are sure that he shows no such distress or decreased ability, delusional disorder is a consideration. However, how do you know? Diagnosing delusional disorder instead of psychotic depression generally gives the patient the risk of the doubt: The risk, in that delusional depression carries a poor prognosis and is less treatable than psychotic depression. Idiosyncratically, *DSM* permits tactile and olfactory hallucinations in delusional disorder but not visual hallucinations. However, the core concept of delusional disorder is that it includes only delusions; extending a diagnosis of poor prognosis to more patients does not give them the benefit of any doubt, but there is doubt in abundance.

Rapid cycling

Rapid cycling refers to patients who cycle between manic episode and bipolar depression with four or more episodes per year. In considering rapid cycling, the bipolar depression must be psychotic, melancholic, or catatonic, but not atypical. Virtually all patients who complain of mood swings several times per week have an anxiety disorder that accounts for these variations. This applies particularly to patients who enthusiastically claim to have rapid cycling; enthusiasm for restitution is a feature of anxiety, not depression. Treating for severe anxiety disorder as described in Chapters 7 and 8 should help avoid antipsychotic tranquilizers in these anxious patients. Some patients will develop an anxiety disorder from the traumatic experiences of psychotic depression or bipolar disorder. The assertion that 10 percent of hospitalized patients with depression or mania have rapid cycling (Liu and Wang, 1992) is best explained by anxiety disorder.

A typology of psychotic depression

According to observations of patients who have psychotic depression, it is clear that there are various types of psychotic depression. The types are elucidated below, but first here is the list:

1 Melancholic psychotic depression
2 Psychosis-dominant depression
3 Catatonic psychotic depression
4 Psychotic-equivalent depression
5 Tardive psychotic depression
6 Drug-induced psychotic depression
7 Coarse brain disease psychotic depression

In addition there are patients with pseudopsychosis and others whose type is unclear. Depending on the type of clinical environment the frequencies of these seven types will vary, but ordinary clinical experience shows that none of these types is rare. The first three types are probably the most common in patients not exposed to medications or street drugs. In addition, psychotic depression and its treatments can induce several other serious psychiatric disorders, which will be detailed separately. Because the *DSM* does not attend to such types of psychotic depression, there is no conflict with it.

Melancholic psychotic depression

The patient appears sickly and slowed, as severe melancholics do, but a probing interview reveals delusions that portray misery. The delusional content is typically of poverty, nihilism, dying, worthlessness, guilt, or body illness. Sickness delusions include organ dysfunction (e.g., bowels do not work), being rotted or full of waste, poisoning, cancer, or infestation. Passivity and apathy are the legs of melancholia, and the details they carry are faint and sparse. Exemplifying the profound slowing of thought processes and emotional expression, these delusions are presented flatly and without drama. So, it is easy to overlook them. Moreover, marked psychomotor slowing may hide psychosis, as the patient does not mention it. Still, the presence or absence of depressive delusions has a strong effect on treatment response. This is a common form of psychotic depression. Some patients with bipolar disorder have episodes of depression that look like this. In *DSM* this would be classified as major depressive episode with both psychotic features and melancholic features.

Several decades ago, melancholia represented an observable depression (Hamilton, 1989), but no longer; with *DSM*, this usage has gone out of style. Melancholia previously identified a sickly persona different from the patient's usual bearing, typically with psychomotor retardation, deficient expression of new thoughts, omega sign ("the raising of the inner ends of the eyebrows," as Darwin put it), and deep-throated groans. In contrast, in *DSM*-IV the melancholia "qualifier" of major depression can represent subjective symptoms alone, such as claims of pleasure deficiency, distinctly depressed mood, greater severity during mornings, early morning awakening, low appetite, or complaints of guilty thoughts. Because these symptoms are not associated with outcome (Nelson and Charney, 1981), their inclusion in melancholia is arbitrary. Because these symptoms are subjective, their assessment is unverifiable and unreliable, and *DSM*-IV-style melancholia includes conditions besides traditional melancholia. Specifically, only 51 percent of patients with *DSM*-III-R melancholic features showed psychomotor disturbance (Parker et al., 1995). This probably explains why the diagnosis of melancholic features has become unreliable (Chelminski et al., 2000). A more reliable diagnosis of melancholia requires objective signs.

Brought by the police with commitment papers completed by her husband, this 28-year-old white female had been agitated for 1 week, talking to the television, stating delusions that her husband is a famous religious icon, threatening him, and battering him. She was unkempt, quiet, and emotionally flat, and she moved little. She spoke slowly, answered "I don't know" to most questions, and reported hearing the voice of a holy man and seeing people who were not there. She occasionally had command hallucinations. With ECT her psychotic depression gradually decreased until after the fifth treatment she abruptly changed into a state of acute euphoric mania. The ECT course was continued and the mania faded progressively until she appeared in the normal range of mood after the fourteenth treatment. She was discharged on lithium. She remained well until discontinuing lithium 18 months later, when psychotic depression reappeared.

Despite receiving potent antipsychotic drugs as an outpatient, this 33-year-old married black female continued to hear insulting voices and to believe she is inhabited by a spirit who has sexual relations with her. She told of decreased sleep and appetite. On examination she was oriented but showed poor eye contact, sadness, marked psychomotor slowing, and poverty of thought and speech. By the sixth ECT, the voices and delusions had quit and she was in a cheerful remission, talking and moving normally.

After 2 weeks of insomnia and anorexia with a ten-pound weight loss, this 25-year-old black male started hearing voices telling him to commit suicide and cut his wrist with a razor. In the past he had heard voices, had taken haloperidol and an unidentified antidepressant, and had been confined in several state hospitals. His first psychiatric symptoms had begun a year ago. On examination he was very quiet, slowed, and withdrawn. After a course of seven ECTs no depressive or psychotic symptoms persisted, and his Mini-Mental State Examination, or MMSE, was 30 out of 30 (100%, a good outcome). He was discharged on bupropion and lithium. Yet his outpatient psychiatrist tapered out the lithium and the patient was readmitted 6 weeks later after a suicidal overdose in full relapse. He remained profoundly hypoactive and withdrawn despite receiving lithium, thiothixene, and bupropion. With another course of ECT he again achieved remission.

Of course these are anecdotes – what the FDA calls "testimonials" – but they convey a feeling for the melancholic form of the illness, which is clearly distinctive.

Psychosis-dominant depression

This might be called mood-neutral psychotic depression because there is little sadness or apathy, but this would be naming according to what is missing. If type #1 above is big depression subtle psychosis, this is big psychosis subtle depression. The patient is assertively psychotic without obvious sickliness, slowing, sadness, or apathy. The delusions typically involve paranoia, contamination, religion, or self-importance. Beside the massive drama of the delusions as the patient describes them, it is easy to overlook, or hard to notice, that the patient is not able to enjoy living. The drama and rationalization of "who wouldn't be depressed by this?" obscures the depression as primary.

There are two subtypes of psychosis-dominant depression: bipolar mixed state and deteriorative. They are treated differently. Some of these patients might be classified as having a mixed manic-depressive episode with psychotic features, as a facet of bipolar disorder. Sometimes the features of mania and depression conflict with each other and summate so that both mania and depression are obscured. Yet simultaneous mania and depression is a problem under *DSM* because for the "mixed" diagnosis *DSM* requires that criteria be met for both manic episode and depressive episode. Unfortunately, in the summation neither manic nor depressive episode might be clearly observable. *DSM* does not contemplate the interaction when mania and depression occur simultaneously. The remaining *DSM* classifications applicable to psychosis-dominant depression are schizophreniform disorder and schizophrenia, depending on episode duration. Because the schizophrenia-related disorders traditionally show marked affective blunting, and psychosis-dominant depression does not, the "schizo-" diagnosis group is a misfit.

Moreover, schizophreniform is an unfortunate name because it inherently suggests use of impairing antipsychotic drugs. It also suggests stigmatization because few people appreciate differences between schizophreniform and true schizophrenia. Schizophrenia itself carries a bad prognosis, obligatory treatment with antipsychotic drugs, and frightening stigmatization; diagnosing schizophrenia is always a last resort. So, we will use the term psychosis-dominant depression. We could as well use the name "affect-laden psychotic depression" in analogy to Karl Leonhard's use of "affect-laden paraphrenia" in subtyping schizophrenia, to emphasize how psychosis-dominant depression is associated with stronger affect than other types of psychotic depression. Leonhard's (1957) nosological system helps identify psychopathology but has been overlooked in North America.

Here is how psychosis-dominant mixed state depression feels: Two months previously, this 57-year-old female took in a stray dog with fleas. The fleas spread to her two cats and three dogs. She became convinced she was infested with bugs, gave her pets away, and boiled her clothing repeatedly. She pestered her family doctor for treatment and twice received Qwell applications for pinworm. She spent virtually all her days trying to exterminate bugs. She became delusional that worms crawl out her rectum and into her genitalia. She had tactile, visual, and auditory hallucinations. She ate nonfood substances to kill bugs and gave herself garlic douches and enemas. On examination she was continuously agitated without any real stimulus. She spoke rapidly and repetitively, with flight of ideas. Her affect was of unhappy irritated concern. Laboratory tests, stool cultures, and examinations were normal. We diagnosed psychotic mixed manic-depressive state and tried giving simultaneous lithium and carbamazepine, but this failed. During a course of six ECTs she became progressively less delusional and more normal in the format and content of her speech, eventually achieving remission. She was discharged on lithium and valproic acid; we used both because we were appalled by her suffering and the risks of these medications together seemed far less than the risks of and from reoccurrence. In this case psychotic behavior was extremely dramatic and prominent; it drew more attention than the flight of ideas or the patient's sadness and loss of ability to enjoy life. However, the psychosis was part of the bipolar disorder and not a diagnosis by itself. This patient did not have schizo-anything. If we had placed her on an antipsychotic drug, she would have been impaired by its adverse effects and by the incompleteness of its benefits for the illness, and we would have done her a disservice.

Following a spontaneous abortion 4 months before admission, this 34-year-old white female began hearing voices, sleeping poorly, and feeling tired and apathetic. She gained weight, spending all her time watching television and ingesting junk food. This contrasted sharply with her "happy-go-lucky" preillness persona. On admission she complained "I can't think" and she was sad. She showed a prominent "omega sign," a protruding hypertrophied muscle just above the nose in the shape of the Greek letter omega (the symbol used to represent ohms of electrical resistance). She showed agitation and assaultiveness for no reason, sadness, and poor eye contact. Speech was slow, there was no flight of ideas, and she had trouble making decisions on mundane questions. She achieved therapeutic lithium levels within 5 days and was discharged in remission on lithium alone in 7 days.

Six months prior to admission this 24-year-old black female began believing that she is dead. She was seen by several psychiatrists and she received separate trials of clomipramine, lithium, and paroxetine, and a combination of bupropion, thiothixene, and clozapine. None of these helped. Recently she had injured her neck with a chain saw. There was localized cellulitis but no serious trauma. She told us this was not a suicide attempt. Rather, she was trying to cut off her head to show other people that she is the living dead, and that she will continue talking and moving the same way with her head off. She was a student of a major profession at an eminent university. Although she claimed depressed mood, on examination she did not appear sad or euphoric. She was able to make jokes about her situation, but she had no insight. Ordinary cognitive skills were intact. She showed mild psychomotor slowing and paucity of spontaneous speech, but this could have resulted from thiothixene and clozapine. MRI and electroencephalogram (EEG) were normal. On the ward she became agitated and irritable at times, and set her mattress on fire. She achieved remission with a course of six ECTs. Discharged on lithium, she returned to school and remained well over a known 2-year followup.

This 30-year-old female complained that people were clogging her thinking by being in her space. She also felt she was losing control of her mind. She had a severe depression 4 years prior, right after giving birth. On examination she was confused and agitated, and she repetitiously complained that people were in her space. Lithium and perphenazine were started. Perphenazine was tapered out in 4 days. After 2 weeks the patient achieved stable remission and was clear, calm, oriented, and logical.

Other patients in this group might be *DSM*-classified as psychosis or depression due to cerebrovascular disease, an example of the deteriorative subtype. These patients have prominent hallucinations, delusions, or other sensory disruptions (such as dizziness) but they do not appear generally sad or apathetic. The affect is different from normal; it might be mechanical or hyperreactive. This change in affect might be noticed as different from normal only by a close and highly observant relative – or only after effective treatment. These patients often have a history of cerebrovascular disease (or signs of one, such as transient ischemic attacks (TIAs) or cerebrovascular deterioration on computed tomography, CT, scan); they may have cardiovascular risk factors such as hypertension, diabetes, smoking, homocysteinemia, hyperlipidemia, hypogonadism, or corresponding family history. Patients with cerebrovascular disease can have psychotic depressions of other types, for example, catatonic.

An archetype is the elderly patient who covers home windows with foil or plastic because of the delusion that the neighbors are directing poison toward him. This was formerly called involutional paraphrenia. Another archetype is the elderly patient with delusional and hallucinatory parasitosis but who otherwise seems reasonably well adjusted, rational, and not depressed.

For example: With a history of 10 years of hallucinations, this 68-year-old divorced white female was hospitalized by her children. She told of being plagued by a 6"-long spirit who lives in her clothing, steals her money, and causes body pain, such as headaches. She had delusions about an agreement to marry a particular man who will rid her of this spirit. She told of sleeping 2 hours nightly for years, poor concentration, low energy, and having no fun in her life. She spent her time looking at television and visiting family. She showed no sadness, agitation, or slowness in thought, speech, or motor activity. She was neatly dressed and groomed, and had good eye contact, neutral affect, and ordinary interactive conversation behavior. Although she was not overweight, cholesterol was 266 (high) and fasting glucose 155 (high). Brain MRI showed cerebrovascular changes in the white matter and mild diffuse atrophy. The mini-mental score was twenty-three out of thirty, suggesting cognitive impairment. The patient received a course of six ECTs (for ECT connoisseurs, she had left anterior right temporal (LART) placement). After her ECTs, the patient reported that the six-inch long spirit had left her for the first time in 10 years. She became noticeably cheerful; in retrospect it became clear that her pre-treatment affect had been blunted, that is largely empty of emotions. She was discharged on bupropion.

Hospitalization was insisted upon by the daughter of this 54-year-old female. After her mother died 2 years ago, the patient gradually developed increasing hallucinations of voices of her coworkers in a government office where she had worked for 20 years. She believed that a device is amplifying their voices, which converse with each other. She talked about her coworkers' attempts to have her fired. She believed her coworkers could read and control her thoughts. She had no insight. She repeatedly asked her psychiatrist (CS) to telephone her coworkers and ask them why they talk to her through an amplification machine; she had no idea that such an inquiry could cause the loss of her job. She believed she is a good person, not depressed, and deserves better treatment. She said she is baffled and puzzled about what goes on between her and other people, so she stays to herself after work, reading magazines and watching television. She has diabetes and hypertension. On examination she was fully alert and thoroughly calm, indeed implacable. She was extremely well groomed and overdressed for being in the hospital.

Although she claimed to be worried, she showed no tension, sadness, irritability, or apathy, even when irritating questions were asked to probe her composure. She was fully oriented and knowledgeable about current events, and she denied difficulty paying attention or concentrating. She spoke with normal rate and rhythm, but her answers to most questions were beside the point and often surprisingly irrelevant. After a couple of sentences her speech would become meaningless and vague. When asked if she would comply with prescribed medication, she was unable to decide, but when it was handed to her she always took it. Formal neuropsychological evaluation reported generally normal cognitive function except for slowness in test performance, mildly impaired verbal fluency, confabulation, and perseveration. An MRI showed hyperintensities in the periventricular white matter, consistent with cerebrovascular disease.

She was started on a low dose (10 mg/day) of loxapine, a mild antipsychotic drug, and ECT was begun. After a week of loxapine and a couple of ECTs, the hallucinations had stopped; she explained that the amplification machine must have been turned off. She felt that she could enjoy life more and had not realized the deficit. Her affect was emotionally reactive and expressive, no longer calm and implacable; this was a large observable change. She was no longer particularly well groomed or overdressed, but was about as casual as the hospital staff, which was more appropriate.

Brought by her family, this 72-year-old female complained that her husband had shot and killed one of their sons, is carrying a gun and intends to kill her. She told of learning this by hearing their voices outside, through the walls. She told of the death of her 9-year-old nephew, which also was not true. She also complained of racing thoughts. She felt she is a good person, and she deserves better treatment and not punishment. She slept poorly. On examination she appeared puzzled and tense, and showed hypervigilance, intense emotionality, lability of affect, and rapid speech, but was easily interruptible. She was fully oriented. On the ward she claimed to have conversations with her sister on the second floor, but there was no second floor in this rural hospital. Laboratory tests were normal excepting mild hyperthyroidism from excessive thyroid hormone dose. Thyroid hormone blood tests fell rapidly with dose adjustment but the patient showed no change in behavior or hallucinations. An MRI showed hyperintensity in the periventricular white matter and brainstem, consistent with cerebrovascular disease. ECT was started. Because of the cerebrovascular disease, stronger temporary cognitive effects were expected from ECT, so right unilateral electrode placement was selected. She was mildly improved after the first ECT, but she experienced an unusual delirium after the second treatment. Although the delirium was not life threatening, waiting for the delirium to pass seemed prudent before continuing ECT. Another ECT 4 weeks later produced another delirium so no further ECT was given. As this confusion faded the patient showed normal behavior and mood, and was no longer psychotic, labile, or tense. She then returned home. Fortunately, delirium from ECT is rare.

According to this 68-year-old divorcee, referred by her family doctor, for the past 4 years people in the neighboring apartment have been manufacturing street drugs for sale to drug dealers. The exhaust fumes from their laboratory have been entering her apartment through the ventilation system intake. She believed that these neighbors frequently broke into her apartment, moved her belongings and damaged them, but rarely took anything. She believed they did this so that her complaints would sound crazy to the police and the landlord. Indeed, after initially showing concern, the police, the landlord, and the FBI dismissed her continuing complaints. Recently she moved, but believes the former neighbors tracked her relocation and continued to break into her apartment. She has been on disability for 7 years because of uncontrolled hypertension, and has severe financial stress, a son with terminal cancer, and several substantial medical problems of her own. She described current insomnia, restlessness, fatigue, irritability, tension headaches, irritable bowels, constant worry, and poor concentration. On examination she was very neatly groomed and dressed, but restless, hyperreactive, repetitive, overinclusive, needy to ventilate, and hypervigilant. Her voice was grating. At times she laughed and grinned, with a clear sense of humor. There was no sadness or apathy, and her cognitive function was intact. Her blood pressure was 159/90 and her heart rate 97. She blamed losing her teeth on sertraline and fluvoxamine, and she announced refusal to take these and similar drugs before anything was offered. She was treated with betaxolol and topiramate to cut her somatic tension anxiety and S-adenosyl methionine 400 mg twice daily as an anti-obsessional. On both of her followup appointments over 3 months, she reported that the neighbors had quit entering her apartment and she could not figure out why. She felt happier, and the agitation, neediness to ventilate, and other signs of somatic tension anxiety were much lower, while her blood pressure was 129/74.

This was a typical response to betaxolol, potentiated by the other two medications. It illustrates that what is classified according to *DSM* criteria as paranoid delusional depression is sometimes the equivalent of an anxiety disorder. It can be obsessive-compulsive disorder, posttraumatic stress disorder (PTSD), or GAD, and it can respond to treatment for anxiety disorder. The term "schizo-obsessive disorder" has been used to describe patients with obsessive-compulsive disorder whose obsessions become indistinguishable from delusions. It is no surprise that antipsychotic drugs are used to manage this subjective and speculative condition (Schulz, 1986), but they still should be reserved as the last resort, after other – and less impairing – treatments are tried, such as we describe here and in the treatment chapters.

This 87-year-old married male was referred by a dermatologist whom the patient had sought out to treat what he believed to be an infestation of his skin by bugs. The referral followed the patient's mention that he might kill himself to escape the infestation. He described the bugs as swordfish-like, about 1/8″–3/16″ long. He saw them and felt them, although sometimes he could not see them. He had excoriated much of the skin on his arms and legs, which bore many dozens of round red lesions from nickel to half-dollar size. It mystified him that his wife was not also infested, and that he had not been able to catch any of the bugs on sticky tape. He showed concern and annoyance about infestation. He denied depression, sadness, apathy, and weight loss. He was well oriented, knowledgeable about current events, and had a consistently friendly manner. In response to quetiapine the hallucinations and delusions disappeared and the lesions faded.

These, then, are a few vignettes from psychosis-dominant depression, where the psychosis seems to overwhelm the accompanying depression, and the skilled psychopathologist must see far beneath the surface.

Catatonic psychotic depression

Basically there are three types of catatonia: episodic, unremitting, and attributable to a medical condition. Catatonic depression is a manifestation of episodic catatonia, while catatonic schizophrenia is unremitting. The vast majority of catatonia is episodic (Fink and Taylor, 2002). Catatonia seems to be the sole syndrome we could identify in *DSM* that is based on observation rather than subjective symptoms, outside of coarse brain diseases such as Alzheimer's disease. Still, interpretation of observations is necessary and movements must be judged as purposeless rather than goal directed, peculiar, or excessive; nevertheless, this can be done systematically and impartially.

Catatonia is observed as a motor disorder that accompanies a major psychiatric illness. (Motor means involving the muscles.) The movements may be abnormally slowed, in the direction of stupor. Alternatively, they may be pathologically quickened, in the direction of manic agitation. Catatonia also includes disturbances of emotion and thought expression, that is, affect and speech. Catatonic patients usually appear puzzled or bewildered, do not say much, do not move much, and stare a lot. What makes catatonic depression usually a subtle – if not overlooked – diagnosis is that the vast majority of patients with catatonia do not have the notorious dramatic signs such as waxy flexibility, bizarre movements, posturing, slap-back negativistic rigidity, or total mutism. Even some of the fairly specific signs of catatonia do not draw attention and can be easily overlooked unless you deliberately check for them, such as echolalia, echopraxia, and mitgehen (involuntary limb movement in response to light pressure, as from a single finger). A detailed clinical explanation of catatonia psychopathology and its differences from other conditions is available (Fink and Taylor, 2002).

Perhaps 20 percent of patients with catatonic depression report delusions or show hallucinatory behavior. Although catatonia usually has a bizarre appearance, when it entails psychotic behavior it is an order of magnitude more bizarre, and we have no good word for that. A catatonic psychotic state is more frequently depression than schizophrenia, but the difference can become moot if the depression is left untreated. If left without effective treatment the catatonia can become chronic, and catatonic depression could possibly become schizophrenia, if what we understand by schizophrenia is chronic psychosis. It is as if the neurotransmitter pattern in the brain mediating catatonia transforms into a structural pattern that is far more resistant to change.

When a patient with catatonia does not speak, you can usually tell if psychosis is present by waiting until the patient does speak. Typically lorazepam (0.5–1.5 mg) by mouth or intramuscularly or oral triazolam will facilitate speech about 50 minutes later. As patients with catatonia improve with ECT, the catatonic symptoms often wane faster than the psychotic and depressive symptoms, and the details of psychosis and depression emerge more clearly until they, too, fade.

After this 71-year-old unmarried white female was found by relatives lying in bed in her own waste, saying little and hardly moving, she was hospitalized. Her history: She had stopped cooking for herself and spent her days lying in bed. Her first psychiatric episode was 1 year ago, when she was anorectic and mute for a week. Over the previous 2 months she had been treated at a local hospital with haloperidol 2 mg/day and paroxetine; this led to remission but she relapsed rapidly when haloperidol was stopped. Restarting the haloperidol produced no improvement. She spoke only a few words but was fully oriented. She moved little. She described command hallucinations that urged her to "lie down on the ground and let the bugs eat me up" and "to kill people." She denied suicidality and homicidality but said "I'm bad" and that she deserved punishment. Blood pressure was 150/60 and the patient had once had a stroke with no known persisting deficit. She returned to normal with a course of six ECTs, and also received antihypertensive medication.

Active suicidality, agitation, withdrawal, severe fearfulness, hopelessness, helplessness, medication noncompliance, and diminished responsiveness led the family of this married 44-year-old black female to hospitalize her. The patient denied these problems. The illness began following surgery a year before. At hospital admission she showed poor hygiene and no rapport, and could not pay attention to or answer most questions. She showed sadness and irritability but otherwise had an unreactive affect and severe psychomotor retardation; yet she paced restlessly at times. In response to lorazepam 2 mg she initially developed near-normal affect and spontaneity. This medication gradually lost effect with continuing doses. Observable signs of illness rapidly responded to ECT, as affect and motor activity became normal. Marked worry about medical illness persisted after ECT. This was probably an anxiety disorder because she had previously survived a mysterious threatening illness that resembled lymphoma but resolved spontaneously, perhaps sarcoidosis.

Six weeks before hospitalization, this 19-year-old black female gave birth to her first child. Two weeks after delivery she became depressed and received fluoxetine, but there was no improvement. On this admission she was brought to the emergency department by police, who found her wandering in the streets, mumbling that she had shot her family. In the emergency department her stupor was so intense that she received intravenous naloxone and dextrose, in case of narcotic overdose or hypoglycemia. With no response and normal laboratory tests she was transferred to psychiatry. She was disheveled, entirely mute, and staring with puzzled and bewildered facies in apparent lethargy. She failed to respond to nortriptyline with triiodothyronine. After lorazepam administration she spoke but was unable to hold a rational conversation; for example, she alternately insisted that she had killed her family and that she had not killed them. After receiving triazolam she was able to converse logically and showed surprise that she had a baby at home. After six ECTs she felt well and remembered her baby. At hospital discharge she appeared quite normal, spontaneous, and witty.

Low mood, difficulty concentrating, weight loss, poor appetite, and hearing laughing voices were described on admission by this 38-year-old black developmentally disabled male. He had recently received fluoxetine, pimozide, and lorazepam without improvement. He spoke only in response, slowly, softly, and no more than one sentence at a time. He appeared confused and sad, with poor hygiene. In response to six ECTs the depression and psychosis lifted, and the patient returned to his usual self.

After locking a nurse in a bathroom and throwing furniture and books around his room, this 65-year-old black male was sent from a nursing home to the psychiatry ward. Twenty years before he had been started on potent antipsychotic drugs and had taken them ever since. He complained of unintelligible voices talking over the public address system in the nursing home, of plots to put cleaning solution in his nose and mouth, and of poisonous gas issuing from the heaters. He appeared puzzled, stuporous, and slow, and he spoke only briefly and in little detail. He was unable to find his way from his room to the ward dining room. In response to lorazepam 1.5 mg intramuscularly he abruptly started speaking normally, socialized with others, moved normally, and frequently showed cheerfulness. The effects of this dose seemed to last for 1 day, then he returned to stupor, and additional doses of lorazepam had no noticeable effect. In response to a course of nine ECTs he was moderately improved but not well. He no longer had psychotic symptoms, and he behaved and responded in an appropriate manner with other people, but he did not initiate conversation. He seemed subdued rather than happy. One week after the last ECT, after returning to the nursing home, he regained spontaneity and cheerfulness. Three years later he remained well on lithium, without recurrence.

For 6 weeks this 22-year-old white female experienced confusion, low mood, disorientation, crying spells, and delusions that people around her were trying to kill her and take her job in jewelry sales. Indeed, she lost her job. On admission she showed confusion, paranoia, and speech blocking. She showed no spontaneous motor, speech, or emotional expression and replied to questions with only a word or two. Lorazepam produced mild improvement, to the extent that she could speak an entire sentence, but initiation remained absent. She told of hearing hallucinated voices but could not understand what they asked her to do. She showed no response to the combination of nortriptyline and triiodothyronine, or to lithium, becoming stuporous and mute. She rapidly improved with ECT and after seven treatments was discharged in remission on lithium.

This 29-year-old black female told of panic attacks with chest tightness and shortness of breath over the past half year in association with financial and family stresses. Over the past month she developed decreased mood, energy, sleep, ability to enjoy herself, and self-worth. She began to feel she deserved punishment and started telling others of plans to drive into oncoming traffic or a truck. She heard the voices of her deceased father and grandmother saying they do not like doctors and they have been praying. On examination she showed psychomotor slowing and sad affect. Nortriptyline 125 mg/day with triiodothyronine 25 μg/day was started, and she responded with rapid and marked improvement. However, she experienced episodes of sinus tachycardia, so the doses of nortriptyline and triiodothyronine were decreased. She immediately relapsed and the original doses were restored; a beta-blocker was added to prevent the tachycardia. She remained compliant with medication.

Two years later she returned to the hospital after a 4-day episode of complete muteness. On admission she initiated no speech and replied only sometimes, and then with only one or two words. She appeared bewildered, showed agitation but otherwise hardly moved, and was unable to spell words or perform any arithmetic. She told of hallucinations as before. After lorazepam she was able to converse briefly and rationally. She responded rapidly to ECT, achieving remission with four treatments and completing the course of six sessions. In these two episodes this patient experienced two different types of psychotic depression. The melancholic psychotic episode responded to the TCA nortriptyline potentiated with triiodothyronine, but the catatonic psychotic episode did not. This corresponds to the different treatment plans associated with these types of psychotic depression.

Readers may be surprised at the large number of African American patients featured in these vignettes. This is simply because one of the authors (CS) practiced for a long time in hospitals with heavily black catchment areas. Surely, similar pathology occurs in all races; these are the vignettes we have. Because we are intent upon giving you, the reader, patient-centered experiences drawn from observed events and not just authority-centered knowledge from journal articles and textbooks, we report what we have seen.

For several months this 78-year-old frail black female spent most of her time lying on the floor of a nursing home, with her brief explanation that she is dead. She hardly moved or talked. She refused to eat or go to the bathroom, but moved her bowels while lying on the floor. When asked any question she would reply, "I am dead" and sometimes pulled a blanket or clothing over her head. She was sent to the hospital because of weight loss and inanition. Trials of sertraline and haloperidol with benztropine produced no benefit. She had a history of receiving ECT for psychotic depression. On the psychiatric ward she continued the same behavior until beginning a course of eight ECTs. These treatments made an abrupt and dramatic improvement. She became spontaneously conversational and took care of her own dressing, bathing, and toileting appropriately. She was discharged without any medication, but she relapsed in 3 weeks. On readmission she did not move or respond at all.

She received eight more ECTs with improvement but not the remission she previously showed. She remained hypoactive and slowed, and she seemed tired. A combination of nortriptyline 60 mg/day and triiodothyronine 25 μg/day improved these somewhat, and the addition of methylphenidate (Ritalin) 5 mg at 7 AM and noon restored her activity and energy to good levels. She was discharged on these medications and remained well several months later.

Tranquilizing drugs such as antipsychotics and benzodiazepines can change a patient's symptoms and signs so much as to prevent a proper diagnosis. After all, we use these drugs to bring about large changes in psychopathology. Accordingly, diagnosis cannot be assigned on the basis of signs and symptoms that occur while the patient is under the influence of substantial doses of an antipsychotic or sedative-hypnotic tranquilizer. Not considering such drug influence is a massive omission in *DSM*. Even a small dose of a benzodiazepine such as lorazepam or triazolam can hide catatonia and continue to do so for several days in some patients. Antipsychotic drugs can diminish symptoms of mania, depression, or psychosis, in differing degrees from patient to patient. In some patients 1 mg/day haloperidol will entirely hide mania; other patients will continue to show severe mania despite 100 mg/day haloperidol or more. Similar variations occur in depression and schizophrenia.

The following case was a porcupine of surprises. This 59-year-old Caucasian woman was admitted complaining of increasing depression and anxiety over the past year, with insomnia, anorexia, loss of pleasure, crying, tension, worry, and suicidality. She had a history of receiving ECT. On examination she was fully oriented, alert, neatly dressed and groomed, interactive, and rational; she did not appear depressed. Her only medication was alprazolam; it was switched to the equivalent but longer-acting drug clonazepam, which was progressively tapered to zero over 10 days. The patient withdrew to her room, then complained that the medical staff was trying to kill her. She then became mute, unmoving, and unresponsive. In response to lorazepam 1 mg she was able to interact with other people and speak. She was given regular clorazepate in expectation that anxiety but not catatonia would respond. On clorazepate she quit eating, talking, moving, and responding. This confirmed catatonia and ECT was started. The catatonic symptoms remitted with the first ECT, but she remained troubled by anxiety and psychosis. She insisted on leaving against medical advice, but when her daughter came to see (and possibly collect) her she kept screaming that this person was not her daughter and we were trying to kill her. She started running through the ward screaming and colliding with the walls. Because this hospital could not accept involuntary patients, she was committed to the state hospital. This patient seemingly had two illnesses: psychotic catatonic depression and an anxiety disorder. Prior to admission both were being inadequately managed with benzodiazepines. To properly treat this patient required commitment for hospitalization and ECT.

This case collides with the limitations of symptom-based diagnosis. After the first ECT, the patient remained psychotic but the catatonia had disappeared. Does the patient then still have depression with catatonic features? Or does the diagnosis change to reflect the changes in psychopathology with partial improvement? From a strictly superficial *DSM* approach, before ECT the patient had both psychotic depression and catatonic depression, and after the first ECT, catatonic depression was relieved and only psychotic depression continued. Having two separate similar severe psychiatric illnesses at the same time is not credible. Changing the diagnosis to reflect psychopathology changes that have been induced by psychiatric treatment is not appropriate. Logically then, the patient continues to have catatonic depression although she no longer shows catatonic features.

Hearing voices in his head for 2 weeks telling him to cut his wrists, this 27-year-old male also told of sadness, anorexia, fatigue, and loss of interest in living. He was taking haloperidol 20 mg/day, clomipramine 100 mg/day, and clonazepam 1 mg/day. He also drank heavily and used marijuana. He had a history of abuse as a child. As an adult he had many brief hospital admissions. He had never been employed. On examination he appeared sad, slowed, and quiet. Speaking was a struggle and he eventually said "I'm confused." He was oriented but unable to perform simple arithmetic. Started on lithium and sertraline, he did not improve. He became stuporous and showed waxy flexibility of arms and head, maintaining his head four inches above a pillow. He showed remission of psychomotor abnormalities after the first ECT and left the hospital against medical advice. On another admission 14 months later, he said that voices told him to steal his sister's bracelet; he did not steal it but felt guilty anyway. He told of sleeping 2 hours per night, and said that he is afraid to sleep because he will awake in hell. He was disheveled, fidgety, and tremulous, but very slow in movements and speech, with no emotional expression and a monotone voice. He declined ECT treatment and was started on lorazepam, depot intramuscular haloperidol, and lithium. Suicidal thoughts and hallucinations faded, and he was discharged 1 week later. In this case the patient's prognosis was low in any case, and he was unable to comply with any course of treatment.

Suicidal drinking of liquid laundry bleach, soap, and skin lotion led to admission of this 45-year-old black female. She described voices telling her to suicide by cracking her head open. For the previous month she had severe insomnia and loss of interest in church activities. Other problems were seizure disorder and marked mental retardation. She took phenytoin and valproic acid for the seizure disorder. In the emergency department she was alert, agitated, irritable, sad, and tearful. Her speech rapidly and repetitiously described thoughts and plans of suicide and of her god deserting her. She received clonazepam and then giggled continuously and would not answer questions. Her anticonvulsant medications were changed to carbamazepine and clonazepam 1 mg/day. She was discharged on this medication after showing behavioral stability and normal EEG on these medications. The abrupt and enormous response to low doses of clonazepam is not typical of either seizure disorder or catatonia, but is possible with catatonia. There are no studies of outpatient or prolonged treatment of catatonia with benzodiazepines, so it is hard to recommend it. Nevertheless, CS has seen several stable remissions with doses of 1 mg/day or less of clonazepam or lorazepam, and none with higher doses. So, if 1 mg/day or less brings remission, together with regular followup it seems a reasonable treatment.

This next patient, a female in her early 70s, was transferred from the medical floor because of refusal to eat or drink. She had been admitted there for congestive heart failure. One year previously she had attempted suicide and was placed on fluoxetine. She had a carotid endarterectomy after TIAs and coronary artery bypass grafts, and she had diabetes and cardiomegaly. Brain CT showed mild atrophy and small pontine lacunar infarcts. On entry to the psychiatry ward, she told of low mood and wanting to die. She was withdrawn, slow, anorexic, and sometimes fully oriented but sometimes obtunded and only minimally responsive. She was delusional that cameras were watching her. She was unable to tolerate nortriptyline. She improved gradually with ECT, becoming consistently alert, oriented, and free of delusions. The fluctuating level of consciousness and refusal of food and drink suggest catatonia rather than melancholia.

These are anecdotes, not statistics. They are suggestive rather than conclusive. Nonetheless, clinical expertise is built on combining observational case experience with conceptual knowledge. Taken together, experience with these cases and many others suggests that catatonic psychotic depression tends to be utterly disabling, invasively unpleasant, easily confused with schizophrenia, and resistant to medications. ECT is the only reliable treatment for catatonic psychotic depression, excepting perhaps the very few patients who show remission with 1 mg/day or less of lorazepam. More on this in the treatment chapters.

Psychotic-equivalent depression

This is depression with reversible dementia, formerly called pseudodementia. Patients have incoherent speech or other marked deficits in using logic, in emotional expression, or in motivation. Problem-solving abilities and appreciation of complexities in human relationships are clearly below the patient's preillness performance. Generally, those with psychotic-equivalent depression are not catatonic, nor do they have a severe melancholic depression. Dementia, of course, is not the same as psychosis. Yet in the presence of seeming "dementia," the alert clinician needs to keep in mind that the underlying problem may be a mood disorder, rather than the inexorably progressive demise of Alzheimer's disease or cerebrovascular dementia.

Depression causing profound cognitive impairment is qualitatively similar to psychotic depression, not only in terms of thought processes, but also in the more pessimistic clinical outcome with antidepressants (La Rue, et al. 1986; Aronson et al., 1988). Elderly patients who become disoriented or temporarily demented during episodes of depression are at high risk of developing permanent dementia such as Alzheimer's disease (Alexopoulos et al., 1993).

Tardive psychotic depression

Tardive psychosis is psychosis and depression that eventually occur in reaction to taking a dopamine-blocking drug, usually an antipsychotic tranquilizer. New-onset hallucinations and delusions were observed in men of ages 65 and 74 years after taking metoclopramide for just 3 and 6 months, respectively. This was to treat gastrointestinal distress, and neither patient had a psychiatric history (Lu et al., 2002). Similarly, in young adults who were taking antipsychotic drugs for nonpsychotic mania, mood-incongruent psychotic phenomena began occurring after 3 years (Downs et al., 1993). This psychosis appeared while the patients were actively taking an antipsychotic drug, not after discontinuation, implying that worsening psychotic symptoms can constitute tardive psychosis, regardless of initial diagnosis; substantial evidence of tardive psychosis has been reported (Swartz, 2004a).

As with tardive dyskinesia, tardive psychosis appears to be a long-term rebound phenomenon. In rebound, a drug that produces a particular therapeutic effect in the short term produces the opposite effect when taken long term. The basic concept of tardive phenomena is that in response to initial dopamine blockade natural homeostatic processes cause dopaminergic supersensitivity; this is seen both neurologically, as the physical deformity of tardive dyskinesia, and psychiatrically as tardive psychosis. Just as antibiotics can provoke superinfections and long-term alprazolam (Xanax) may induce panic, antipsychotics can cause tardive dyskinesia, tardive psychosis, and tardive depression. This basic concept does not manage to explain why tardive phenomena are irreversible and persist whether the antipsychotic drug dose is raised or discontinued entirely. These persisting effects point to brain deterioration from the antipsychotic drug, as has been observed in animals (Naidu and Kulkarni, 2001; Andreassen et al., 2003).

The time courses of tardive dyskinesia and tardive psychosis are presumably similar, that is, they develop gradually and with increasing frequency after several years. With drug discontinuation and with time they can improve somewhat, but they are often chronic and largely irreversible. Recent data suggest that tardive psychosis might affect over 50 percent of patients who take antipsychotic drugs for an average of 13 years (Swartz, 2004a).

Because of tardive psychosis, it is wise to avoid abruptly discontinuing even tiny long-standing doses of neuroleptics, for example, 25 mg/day of thioridazine for 20 years. Abrupt-onset tardive psychotic depression may be the unwished result, accompanied by marked symptoms of both psychosis and depression.

It was demonstrated in a 4-year followup study that antipsychotic drug use during a first episode of illness predisposes to long-term antipsychotic use, and ensures the continuing diagnosis of schizophrenia (Whitty et al., 2005). In this study, of fifteen patients initially diagnosed with schizophreniform illness, ten were rediagnosed with schizophrenia; six of twelve patients with delusional disorder were also rediagnosed with schizophrenia, as were all three patients with psychosis not otherwise specified. Complementing this, seventy of seventy-two patients initially diagnosed with schizophrenia continued unchanged. What applies to all these groups of patients is that the syndrome of schizophrenia is the final common pathway. The simplest explanation for this is that antipsychotic drugs cause symptoms indistinguishable from schizophrenia, namely tardive psychosis, and that, as with tardive dyskinesia, these symptoms are persistent.

Analogous to tardive dyskinesia, gradual withdrawal of antipsychotic drugs may lead to less relapse than does abrupt withdrawal. Also similar to tardive dyskinesia, gradual withdrawal of antipsychotic drugs is followed by less relapse than abrupt withdrawal (Viguera et al., 1997). Yet some patients will show tardive pathology regardless of how the antipsychotic drug is withdrawn, particularly those who have taken the drug longer and at higher dosage.

Culprit drugs include all antipsychotics excepting quetiapine (Seroquel) and clozapine (Clozaril). Also included are dopamine-blocking antinausea drugs such as prochlorperazine (Compazine) and some miscellaneous drugs such as metoclopramide (Reglan). As with tardive dyskinesia, sometimes the symptoms of tardive psychotic depression appear not only when the dopamine-blocking drug is discontinued, but also when the drug is taken regularly.

By omitting mention of the various effects of psychotropic drugs, the *DSM* implicitly suggests that there is no need for psychiatrists to consider tardive psychosis. As with *DSM* in general, this is a physician-centered consideration, one that provides pharmaceutical firms with the benefits of the doubts. So, if antipsychotic drugs are to be prescribed for longer than 3 months, it seems appropriate to discuss the risks of tardive psychosis as well as tardive dyskinesia with patient and family. There follow two of the many illustrative cases we have seen; there are others (Swartz, 1995).

Obscene derogatory auditory hallucinations had persisted for a month despite lithium and increasing doses of fluphenazine (a dopamine-blocking antipsychotic) in this 44-year-old black female patient. She told of low mood, restlessness, agitation, and pacing. In the hospital the patient was placed on lithium alone. She rapidly improved, became asymptomatic, and was discharged in 8 days on lithium alone. After 2 months she stopped the lithium and the hallucinations returned.

This 30-year-old black female, referred for hospitalization by outpatient psychiatrists, had experienced for a week weakness, insomnia, anorexia, hearing voices urging suicide, and seeing snakes and dogs attacking. The patient feared she might kill her 11-year-old daughter. She had her initial psychiatric illness 4 years ago, with the same symptoms, and had received antipsychotic drugs ever since. Lately, she had been given fluphenazine 20 mg/day, a large dose, and there were three previous psychiatric hospitalizations. Again, chronic use of a dopamine-blocking agent is apparent. On examination she showed immobility, staring, sad facies, flat affect, no speech initiation, slow whispered monotonous speech in response, and extreme poverty of thought, but full orientation. She showed no response to lorazepam. Nortriptyline 75 mg/day, triiodothyronine 25 μg daily, and lithium were started. Within 2 days the hallucinations disappeared, her speech normalized, and her complaints faded. She was discharged on these medications after 8 hospital days, without antipsychotic drugs.

Drug-induced and hormone-induced psychotic depression (including postpartum psychosis)

Corticosteroid administration, rapid withdrawal of androgenic or estrogenic steroids, thyroid hormone deficiency, and amphetamines can induce a psychotic depression that persists long after the drug or hormone is discontinued. Surely many other drugs and hormones (or their discontinuations) can do likewise, but the evidence is less clear. We will include postpartum psychosis in this category because of the large fall (about 95%) in female steroid hormones at the time of parturition. Such decreases include the psychoactive female hormones estrogen, pregnanolone, and allopregnanolone, although none of these is known to be specifically involved in psychotic depression. What applies to postpartum psychosis applies as well to postabortion psychosis. The cause of a psychosis is a biological change in body physiology such as hormonal status. The grievous personal stresses from the loss of a pregnancy can provoke profound dissatisfaction, unhappiness, and tension, but psychological experiences are not the basis for psychotic depression just as psychological therapies are not effective treatment.

Severe psychiatric reactions have been said to occur in 5 percent of steroid-treated patients, primarily consisting of depression, mania, psychosis, and mixtures of these (Lewis and Smith, 1983). This 5 percent figure is probably true of patients who receive high doses of corticosteroids or have a personal history or strong family history of depression, mania, or psychosis. Surely it does not include patients who receive corticosteroids from primary care doctors. About 5 percent of anabolic steroid abusers experience mania-like symptoms, and likewise 5 percent experience depressions when they halt these hormones (Pope and Katz, 1994).

We began this book with the story of Andrea Yates, which attracted national publicity. In an episode of postpartum psychotic depression she murdered her own children. Postpartum psychotic depression is far more debilitating than the much more common postpartum blues and postpartum anxiety, but fortunately rare. It occurs once in a thousand births and particularly in women with personal or family history of serious depression or bipolar-I disorder. The onset is usually within 1 month but can be longer (Kendell et al., 1987). Swartz: One of the most painful experiences of patient and family that I have seen is of a woman in her mid-20s who had screamed continuously for a year in postpartum psychosis, until she received ECT and returned to a normal appearance. Here is the story.

Shortly after admission to the state university hospital, this patient's terrifying shrieks intruded on everyone, staff and patients alike. Everyone was quiet, intimidated by the unworded speech of horror. Even a minute in her proximity was painfully long. It was common knowledge that this state university hospital was expert and patient friendly. Yet how could the family have endured this for a year without obtaining effective treatment? Only fear could provide such endurance and allow people to blind their eyes and deafen their ears to the agony of untreated illness. How else could they deny that the illness should urgently be treated in some other way? Such insensitive behavior has the effect of blaming the sick person for being ill. This blame is medieval and stigmatizing. With ECT this patient became normal, but I shiver when I imagine the effects of the long painful experience that she, her husband, their parents, and the infant had experienced. We are humbled by the face of unrelieved suffering from illness, and we respect the need for prompt relief. Allowing postpartum psychosis to continue without prompt effective treatment provokes the development of chronic PTSD, which itself causes much additional painful suffering, interpersonal friction, and impairment. This is all in addition to the interference in family relationships and proper mothering caused by the psychotic depression.

Drug- and hormone-induced depressions can be serious and life threatening. These drugs can also cause serious autonomous psychoses that are not depressive. Tardive psychotic depression is perhaps another hormone-induced depression, but it is so underappreciated that it deserves separate recognition.

Coarse brain disease psychotic depression

The term coarse brain disease refers to illnesses that include brain lesions observable through such means as EEG, brain imaging, angiogram, or definite abnormal neurological signs on physical examination, for example, spastic paralysis. Some examples of coarse brain disease are epilepsy, cerebral lupus erythematosis, Alzheimer's disease, cerebrovascular disease, multiple sclerosis, neurosyphilis, Huntington's chorea, and Parkinson's disease. Patients with coarse brain disease are at risk of psychoses and depressions, including psychotic depression. Risks of psychosis and depression increase with greater severity of the neurological illness, especially with concomitant dementia and advancing age (Sanchez-Ramos et al., 1996).

In patients with Parkinson's disease that has advanced into dementia, 36 percent had hallucinations, delusions, or both (Naimark et al., 1996), and they required greater supervision. Over all Parkinson's patients, the prevalence of psychosis is 5–20 percent (Pollak et al., 2004). It is unclear how much psychosis and depression derive from the Parkinson's disease itself and how much from the medications used to treat it. In advanced Parkinson's disease with dementia 40 percent have psychosis, and visual hallucinations are the most common psychotic symptom (Aarsland et al., 1999). Delusions usually involve paranoia and focus on a single theme.

Depressive symptoms are at least as common in Parkinson's disease as psychosis. In one study 40 percent of Parkinson's patients with psychosis also had depression (Marsh et al., 2004). This poses the unusual challenge of distinguishing between psychotic depression on the one hand and coincident depression and psychosis on the other. The *DSM* provides no guidance in making this distinction, but it is important because treatment selection depends on it. The Parkinsonian symptoms make the assessment even more difficult because they overlap with melancholia. If the depression and psychosis began about the same time, or if the patient shows intense concern about the psychotic symptoms, psychotic depression is more likely. If the patient has only visual hallucinations with accurate insight that they are hallucinations, psychotic depression is less likely.

The occurrences of psychosis and depression in Alzheimer's disease resemble those in Parkinson's disease, except that delusions are more common than hallucinations. Delusions occur in about a third, hallucinations in a sixth, and either in 40 percent. Psychosis is associated with particularly rapid progression and perhaps older age and longer duration (Ropacki and Jeste, 2005). Cross-sectionally, a quarter of Alzheimer's patients have major depression, another quarter have minor depression, and delusions were most common in those with major depression (Starkstein et al., 2005). Parkinsonism was also most common in those with major depression.

There are basically two groups of psychotic depression in these circumstances, the dependent group and the autonomous group. Dependent psychoses and depressions are direct sequelae of the disease or its treatments; as the disease fades, the dependent condition fades. On the other hand, an autonomous depression would continue despite remission of the underlying coarse brain disease, and would require separate treatment independent of the disease. Autonomous nature is usually presumed rather than proven. Sometimes an autonomous condition is diagnosed because there is no clear relationship between the coarse brain pathology and the depression. Sometimes the distinction between dependent and autonomous is only hypothetical because there is no substantial treatment for the coarse brain disease, as with Alzheimer's.

Usually regarded as autonomous are psychotic depressions and other psychoses that accompany dementing illnesses or Parkinson's disease. Treatment for them corresponds to that of similar types of psychotic depression (see Chapter 8). Of course, the goal of returning to baseline function is vastly different in these patients than in other patients who do not have dementia. In other words, antipsychotic tranquilizers are less likely to cause substantial impairment of psychological performance because the patients are already greatly impaired. Nevertheless, most antipsychotics substantially increase risks of impaired mobility, falling, pneumonia, and other medical conditions provoked by physical weakness and abulia. (Quetiapine and clozapine are relatively desirable because of the absence of Parkinsonian side effects. Typical starting doses of these are 6.25–25 mg/day, and maintenance doses 25–100 mg/day; Pollak et al., 2004.) In a depressed demented patient with problematic agitation or inanition who is resistant to antipsychotics, ECT is the appropriate treatment. Effective prevention of aspiration pneumonia from ECT in elderly patients taking an antipsychotic drug generally requires administration of an atropinic agent and use of an anesthetic agent other than propofol (Swartz, 2005).

When a seizure disorder causes psychotic depression, it is usually a dependent type depression. Complex partial seizures can produce serious behavioral disruptions. This condition was formerly called temporal lobe epilepsy or psychomotor seizures. It does not necessarily involve specific convulsive movements. The movements that occur can manifest merely as smacking of the lips, appearing dazed or vacant, behaving confusedly, showing automatic behavior, or showing virtually any psychiatric symptoms. When untreated or undertreated, complex partial epilepsy can cause the entire picture of melancholia, psychosis, or psychotic depression.

Symptoms of depression are described by up to two-thirds of patients with intractable epilepsy. Complex partial seizures that involve the temporal lobe or the dominant hemisphere (usually left) are thought to be particularly depressogenic. Paranoid delusions and paranoid auditory hallucinations are common. Among the treatments of epileptic psychotic depression might be mentioned the adjustment of the anticonvulsant medication, the addition of antimelancholic drugs, and ECT. TCAs and bupropion tend to make epilepsy worse and should be avoided; drug-induced seizures generally follow dose additions (Lambert and Robertson, 1999). Venlafaxine is probably the first-choice antimelancholic drug for these patients.

Identifying active epilepsy is crucial in the diagnosis. These cases come to psychiatrists because neurologists have either missed an atypical seizure disorder or are not handling its psychiatric effects. Atypicality means that the EEG does not demonstrate seizure, and might show no hint of seizure. The EEG is sensitive to only the outer 15 percent of the cerebral cortex, and depth electrode studies have proven that limbic seizures can occur with a normal standard EEG. Methods that can go beyond standard and sleep-deprived EEGs include drug-provoked EEG (e.g., with promethazine, promazine, or loxapine), serum prolactin level monitoring, positron-emission tomography (PET) brain imaging, and anticonvulsant drug trial. Serum prolactin level monitoring is most useful when the patient has episodes of behavior disturbance, such as diminished responsiveness or apparent confusion. The serum prolactin level should be drawn within 30 minutes of onset, and a comparison serum prolactin drawn after at least three continuous hours free of the behavior disturbance. Because antipsychotic drugs (except quetiapine and clozapine) can raise serum prolactin levels, this testing cannot be done in patients who received any antipsychotic drug within the previous 7 days.

A 56-year-old man with a decade-long history of epilepsy was hospitalized for believing that witchcraft is killing him and in response to annoying staff at occult bookstores, who called the police. He attempted to dispel evil spirits by sitting in Epsom salt baths for hours every day. Under the care of a neurologist he was taking carbamazepine. He carried around a yellowing to-whom-it-may-concern letter from a neurologist stating that the psychiatric disturbance was not a result of epilepsy. On the ward, for 3 days he remained sad and subdued. Yet within 1 day of adding a second anticonvulsant (primidone), his depression and psychosis were gone, leaving only a suggestion of superstitiousness. He became outgoing, cheerful, and sociable, and he happily noticed the difference. Besides the patient, the nursing staff mentioned surprise at the rapidity and amount of improvement.

A 46-year-old African American woman was hospitalized for depressive symptoms with unpleasant visual and auditory hallucinations that urged her to commit suicide. She showed pained concern, impoverished thought and speech, agitation, and sickliness. A seizure disorder had begun during childhood for which she received phenytoin, but she had not taken any anticonvulsant for 10 years. Rather, she took potent antipsychotic drugs prescribed by outpatient psychiatrists at St. Louis University. With olanzapine but not haloperidol, hallucinations disappeared. An EEG showed abundant epileptiform discharges "compatible with complex partial epilepsy of the left anterior temporal area." In response to phenytoin all signs and symptoms of depression and psychosis disappeared in 1 day. Unfortunately, her misadventure did not end there. After hospital discharge outpatient psychiatrists discontinued the anticonvulsant and restarted olanzapine. The patient gained 30 pounds in 1 month and discontinued olanzapine. A different antipsychotic drug was started but the patient did not return for followup. The outpatient psychiatrists treated hallucinations as if they were a primary psychotic illness rather than as a symptom of epilepsy. Epilepsy remained untreated. Nothing is specific to schizophrenia; it is a diagnosis of exclusion that requires that all other explanations for the symptoms do not apply.

A 15-year-old high school student from a tiny farming town was hospitalized after 6 months of fixed delusions that he leads a gang of a hundred teenage males in a war against a similar gang. He was terrified that he would be killed. His school grades had fallen. He was so convincing that we telephoned the town's police chief, who laughed hard at the question. A batted baseball had hit the side of the patient's head 2 years ago. He lost consciousness briefly and felt occasional headaches at the spot. The delusions remained unshaken after 4 calm days in the hospital, with abundant counseling and normal EEG, CT scan, and laboratory tests. As we watched, an hour after taking loxapine 10 mg, the only dose of antipsychotic drug he ever received, he began throwing furniture around the psychiatry ward. He would not speak. A prompt EEG showed complex partial seizures. Two days later a repeat EEG was normal; still, the delusions remained. Within 1 day of starting phenytoin all delusions and distress disappeared. He relaxed and in retrospect it became clear that his affect had been abnormally mechanical before treatment. At followup 6 and 12 months later he remained well and was performing well in school.

This 25-year-old black male told of feeling depressed and suicidal, and of auditory and visual hallucinations about his ex-girlfriend. Following a romantic breakup and an aunt's death 6 months prior, he lost 15 pounds and had typical adjustment symptoms similar to anxiety or depression. He had been taking medication for seizure disorder, and a day before admission experienced a seizure witnessed by a psychiatrist. On examination he was dirty, unkempt, hypoactive, uncooperative, and intent on listening to his pocket radio throughout. What little he said was only in response to insistent questioning. EEG revealed abnormally low amplitude brain electrical activity but no seizure activity. In response to pimozide the patient showed improved affect and somewhat decreased hallucinations, but was far from remission. After a course of six ECTs the patient showed a bright cheerful affect and was free of hallucinations. The seizure he had experienced was apparently psychotogenic. Seizure is the only identifiable precipitant of catatonia that author CS has seen repeatedly, but only in a few percentage of patients with catatonia.

In brief, the clinician needs to remember that psychotic depression of any type can be caused by seizure and seizure disorders. Seizure-induced psychosis is common and does not represent evidence of schizophrenia. Past seizure and possible traumatic brain injury are necessary parts of history taking for every patient with psychosis or major depression. An EEG should help make the diagnosis and it is the province of the psychiatrist to order it when seizure-induced psychopathology is possible.

Pseudopsychosis, or false psychotic depression

Several conditions can easily be called psychotic depression yet are not depressive or psychotic. The distinction is important because these conditions require their own particular treatment to achieve remission. Patients with delirium suffer hallucinations, delusions, or incoherent speech or behavior that appears guided by hallucinations or delusions. These hallucinations and delusions should be considered delirious rather than psychotic. The clinical appearance of such delirium can be indistinguishable from catatonic psychotic depression, but the distinction can be made with information from the history, an EEG, laboratory tests, and perhaps brain imaging. After several days of sleep deprivation, experiencing visual hallucinations is expected, and not reflective of psychiatric or medical illness. With a good night's sleep assured by hypnotic drugs, the patient with simple sleep-deprivation hallucinosis awakens free of hallucinations. Patients without depression can suffer such insomnia because of an anxiety disorder or adjustment disorder, and these should be specifically inquired after. Of course, other possibilities for causing sleep-deprivation hallucinosis are legion, for example, stimulant abuse, substance withdrawal syndrome, endocrine disorder, or neurological illness, to mention a few.

Patients with severe anxiety or personal stresses can experience dissociative symptoms or conversion reactions that some might call psychotic. These patients commonly claim to be depressed and there is little doubt they are suffering; still, all psychological suffering and dissatisfaction with mood are not depression. When an agitated patient who claims to be depressed and thinking a lot about death tells of hearing the voice of the devil, seeing the letters "KILL," or feeling that his food is being poisoned by his roommates, psychotic depression is the easy diagnosis to make. Yet it is not always the right one, and the full picture is needed. Psychotic depression might be the wrong diagnosis because the voice and visualization can be conversion reactions, and the poisoning a contamination obsession. Because these are subjective symptoms, the distinction between psychosis and pseudopsychosis is made according to the context: what does the rest of the clinical picture fit?

Similarly, patients with PTSD commonly experience hallucinations of the traumatic event, called flashbacks. These are considered dissociative phenomena, not psychosis. The agitation, affect disturbances, and anger that patients with PTSD display often challenge their caregivers and can goad them to refer to the patient as depressed or psychotic. Yet here depression and psychosis do not apply in their specific professional meaning. Ironically, severe PTSD accompanied by pseudohallucinations and nondelusional paranoia is probably more difficult, time consuming, and costly to treat than is psychotic depression with hallucinations and delusional paranoia.

That these patients are not psychotic does not diminish the credibility of their illnesses or their sufferings. Because of the need for specificity in diagnosis and treatment, it is important to avoid unnecessary use of antipsychotic drugs or other treatments that expose patients to needless adverse effects.

Patients with Briquet's syndrome, or chronic polysymptomatic somatoform illness, commonly tell of auditory hallucinations and mood disturbances and even show hallucinatory behavior. These hallucinations are dissociative, not psychotic. In *DSM* terms, Briquet's syndrome is concurrent somatization disorder and dissociative disorder, perhaps also with borderline or histrionic personality disorder. Patients with antisocial personality disorder similarly claim hallucinations and mood disturbances. Their hallucinations can result from traumatic brain injury, PTSD, abusive substance toxicity or withdrawal, or dissociation; they can also represent blunt manipulative factitiousness.

How would you treat a patient with clear borderline personality disorder who describes a severe depression with hallucinations and delusions? Before a consensus conference on psychotic depression, 64 percent of attendees said they would treat them in the same way as other patients. After the conference this percentage dropped to 34 percent, in response to "learning that patients with borderline personality disorder have stress-related ephemeral delusions or hallucinations," in addition to the usual borderline symptoms. Such patients also do not show psychomotor disturbance, such as motor retardation or poverty of thought (Finlay-Jones and Parker, 1993). Apparently the patients described as borderline in this consensus conference were also symptomatic of a dissociative disorder.

Referred by a neurologist for violent behavior, this 16-year-old married patient described 6 months of insomnia, anorexia, fatigue, loss of pleasure and libido, decreased speech, thoughts of death, and slowness in getting dressed. Dressing took an hour rather than the usual 10 minutes. He was delusional or severely obsessed that his wife is unfaithful, sometimes angrily awakening her from sleep. The patient's wife said he has no control over irritability. Two months prior he was started on risperidone 2 mg/day, which made him worse. The patient had symptoms of Parkinson's disease since age 12 and was taking Sinemet (L-DOPA with carbidopa). The Parkinsonian symptoms recently worsened, but it was unclear how much risperidone had contributed to this. An MRI taken a month ago revealed megacephaly with congenital hydrocephalus and subluxation of the cervical spine. In the hospital we discontinued risperidone and started the beta-blocker betaxolol to diminish somatic tension anxiety. We also started biperiden, to reverse suspected risperidone-induced exacerbation. The patient improved rapidly and after 3 days was no longer irritable, depressed, or suspicious about his wife. The patient was discharged 5 days after admission. Although the beta-blocker betaxolol effectively decreases somatic tension anxiety (e.g., irritability, agitation), it does not diminish true psychosis, and likewise for biperiden. By his presentation this patient might have been psychotic; the response to medication revealed that there was no psychosis.

This patient shows how antipsychotic medication can make tension anxiety worse. When an antipsychotic medication is prescribed to treat a condition that is not psychotic, there seems to be an intrinsic illogicality. Yet antipsychotic drugs are not specifically antipsychotic. Their action of diminishing psychosis is only incidental to their primary effect, which is to simplify and decrease thinking. This is theoretically useful for people who have "too many thoughts." Antipsychotic drugs are not specific to psychotic thoughts; they decrease a wide range of thoughts and thereby diminish the ability to appreciate complexity.

Admitted to the hospital because of personal conflict, this 16-year-old female said the devil lives in her house. She told of hearing the devil's voice within the sounds of the ventilation system and feeling fearful from these sounds. She also said god talks to her and this makes her happy. Her mother has a dissociative disorder and is noncompliant with prescribed medication. In the hospital the patient said she is fearful that her food has medicine in it. She was worried, irritable, easily upset by small things, and hypervigilant, but she showed no sadness, apathy, or anhedonia. Rather, she was highly attentive, interactive, and alert, frequently asking questions and claiming to deserve better treatment from other people. Her blood pressure was also labile, but not clearly excessive. Working under the diagnoses of anxiety disorder and conversion disorder, we started the beta-blocker betaxolol, along with the antiobsessional drug fluvoxamine. In response to betaxolol, by the next day the hypervigilance, hypertalkativeness, and tension had faded, and the patient was more relaxed. She was still worried and dissatisfied, and it was expected that fluvoxamine would take about a month to mitigate that.

Unclear circumstances

Sometimes it is simply unclear what is going on. If you are unable to make a diagnosis, it may be because you are dealing with an atypical form of the illness, or because you are confronting a syndrome not yet well characterized. Perhaps the patient is showing unfamiliar psychopathology, which deserves further study.

This category includes the patient who appears so deteriorated, unrelated, or otherwise peculiar that you do not want to diagnose catatonia and you do not want to give ECT. The challenge to professionalism starts with giving the patient the "benefit of the doubt," and recognizing the possibility that your own low expectations will inhibit you from administering a helpful treatment. The challenge continues with stating high expectations and treating accordingly. Conferring with colleagues and seeking others' opinions can help. Here are a couple of diagnostic challenge cases from Conrad Swartz's practice:

A 29-year-old male with a head shaped like a football was referred to me for ECT by another psychiatrist, with the diagnosis of psychotic depression. The skull malformation resulted from premature closure of one suture, of a type that does not cause mental retardation. The patient had been in the veterans hospital for 10 consecutive years, initially admitted for depression. On interview the patient showed an unrelated affect and incoherent mumbling speech. He looked at the ceiling lights as he spoke, as if conversing with them. He showed no recognition that

I was present and trying to hold a conversation. We could see no sign of depression or mania, only severely disorganized speech and behavior. Giving the patient the benefit of the doubt, we took the past diagnosis of depression as the present diagnosis, albeit psychotic depression. After the second ECT he was well related, coherent, affable, and in a state of typical euphoric mania. He achieved remission with a few more ECT treatments. In retrospect the diagnosis was bipolar disorder with mixed manic-depressive episode and catatonic features. Perhaps the concurrent mania and depression obscured each other and produced the signs of catatonia.

Anorexia and insomnia began a year prior to admission for this 41-year-old white female. After 9 months she felt irritated by everyone else and she withdrew. She received lorazepam 2 mg/day and trazodone at bedtime but began having visual hallucinations of "evil dark beings in the corners of rooms" and nonthreatening auditory hallucinations. Her hospitalization was precipitated by an overdose with suicidal intent, which she slept off. As a child she suffered physical and sexual cruelty. As a young adult she abused various street drugs including heroin and was an urban streetwalker. Over several decades she has had several periods when she would feel particularly well and energetic, even hyperactive lasting a day or two, occasionally a week. Over the past 10 years she used marijuana occasionally. On examination she was agitated, fidgety, and consistently sad, crying occasionally, yet at the same time she was friendly. Speech was rapid, spontaneous, and overly detailed. She was fully alert and interactive. Because of the reported hallucinations and the 3-month period during which she differed from her usual (although anxious) persona, she received a course of six ECTs. She responded rapidly, maintaining full cognitive function but no longer feeling suicidal or unhappy. Our impression was that this patient had both melancholia and PTSD, two separate illnesses with some similar symptoms. We never knew if the melancholia was psychotic or if it had exacerbated the PTSD so as to provoke dissociative nonpsychotic hallucinations. Patients with chronic PTSD have been observed to have discrete episodes of melancholic major depression; the two conditions can be separately diagnosed and treated (Swartz and Guadagno, 1998).

This 39-year-old white male told of hearing voices from the devil telling him to suicide by overdose. He reported low mood and recent crying spells, but no insomnia, anorexia, or fatigue. He had overdosed 6 weeks before, had many past hospitalizations, and was taking high doses of the potent antipsychotic drug thiothixene (Navane), moderate doses of diazepam, and theophylline for asthma. He had a 15-year history of depression, hallucinations, and stimulant abuse. On examination he was alert, tearful at times, and well oriented. Maintained on the same medications, his suicidality and hallucinations rapidly faded and he was discharged in 2 days. At that time it seemed that the diagnosis was obscured by his medications. He was readmitted 5 months later after cutting his wrists, citing financial pressures and personal conflict. He was hallucinating and had continued taking the same doses of theophylline and thiothixene. Lithium and bupropion were added and he was discharged 3 days later. The diagnosis remained undetermined. With the patient under the influence of thiothixene, we were deprived of seeing the psychopathology of his illness. Moreover, theophylline can be psychotogenic, and the history of stimulant abuse suggests the possibility of undisclosed street drugs.

The bottom line is that psychopathology is complex, and a simple criterion-based approach is not reliable enough to provide a relevant and proper diagnosis. Laboratory measurements are similarly complex and nonspecific. Cortisol levels in the dexamethasone suppression test have served only to tease us with results that are clearly positive at the level of groups – indicating the biological nature of psychotic depression – but so variable among individuals as to have unclear clinical reliability and value on specific patients. After almost a hundred years of psychoanalysis, and twenty-five of the metascientific yet authoritarian-derived *DSM* schema, psychiatry has not progressed far in its ability to delineate clearly circumscribed illness entities or to inventory, classify, and apply the evidence that is available. Psychotic depression is about as close as psychiatric diagnosis approaches to an evidence-based medical diagnosis such as measles or left bundle-branch block.

Psychotic versus nonpsychotic major depression

Many publications have considered the question of whether psychotic depression is distinctly different from nonpsychotic major depression. An initial obstacle in the road is the nature of *DSM*-compliant "major depression," its components indistinct and the boundaries between them vague. The diagnosis of major depression has long been used in widely different ways. Some practitioners apply it only to patients who have the slowed-down depression that comes from within, meaning without relation to real-life events; this would be an endogenous or obviously biological depression. Other practitioners mostly use "major depression" with patients who express severe or persistent distress or suicidality about current actual events in their lives, a hyperreactive depression. Before we even consider psychotic depression as such we have to deal with two starkly different depressive conditions. The relevant question then becomes Does the psychosis of psychotic depression itself indicate that this condition is distinctly different from precisely the same depression without psychosis? Once we recognize that psychotic depression itself has several distinct types, the question becomes far more complex.

Proper study of the question requires subtyping psychotic depression and comparing psychotic and nonpsychotic patients of each subtype, for example, melancholic nonpsychotic against melancholic psychotic patients, and catatonic nonpsychotic against catatonic psychotic patients. Most studies that describe types include only melancholic. For example, in one study 36 percent of psychotic patients met *DSM* melancholia criteria, but only 19 percent of nonpsychotic patients did (Maj et al., 1990). In another study, patients with psychotic depression had more severe symptoms of melancholia than did nonpsychotic patients with melancholia (Parker et al., 1997). This indicates that severe melancholia is more often psychotic than mild to moderate melancholia is. It does not imply that psychotic depression is specifically a severe form of melancholia, as some have suggested.

In the absence of verifiable evidence or subtyping, it is no surprise that many studies have not discovered differences between psychotic and nonpsychotic depressions, regarding intensity of symptoms, familial incidence (Bellini et al., 1992), age of onset, duration, social status, and physical health (Kivela and Pahkala, 1989). In other studies, patients with delusional depression were more severely ill on admission (Maj et al., 1990; Kuhs, 1991), showed more severe psychomotor disturbance and constipation, and lacked the circadian variation cited by DSM as part of melancholia (Parker et al., 1991a). However, the subtypes of psychotic and nonpsychotic depression must be delineated. For example, there is no point to comparing melancholic psychotic depression with reactive atypical nonpsychotic depression; they are two utterly different conditions. By extension, there is nothing specific to be learned about a group including some psychotic depression in comparing it to a group including some atypical depression; there is simply too much irrelevant variation. The existence of different types of psychotic depression is not consistent with assertions that psychotic depression is a distinct clinical entity on its own (Glassman and Roose, 1981; Schatzberg and Rothschild, 1992); rather, it is a group of separate entities. In this way it is analogous to depression itself. Melancholic depression, catatonic depression, and atypical depression are each a single entity. In contrast, psychotic depression is the only subtype of major depression that is a group of several different entities.

Family studies (Weissman et al., 1984) and higher serum cortisol levels (Carroll et al., 1976) suggest that psychotic depression is distinctly different from nonpsychotic depression and more frequently symptomatic of bipolar disorder. Patients with delusional depression have more cerebral atrophy than do other patients with depression and normal controls, as shown by both ventricle to brain ratio and cerebral atrophy ratio (Shiraishi et al., 1992). A variety of evidence, therefore, shows that psychotic and nonpsychotic depression are not the same entity.

Depression-induced anxiety disorders

There are risks associated with not obtaining prompt and effective treatment of psychotic depression. They include extended suffering, suicide, interrupted career, isolation, financial stress, stigmatization, pulmonary embolus, pneumonia, osteoporosis from starvation, myocardial infarction (heart attack), and sudden death. Besides these are medical, social, personal, and psychiatric problems caused by antipsychotic tranquilizers sometimes used in managing psychotic depression. Not included on these lists is one routinely overlooked but portentous consequence of undertreating psychotic depression. Specifically, the suffering in experiencing psychotic depression can cause another psychiatric illness, PTSD. About a third of patients with psychotic depression that first began by age 50 suffer from de facto PTSD. This is apparently from the personal stress and menace of their illness. A few words about this and other anxiety disorders will close this chapter. We describe more on these issues in the treatment chapters.

PTSD is the condition that causes persisting mental anguish to many survivors of war prisoner camps, concentration camps, military combat, and sexual abuse. Its definition includes many of the same symptoms that are called in *DSM* "major depression," including sadness (intense distressing feelings), anhedonia ("diminished interest or participation" and "estrangement from others"), apathy ("unable to have loving feelings"), hopelessness ("sense of foreshortened future"), insomnia, poor concentration, low energy, agitation ("irritability, outbursts of anger"), guilty thoughts (self-blaming), and suicidality. Nevertheless, major depression and PTSD are two separate disorders, and they can be experienced together or separately, and then treated separately (Swartz and Guadagno, 1998).

By definition, PTSD includes exposure to a threatening event in which the patient experiences intense fear, helplessness, or horror. The essence of meaning of the "T" in PTSD is threat. In *DSM* the "T" stands for "trauma" and "emotional trauma" but this is unfortunate because it confuses cause and effect. The cause is the threat to the patient. The consequent psychiatric effect is the emotional trauma, which can include PTSD, acute stress disorder, and adjustment reaction. The terminology confusion is important because it probably contributes to overlooking and underdiagnosing PTSD, especially in patients with past or present psychotic depression and related conditions.

PTSD is severely underdiagnosed (Schwartz et al., 2005). It is more than severely underdiagnosed in psychiatric patients with severe mood disorders or chronic psychosis. In the latter the actual incidence of concurrent PTSD was 43 percent but it had been recognized in only 1 percent, which was 2 percent of those with PTSD (Mueser et al., 1998). Moreover 98 percent of the entire group of patients had been exposed to at least one threatening potentially traumatic event – and these patients were living New Hampshire, a relatively nonviolent region.

PTSD explains an otherwise mysterious conflict between what we could see and what the patient said in a Discovery Channel program that ran in 2002 and 2003, "Shock Therapy: The Last Resort." The patient, a 30-year-old mother of two, looked healthy and well, yet told of suicidal intent and morbid thoughts that arose shortly after her first child was born. These problems persisted for 5 years, despite six therapists and eight antidepressants. There were three suicide attempts. (At least, according to the video. Actual circumstances of the patient might have differed from the cinematic portrayal.)

During the program we saw this patient receive ECT in good form. Still, within 5 days of her last ECT treatment she reported, "All I could think about was how I could kill myself with pills or with a gun." As her mother-in-law explained the patient's mysteriously persisting symptoms: "Life is diapers, dirty dishes and dinner, face it, for everybody." To these two mentioned possibilities of resistant major depression and narcissistic disillusionment we add PTSD, as a consequence of under-treated postpartum psychotic depression.

The television program reported that this patient had experienced a profound postpartum depression. Until childbirth, she had been "outgoing" and "happy-go-lucky." Then she began "crying all the time" and "couldn't figure out why." She stayed in bed and did not clean her home. This childbirth was 5 years prior to the program, however, and her condition during this previous time was not shown. Rather, we saw her only as she was shortly before, during, and after ECT.

We saw her fishing with her husband, and smiling and laughing while walking normally with family members. She looked as healthy as they seemed. There was no noticeable fatigue, slowness, weakness, apathy, sadness, motor retardation, or poverty of thought or of emotional expression, symptoms that are typical of psychotic depression and other severe depressions. The young mother spoke without hesitation, with normal rate and rhythm of speech, and with appropriate affects of concern, sincerity, and frustration. Her husband stated his own frustration: "Sometimes you feel she's just making it up to avoid responsibility." No noticeable difference was shown after ECT. Yet because she looked normal before the treatment, there was no room for improvement.

Her present condition was different from staying in bed and crying all the time, which was the nature of her severe depression while postpartum. The use of ECT can be justified by persistent suicidality with postpartum onset; this was not an issue at the moment of filming. Our concern is what, if anything, is still wrong with this patient's health.

The point is that while psychotic depression can eventually fade through time and medication, the personal threats experienced during it can injure the patient. By uniformly identifying psychotic depression as severe, *DSM* recognizes that it can be a life-threatening, emotionally intense, unpleasant, and stressful experience. These are the particular characteristics of events that can trigger PTSD. Because psychotic depression came first, the PTSD could be called "secondary"; however, all PTSD is secondary to serious threat.

The central issue here is that experiencing psychotic depression or similarly serious psychiatric illnesses can cause anxiety disorders and adjustment disorders, and when it does, separate treatment plans are needed. PTSD can result from overwhelming stresses that threaten life or personal integrity; it can also emanate from influences such as heightened emotional awareness and intensity; unpleasantness; stigmatization; intimidation; activation of the sympathetic nervous system; and losses of independence, job, stature, financial security, and family. Moreover, psychiatric hospitalization itself can be a troubling experience. In a survey of 142 randomly selected adults who had been discharged from a psychiatric hospital, 31 percent complained of physical assault, 8 percent of sexual assault, and 63 percent of witnessing threatening potentially traumatic events. Moreover, 59 percent reported experiencing seclusion, 34 percent restraint, and 65 percent transport in handcuffs. Previously 87 percent had been exposed to threatening potentially traumatic events, including sexual assault in 33 percent, and 19 percent of the group probably had PTSD (Frueh et al., 2005). Obtaining prompt remission to minimize agitation and hospital stay will help to decrease and prevent such experiences.

Unfortunately, these events figure among the ordinary risks or consequences of illness, and often occur in episodes of biogenic-endogenous mood disorders and psychotic illnesses. Of course, an acute life-threatening medical illness can cause PTSD. When a patient is said to be depressed from developing cancer, if the depression results from the threatening stresses rather than directly from pharmacological, endocrine, or physiological processes of the disease, it might be PTSD, acute stress disorder, or adjustment disorder.

The enormous comorbidity of anxiety disorders among patients with mood disorders (Brown et al., 2001; Zimmerman et al., 2002) is more than can be attributed to coincidence or genetics. Alone, these explanations overlook the psychological and physiological stresses experienced by patients with psychotic depression. Moreover, the high incidence of anxiety disorders in patients with bipolar-I disorder who are not presently in an episode of mania or endogenous depression indicates a separation between the mood disorder and the anxiety disorder. Identifying the mood disorder itself as a threatening and potentially traumatic stress helps us to recognize the anxiety disorder as PTSD. Because this is generally not done, panic disorder or GAD is diagnosed instead.

PTSD is more likely with exposure to larger numbers of threatening stresses. Accordingly, symptoms of PTSD should be milder and less likely to occur if the experience of psychotic depression is shorter and less stressful. Because ECT treats appropriate cases of depression rapidly and effectively, PTSD should be diminished by the early use of ECT on suitable patients. This is a race against the clock. A similar strategy has been suggested for the initial treatment of schizophrenia, in which some investigators have found that a shorter duration of untreated psychosis is associated with lower anxiety levels and better outcomes (Malla et al., 2002). Nevertheless, once PTSD has become established and the symptoms of the psychotic depressive episode are only a memory, as with this case on the Discovery Channel, the treatment plan might best focus on diminishing PTSD and preventing reoccurrence of psychotic depression.

The terms minor depression, residual symptoms of depression, nonresponse to treatment, and double depression have been offered to account for depressive symptoms that continue after treatment. Residual symptoms are ascribed to incomplete treatment (Bakish, 2001). Minor depression (or subsyndromal depression) is said to be a distinct phase of illness (as mania is distinct from depression) rather than a milder episode of major depression (Judd et al., 2002). Several proponents of "minor depression" have asserted that "[t]rue remission or recovery from a major depressive episode occurs only with abatement of all ongoing residual symptoms" (Judd et al., 2000). The existence of depression-induced PTSD contradicts this assertion. Of course, abatement of all symptoms represents remission, but persisting depressive symptoms from PTSD or another anxiety disorder do not indicate absence of remission from major depression. They indicate the presence of PTSD. A common clinical example is the female patient whose observable signs of psychotic depression (e.g., motor retardation) and psychotic symptoms disappear with ECT or a TCA. However, the patient then complains of persistently recurring depressive thoughts, and on examination the clinician discovers a long-standing PTSD with a history of sexual or physical abuse that had been previously obscured by psychotic depression or antipsychotic drugs.

Nonresponse to treatment might seem the simplest explanation for depressive symptoms that continue after treatment, but evaluation for an anxiety disorder is needed before nonresponse can be pronounced. This is particularly important when a "depression rating scale" (e.g., Hamilton Rating Scale for Depression (HAM-D)) is used to assess the degree of response, because anxiety disorders and some personality disorders can produce elevated depression ratings (Lesser et al., 1989; Simeon et al., 1992). Patients with schizophrenia are said to have depression as part of the syndrome of schizophrenia, that is, depression is intrinsic to schizophrenia. However, their "depressive symptoms" are readily explainable as an anxiety disorder, particularly PTSD. Antipsychotic tranquilizers surely interfere with these patients' ability to describe symptoms; such drugs also make the anxiety symptoms less recognizable; the same applies to psychotic depression patients who receive antipsychotics.

Differences among these explanations for resistant depressive symptoms should correspond to differences in treatment plans. There is little in common between PTSD and psychotic depression in their nature and their appropriate treatment, but the symptoms – "recurrent thoughts of death, insomnia, feeling tired all the time, trouble concentrating, poor appetite, and feelings of worthlessness" (Rapaport et al., 2002) – overlap with each other. Patients with a history of a serious major depressive episode or manic episode who have intermediate depression ratings were said to be in a phase of minor depression, but consideration of anxiety disorders was not mentioned (Judd et al., 2000, 2002).

Diagnosing (or ruling out) an anxiety disorder while a patient is in an episode of psychotic depression is somewhere between exacting and uncertain because anxiety is an ordinary symptom of severe depression. With effective treatment, depression-dependent anxiety recedes with the rest of the psychotic depression. Once the psychotic symptoms and observable signs of depression have completely faded with treatment (not counting tranquilization), so have all symptoms of psychotic depression. Any remaining symptoms are attributable to something else, whether medication side effects, anxiety disorder, medical or neurological condition, adjustment disorder, or personality problem. Admittedly, applying the diagnosis of an anxiety disorder can be challenging, as with defensive patients who angrily assert that they are depressed, not worried, and that they feel worthless, although they deserve better. As with any PTSD, depression-induced PTSD can hide under many guises, and resistant major depression is one of them.

4

Patients' Experience of Illness

According to his journals, as an adolescent Scott Kiser had experienced a bout of depression. When around his twenty-second birthday he underwent a second attack, he had an inkling of what was coming. "This second episode of severe depression, which rapidly progressed to psychosis, was for me all the more terrifying precisely because I recognized exactly what was happening when I began to go mad." Again, he felt "the crushing sense of panic." Yet he was paralyzed: "When the wasteland of nothingness came to claim me yet again, I was utterly helpless and undone in any attempt to free myself from its grasp."

He was an undergraduate in the first semester at a college far away from home. As his symptoms submerged him he tried to reach out to his few new friends, who were clueless. He talked to a school counselor. "I'm not sure what sort of counselor he was; he said that in counseling more than 700 students in his career, he had never seen anyone in my condition. Upon hearing that, my panic increased, and I sank deeper into hopelessness." The director of the counseling center asked him if he had ever been a victim of satanic ritual abuse? Or perhaps Scott was having a stress reaction to having seen a murder? "In response to this, I was completely exasperated and nearly hysterical. What was wrong with these professionals?"

Scott locked himself into his dorm room for hours, fantasizing about ways of killing himself. Then he settled on a plan, "wandering out into the snowy woods and freezing to death."

The last thread holding him to reality snapped. He had been studying for a final exam, reading and rereading the same paragraph. "I suddenly realized that I was right at the edge of losing my mind, and I could see it approaching. For a brief instant, the awareness came over me, and then it was as if I felt a small, frail branch or twig snap, and then a cracking, a breaking, an agonizing severance. I literally saw, as my mind was disintegrating, the image of a descending and chaotic spiral, and I felt my being recede and vanish into this black abysmal whirlpool." He became unable to speak, hear, touch, or taste.

The counselor drove him to the airport. His fellow passengers looked at him nervously. Back at his parents', "I underwent experiences that previously I would never have thought possible: delusions of guilt, persecution, physical decay, and impending death; visual hallucinations and perceptual distortions .... I saw accounts on the news of abandoned babies found in dumpsters, natural disasters, atrocious crimes committed, and I was responsible somehow; it was my fault that they occurred."

He tried to sleep but awoke quickly with "an agonizing sensation that I was suffocating and couldn't breathe." He lay groaning and writhing in his bed. He became catatonic, "stand[ing] still for hours in the same spot, watching the headlights of cars pass, trying futilely to make a meaningful connection with something, anything." Finally he believed he was dying, convinced that "my skin was melting away and my vital organs dissolving." He shouted for his mother to call an ambulance. "She was beside herself, and not knowing what to do, she took me to a local private mental hospital."

It is an interesting comment that Scott Kiser had by then been experiencing severe symptoms of psychotic depression for at least 3 weeks and no one, not his college counselors, his parents, or his parents' friends, had an inkling of what was going on.

Nor were the hospital doctors at first a big improvement. They thought he was on a bad drug trip as he stood, staring into a mirror "and my reflection appeared ... to be horribly distorted, like the image of a devil or demon. I began to wonder if I was becoming possessed by some evil power, perhaps by Satan himself." So, incredibly, his clinicians administered to him the Minnesota Multiphasic Personality Inventory.

He was put into a therapy group, where he sat "vacant and inert, ashamed and embarrassed about my condition. I waited in mortal dread as I saw my turn to speak approaching. When it came, I felt extremely anxious because there was nothing there to give or 'share.' I felt an expansive void open out from me into the room." The other patients in the group looked uneasy. "They were scared. Scared of me."

Finally, after about 2 weeks of this in the hospital, he began to get better, apparently in response to treatment, for he tells us that some nurse "stuck a needle in my arm" (Kiser, 2004).

If Scott had not been treated, he could easily have continued these symptoms, the delusions and hallucinations, "standing fixed and rigid like a stone statue" in his room, for another 8 months until Nature finally pulled him from his ordeal.

***

Barbara Field Benziger, a married New Yorker with four children, was cared for soon after she fell into a psychotic depression at some point in the 1960s. After some initial misadventures she was treated with ECT, apparently at the New York State Psychiatric Institute – she warmly thanks staff psychiatrist William Horwitz in the preface of her memoir – and recovered. But of interest is what she calls her "pain." "How could I convey, to some degree, some of the pain, the actual physical searing pain, which is impossible to describe wholly, that is ever present, as if your body were a reflection of the broken and tormented mind it contains." During her illness, in her journal she wrote,

> My mind is dying and I want to die with it.
> The pain is too much to bear
> Even my body hurts.
> My terrors are crushing me, smothering me. I can't breathe.
> (Benziger, 1969)

Pain, really?

Pain not sadness

People often think that the core symptom of severe depression is sadness. It is not. Although physicians see the essence of melancholia as a pathological slowing, or a mood that stays unhappy regardless of external events, this is not what it tends to feel like. Subjectively for the patient, among the chief core symptoms of endogenous depression is pain. "Depressive illness is probably more unpleasant than any disease except rabies," said one English psychiatrist. "There is constant mental pain and often psychogenic physical pain too . . . Naturally, many of these patients commit suicide. They may not hope to get to heaven but they know they are leaving hell" (Price, 1978).

It is this curious kind of almost indescribable pain in psychotic depression that gave rise to the clinical convention of identifying a "distinct quality" of depressive mood: Clinicians as early as the great German nosologist Emil Kraepelin and Ronald D. Gillespie of Guy's Hospital in London recognized that patients with psychotic depression experienced an almost unique kind of aversive or anguished sensation, which was difficult for them to convey to others. In 1926, in a discussion of whether there were really two depressions or one, Gillespie said that in the depressed phase of manic depression the feelings of these patients were indeed "formless," as another psychiatrist had attempted to dismiss them. "This was precisely the point. The feeling that was called depressive in these patients was often 'formless' – there might be neither 'morbid dissatisfaction' nor 'dissatisfaction with the self or circumstances,' but only something vague and very unpleasant in tone. From this arose the difficulty that these patients so frequently had in expressing their condition to the physician" (Gillespie, 1926).

More recently, Bernard Carroll at the University of Michigan makes "central pain disturbance" an important part of his model of endogenous depression, combined with an inability to experience pleasure. He puts it as a "disinhibition of central pain regulation" (Carroll, 1983). On one occasion Carroll was discussing his psychic pain idea at a seminar. Sam Guze, one of the leading figures in the "St. Louis school" of psychiatry – a group that introduced biological approaches to American psychiatry after World War II – spoke up. Guze was a bit dubious about the pain notion as such. Perhaps, he said, it was more a metaphor?

Not at all, Carroll responded. "I was not being metaphysical when I used the word 'psychic' pain. I was being phenomenological. It is a truly aversive, painful experience. If you doubt that, just ask your patients and they will tell you precisely about that aspect of it. It is no less real than any other type of pain is."[1]

Indeed, in patients' experience of illness the overwhelming impression that emerges of psychotic depression is the pain in which they find themselves. Novelist William Styon said of his episode of psychotic melancholia, "I was feeling in my mind a sensation close to, but indescribably different from, actual pain." Yet even Styron with his literary gifts was unable to describe the exact quality of the pain; he realized that many other patients as well were unable to convey "some of the actual

1 Bernard Carroll, in discussion of, Carroll. 1991. Psychopathology and neurobiology of manic-depressive disorders. In B. J. Carroll and J. E. Barrett (eds) *Psychopathology and the brain*. New York: Raven Press, pp. 265–85, at pp. 283–4.

dimensions of their torment, and perhaps elicit a comprehension that has been generally lacking."

"For myself," Styron continued, "the pain is most closely connected to drowning or suffocation." Once while traveling in Europe, after a nightmarish day in Paris on display in public, he made it back to his hotel room, fell on the bed, "and lay gazing at the ceiling, nearly immobilized and in a trance of supreme discomfort." He had to return to a gala dinner that night and give a speech! "The ferocious *inwardness* [emphasis in the original] of the pain produced an immense distraction that prevented my articulating words beyond a hoarse murmur; I sensed myself turning walleyed, monosyllabic, and also I sensed my French friends becoming uneasily aware of my predicament. It was a scene from a bad operetta by now."[2]

Even the psychiatrists sometimes cannot stand their patients' pain, and refer them to their residents' outpatient clinics or give them a diagnosis of personality disorder, rationalizing that inadequate improvement from treatment stems from personality flaws rather than illness; it is thought that patients with those kinds of disorders do not suffer so much.

To be sure, various psychological planes cut through the experience of depression. There is the isolation that Sylvia Plath captured in the image of the bell jar (Plath, 1996). There is the embrace of escape through suicide that Susan Walen etches in her classic essay, "It's a funny thing about suicide" (Walen, 2002). Yet in psychotic depression one of the pathological facets that glistens most arrestingly is pain. Edwin Shneidman at the UCLA Neuropsychiatric Institute describes the pain as "psychache," or "intolerable psychological pain" leading possibly to suicide.[3]

2 William Styron. 1990. *Darkness visible: A memoir of madness*. New York: Random House; reprinted from an article in *Vanity Fair* in 1989, pp. 16–20.

3 E. S. Shneidman. 1993. Suicide as psychache. *J Nerv Ment Dis* 181: 145–7; see also M. T. Berlim et al. 2003. Psychache and suicidality in adult mood disordered outpatients in Brazil. *Suicide Life-Threat Behav* 33: 242–8; E. S. Shneidman. 1999. The psychological pain assessment scale. *Suicide Life-Threat Behav* 29: 287–91.

Arthur Christopher Benson, later a noted English poet, describes a depression that overcame him in the early 1880s – the first of many during his life – when he was a student at King's College, Cambridge. (He writes about it in the third person.) "One night he went to bed late, and found it difficult to sleep; thoughts raced through his brain, scenes and images forming and reforming with inconceivable rapidity." He attempted to read in bed but "a ghastly and poisonous fear of he knew not what seemed to clutch at his mind." This was the beginning.

Benson dwelt on the pain aspect: He should have gone to a doctor, he said, "but the suffering appeared to be of so purely mental a character that he did not realise how much of it was physical." It lasted for weeks as "he tasted, day by day, the dreary bitterness of the cup of dark and causeless depression, and laboured under an agonising dejection of spirit. This intensity of suffering seemed to shake his whole life to its foundation."

This first depression for Benson was psychotic, delusions bearing on his religious life. "He became possessed by a strong delusion that it was a punishment sent to him by God for tampering with freedom of thought, and little by little a deep moral anxiety took hold of him. He searched the recesses of his heart, and ended by painting his whole life in the blackest of colours." Finally "Hugh," as Benson styles himself in this thinly fictionalized account, swam spontaneously up from the depths – as indeed there were no treatments – and "came back gratefully and wearily to his old life, his old friendships."[4]

So from the patients' view point, pain was a big accent in psychotic depression. In terms of how depression is conventionally described, psychic pain is usually not on the checklist. A brief screen for depression was published in the *New York Times* in 2005 (Santora and Carey, 2005): What you as a patient or as a family physician should look for. The nine

4 Arthur Christopher Benson. 1907. *Beside still waters.* London: Smith, Elder, pp. 48–50. For details of Benson's life and repeated depressive illnesses, see David Newsome. 1980. *On the edge of paradise: A. C. Benson: The diarist.* London: John Murray, passim.

items included "little interest or pleasure in doing things," or "feeling tired or having little energy," the symptoms associated with the kinds of "depressions" that seem today to be spreading with epidemic rapidity. Yet mental and physical agony are simply not on the list, not on the radar of the depression screeners, attuned as they are to low self-image and fatigue. But it is a core subjective symptom of melancholia, and the screeners might miss the psychotic blackness of the illness.

Describing the pain of psychotic depression as somehow psychosomatic does not diminish its seriousness, and in homage to the patients and their families who may be reading this, we try to understand it. In our estimation, this pain is an expression of body tension anxiety, which is a common feature of many psychiatric conditions, including melancholia, anxiety disorders, psychotic depression, and even catatonia.

Body tension anxiety can be generated by akathisia, a feeling of compulsion to move. Body tension anxiety includes restlessness and motor agitation and it represents an activation of the sympathetic nervous system – the fight-or-flight reflex – and can be a symptom of an illness or a side effect of drugs that excite or irritate that system. Although body tension anxiety is based in the brain, it is closer to the body-based brain than the mind-based brain.

The body-based brain: Let us analogize to how breathing is controlled by the brain. If we focus our attention on breathing we can manipulate its rate and depth, but in the ordinary conduct of our lives we do not control it psychologically nor can we expect to. Psychiatrists, psychotherapists, and probably most people have come to believe that decreasing worry will decrease body tension anxiety. This might occur if the tension is mild or brief, but if the tension is strong and persistent it becomes a permanent fixture, continuing even if worrying ceases. Severity or persistence of body tension anxiety transforms tension from symptom into illness.

The signs of tension we can observe in other people may include restlessness, jumpiness, agitation, an insatiable neediness to express the agony by spreading it around or at least telling others about it, hair-trigger distress from small things that really should not bother, panicky feelings, muscle tension pain (headaches, chest pains, muscle tightness), irritable bowels, fidgeting, insomnia, and easy anger. This uncomfortable tension drives suicidality, homicidality, rampages, and indulgences. Of course, mild-mannered people can experience body tension anxiety too, but their disciplined courtesy understates their suffering.

Add this body tension to the other symptoms of psychotic depression and what results is the pain our patients experience. In psychotic depression, body tension anxiety is set off by the depression itself. There need be no irritating experience from other people or the environment, the patient's thoughts are themselves grating. At the same time, the hyperreactivity of body tension amplifies and accelerates the emotional reaction of irritation into constant pain.

Patients with body tension anxiety alone, without psychotic depression, are distressed out of proportion by experiences that should be too small to bother. Of course this is not good, but patients with anxiety disorders can at least identify irritating environments (e.g., shopping) and try to avoid them. Patients with psychotic depression cannot do that because the irritant is their own body. Both the irritant and the entity being irritated are the same – the patient. At the same time, psychotic depression prevents patients from expressing their tension as other nondepressed people with anxiety do, such as feeling the need to scream out but being unable to. Body tension anxiety is a discomfort normal people experience in times of great stress. Remembering it should give us some feeling for the enormous discomfort of psychotic depression.

Delusional content

A second issue in the phenomenology of delusional depression is the nature of the delusions themselves. What is actually going through the patients' minds? In order to determine the content of the delusion,

Aaron Beck at the University of Pennsylvania interviewed 280 psychotic patients with varying degrees of depression (Beck, 1967). The themes were age-old: Of those patients with severe depression, 48 percent believed themselves worthless. As one patient said, "I must weep myself to death. I cannot live. I cannot die. I have failed so. It would be better if I had not been born." Another said, "I am totally useless. I can't do anything. I have never done anything worthwhile."

Forty-six percent of these severely depressed patients believed themselves to be terrible sinners or criminals. Punishments such as torture or hanging surely awaited them, they believed. Many patients believed they were being punished and that the hospital was a prison. One wailed, "Will God never give up? Why must I be singled out for punishment?" "My heart is gone. Can't He see this." Fourteen percent of these patients believed themselves to be the devil.

Ten percent of the patients had nihilistic delusions, a syndrome first described by Parisian psychiatrist Jules Cotard in 1880. Beck's patients said, "All is lost. The world is empty. Everybody died last night." Ten percent of the patients also believed they were dead. Many thought they had organs missing or that their viscera had been removed.

Finally, 24 percent of these severely depressed patients believed that their bodies were decaying, or otherwise in disarray. Beck gathered statements such as, "I haven't slept in six months." Or, "My intestines are blocked. The food can't get through." These were patients in a major American city in the 1960s.

It is curious how little has changed historically in the content of depressive delusions. Heinrich Kranz compared the charts of patients with "cyclothymia," by which he meant bipolar MDI, from the Heidelberg University Psychiatric Hospital for the mid-1880s and 1946. He found virtually no changes in delusional themes, despite starkly differing economic circumstances: the 1880s were a time of great prosperity for Germany, 1946 a time of misery and ruin. Yet the share of patients reporting delusional anxieties about impoverishment remained the same. "The cyclothymics seem not at all plugged into circumstances.

One would suppose that especially the depressives would be sensitive to contemporaneous events. That is not the case" (Kranz, 1955).

In 1875 a psychiatrist undertook a community survey of mental illness in the Swiss canton of Fribourg, just before the opening of the first cantonal mental hospital – the point of the survey being apparently to assess need. Of the 164 individuals in which the expert detected substantial psychiatric illness, 28 were depressed and virtually all psychotic. Fribourg canton was at that time poor and very rural. The Zurich psychiatry professor who retrospectively exhumed these 164 charts from the archives, Klaus Ernst, was struck at how little the clinical picture in depression had changed from then to now. "With melancholia and (uncommon) mania, the coincidence with the symptom picture of today is so complete that a detailed discussion is unnecessary. ... The ideas of sinfulness that dominate the self-loathing of the depressives are perhaps somewhat more frequent than today, but even that is not certain" (Ernst, 1983).

It probably is certain. The one idea in psychotic depression to have diminished is sinfulness. A number of statistical studies point to a decline in delusions about sinning against God, as do more seat-of-the pants' assessments by veteran observers. In 1926 Giovanni Mingazzini, professor of psychiatry in Rome, looked back over a long career.

> You used to see melancholics, men and women, seized by anxiety because they were convinced they had committed sacrilege, having spit on the sacramental host, or cursed the Lord God and thus believing they deserved eternal punishment in hell without hope of redemption. Today by contrast it is unusual for such delusions of self-reproach to have such a pronouncedly religious character (the so-called religious manias of the laity). The patients find the source of their purported sins in the belief that they have committed imaginary forgeries, infected the children with syphilis, although they themselves had never acquired syphilis, or stolen money from friends or employers, although they themselves are law-abiding individuals. (Mingazzini, 1926)

Of five statistical studies comparing different periods, three support this shift from sin to crime, or at least away from sin, as the principal change in depressive delusional content: One study finds no change (Robinson, 1988); one finds a rise in hypochondriac preoccupations as the main trend (Eagles, 1983).) At the Austrian asylum Niedernhart, it was found during the first half of the twentieth century that the presence of "guilt ideas" declined from 70 to around 50 percent of all patients (Lenz, 1967). Among melancholics at the Basel University Psychiatric Clinic in the years 1878–951, "ideas of sinfulness" declined in men from 61 to 29 percent, and in women from 71 to 50 percent (Von Orelli, 1954). In a Finnish study, "strong manifest guilt" fell off from 20 percent of all "depressive psychoses" in 1880–9 to 5 percent in 1960–9; "religious symptoms in abundance" declined from 13 to 2 percent (Niskanen, 1972)

How melancholic patients derive their particular set of delusional ideas is clearly complex. Obviously you will not develop delusions about ideas you have never been exposed to, and in such a thoroughly secular society as Finland today, it does not surprise us that only one seriously depressed patient in fifty is delusional about religion. When in Texas in 2001 Andrea Yates drowned her five children in the belief that she was saving them from the fires of hell, she expressed a belief that she might not have acquired had she grown up in a more secular setting. There clearly is some relationship between the outside world and the patient's expression of delusional depression, but it is probably not a close one. Internal hell has its own rules.

Prognosis

The one thing that the patient and his or her family want to know is, "Am I going to get better?" The answer is, "Probably, but you're going to have to be careful." We did not say "yes," although that was the answer that springs most readily to the lips because honest physicians are not allowed to promise, nor should they. The patient could die from suicide, pneumonia, or heart attack, or by unintentional suicide from an action that was absent common sense.

The good news in dealing with serious depression is that one eventually recovers, even when untreated. The bad news is that the patient is the worse for wear. The experience of psychotic depression is life threatening; it is comparable to – and more persistent than – the traumatic experiences that produce lifelong PTSD. Once a patient develops psychotic depression, there is a real race against time, in which effective treatment needs to be given soon enough, or PTSD will develop. Fortunately, not all people are susceptible to PTSD, but about 40 percent are.

Let us also be realistic about treatment. Treatment does shorten each episode, although a Danish study found that previous treatment does not diminish the likelihood of recurrence. We have long known that medications and ECT work, and also that depressive patients are subject to relapse on a lifelong basis. Lars Kessing, who put together followup data on the life histories of patients with mood disorders admitted to Danish mental hospitals between 1971 and 1993, concluded that serious depression seems to take on a kind of rhythm of its own: Apparently regardless of treatment, every new episode means that the risk of yet another episode increases.[5]

The presence of delusions and hallucinations worsens the prognosis. In 1930 Edward Strecker and colleagues in the psychiatric service of Pennsylvania Hospital in Philadelphia followed-up 100 patients with "manic-depressive reactions" admitted between 1917 and 1920; they compared fifty who had recovered from their illness with fifty who had not. Paranoid delusions were present at admission in 50 percent of those who had not recovered, in 34 percent of those who had; 46 percent of the unrecovered had had hallucinations, 30 percent of the recovered.[6] (Again, lack of recovery sometimes results from PTSD caused by the

5 Lars Vedel Kessing. 2001. *Course and cognitive outcome in major affective disorder*. Copenhagen: Laegeforeningens Forlag, see especially p. 27.

6 E. A. Strecker et al. 1931. The prognosis in manic-depressive psychosis. In William A. White et al. (eds) *Manic-depressive psychosis: An investigation of the most recent advances*. Baltimore: Williams & Wilkins; Proceedings of the Association for Research in Nervous and Mental Diseases, December 29–30, 1930, pp. 471–538, see p. 503.

terrible experience of psychotic depression, rather than by residual symptoms of depression itself.)

In one of the classic followup studies of psychiatry, in the late 1970s William Coryell and Ming Tsuang at the University of Iowa selected for followup 525 patients with all kinds of diagnoses admitted to the university psychiatric hospital (then called the "psychopathic hospital") between 1935 and 1940. Of these "Iowa 500," 225 had unipolar depression, and 212 of them were located 40 years later and rated (for many who were deceased, the relatives were interviewed). The balance between psychotic and nonpsychotic depression at admission was about equal. Of the nondelusional patients, 56 percent were well at the end of the first year, only 28 percent of the delusional. So the presence of psychosis (and the absence of treatment in the late 1930s) clearly disposed to a poor short-term outcome.

Yet 10–20 years later, there was little difference between the two groups: 100 percent of the nondelusional were well, 88 percent of those who had been delusional at admission (Coryell and Tsuang, 1982). Thus serious hospital depression was an illness from which one clearly recovered in the long term, yet being psychotic worsened one's experience of illness in the short term. (They were apparently not assessed for anxiety disorders such as PTSD, which is why so many could be said to be well.)

There was one more finding of relevance. Of the 222 unipolar depressive patients whose mortality status the researchers were able to determine in 1974, 64.8 percent of the nondelusional patients were dead, 82.6 percent of the delusional. The difference was not owing to suicide (about one in ten in each group) (Coryell and Tsuang, 1982). Of the depressed patients altogether, within nine years of admission their "mortality ratio" was 2.3 times higher than that of the Iowa population in general (less thereafter) (Tsuang, 1979). If the findings of the Zurich study of Jules Angst and associates are applicable here, the majority of deaths in both groups would have been owing to cardiac causes (Angst et al., 2002).

Just how dangerous are melancholia and its psychotic variety? They are fearful illnesses partly because they predispose to suicide: The depressed inpatients in Jules Angsts's study of Zurich had a suicide rate 18 times higher than that of the general population. Yet the suicide rates for delusional and nondelusional seem about equal.[7]

These illnesses are also dangerous because they put the sufferers at risk of other potentially fatal bodily ailments, such as heart attacks (one and a half times higher in Zurich than in the general population), as well as accidents and fatal inebriation (twice as high in Zurich). The mechanism of this surplus mortality is obscure. Indirect evidence points to body tension anxiety. Such tension causes coronary vasospasm, which means narrowing of the blood vessels bringing oxygen to the heart. Habitually tense people are documented to die prematurely from coronary vasospasm. It is likely – though unproven – that psychotic depression and the anxiety disorders it causes provoke such tension and premature heart-related death. Thus, sufferers and their families need to pay careful attention to such issues as reducing anxiety, diet, exercise, and the other components of a healthy lifestyle. Also, they should be mindful that they are dealing with an illness that predisposes sufferers to more chaotic life experiences than most people have.[8] They need to be watchful!

There is one piece of good news: Patients who adhere scrupulously to a maintenance regimen of antimelancholic medication (AMM) (or to maintenance ECT – see Chapter 7) will likely do very well. One of us

7 This point is controversial. On the view that psychotic depressives are not more suicidal than nonpsychotic depressives, see M. Wolfersdorf et al. 1987. Delusional depression and suicide. *Acta Psychiatr Scand* 76: 359–63; D. W. Black et al. 1988. Effect of psychosis on suicide risk in 1,593 patients with unipolar and bipolar affective disorders. *Am J Psychiatry* 145: 849–52. For the view that suicide is higher in psychotic depression, see S. P. Roose et al. 1983. Depression, delusions, and suicide. *Am J Psychiatry* 140: 1159–62.

8 See George Winokur and Ming T. Tsuang. 1996. *The natural history of mania, depression, and schizophrenia.* Washington, DC: American Psychiatric Press, especially pp. 204–9 on later disability status of the patients with depression.

(CS) looked at long-term outcomes after ECT in a group of patients with catatonic depression, a kissing-cousin to psychotic depression. Of thirty-seven depressed patients with catatonic features seen in an inpatient psychiatric service from 1992 to 1996 (and followed-up in 1999), he was able to track nineteen: thirteen were discharged on AMMs such as TCAs, lithium, bupropion (Wellbutrin), and high-dose venlafaxine (Effexor); six had various regimes of nonmelancholic medication, such as SSRIs. Of the six patients not given AMM, all had poor outcomes and three died of cardiac illness. Of the thirteen on antimelancholic remedies, ten had good recent function and all were alive. The study was not large, though the results are significant statistically (Swartz et al., 2001). But it shows that given appropriate care, a diagnosis of melancholia is not tantamount to a sentence of doom.

5

Treatment in Historical Perspective

An illness that awaits good news

It is October 1879. We are in St. Andrew's Hospital for Mental Diseases in Northampton, England. Consider the treatment options for Miss X, age 31, who had been admitted suffering from melancholia. "On admission the patient was somewhat depressed, and expressed a wish to destroy herself. During the night it was found that she had tied the cord of a window-blind round her neck." In the weeks ahead, her mood seemed to lighten, yet she persisted in "the delusion that she would ruin the place if detained." By early December she was deemed well enough to be taken on a skating party on a neighboring meadow, but at the first opportunity she "threw herself into a hole in the ice, from which she was rescued with some difficulty."

In January, still highly delusional and suicidal, she swallowed a number of straight pins and knitting needles. The next several months of her clinical care focused on giving her laxatives as she slowly, and painfully, passed them in her stool. Finally, she began to recover spontaneously from her depression and was discharged well in September 1880.

What treatments did her medical attendants provide? There were options. "The treatment of the local symptoms at first consisted in the administration from time to time of castor oil," her physician said. Her abdominal distress from the pins and needles was addressed with "poultices and fomentations." The staff prescribed opium for her mood disorder, opium being a specific for depression a thousand years old. "Later chloral was the principal agent employed to allay restlessness and procure sleep." None of these remedies, save perhaps opium – which is highly addictive – touched her underlying psychosis or depression. Yet she recovered on her own after much travail. So medicine has never been entirely helpless in the face of an illness like psychotic depression. Yet Miss X was in a mental hospital for a year, much of which was spent in misery following her suicide attempt with the needles, to say nothing of her suffering from the melancholia itself, from which she long sought the relief of death (Bayley, 1881).

Yet within sixty years after 1880, the travails of the Miss Xs of this world would be greatly meliorated. The modern era of the treatment of psychotic depression began in the early twentieth century.

From the earliest days of interest in the endocrine system there had been efforts to treat psychotic depression. As the endocrine system seems heavily implicated in melancholia in general – not just in its psychotic variety – hormonal treatments have a surprising record of success. One must be careful to sort out genuine results from the kind of misogyny with which psychiatry, and society in general, was infused in those days. Endocrine often meant "ovarian," on the assumption that women's behavior was driven by disorders of the reproductive system far more than men's. Yet some of this work is interesting.

Since the late nineteenth century, physicians had attempted to relieve mental symptoms in "menopausal" women – read women from their late 40s to their early 60s – with ovarian extracts. Thus, in 1922 Edward

Strecker and Baldwin Keyes from the department for mental and nervous diseases of Pennsylvania Hospital in Philadelphia administered to fourteen female patients with "involutional melancholia" injections of "ovarian substance." Of the fourteen, four were "remarkably improved"; this following an average hospital stay of 7½ months; another four showed "definite improvement." Of the fourteen, eleven were psychotic. Of the three nonpsychotic melancholics, two failed to improve.[1] Ovarian extract therapy thus showed some differential effectiveness in the psychotic variety of melancholia. The study was too small to be really meaningful; there was, of course, no placebo control group: in 1922 nobody had yet heard of such a thing. We are not making a serious plaidoyer for treating patients today with ovarian extract. Yet the trial demonstrates a certain therapeutic questing, a desire to undertake something in the face of an illness that left men and women such as these wretched until a spontaneous recovery finally eventuated.

Then in the 1930s real progress began. The history of treatment of delusional depression after the 1930s is a history of steadily accumulating good news, at least for the short-term prospects. Today, the symptoms of delusional depression can be largely relieved. As English psychopharmacologist Alec Coppen said in 1975, "Paradoxically, with depression, the more severely depressed you are the better your prognosis. I think the mild cases of depression ... have probably the worst outlook. But really severe psychotic depression has on the whole an extremely good prognosis. It is the mild, if you like neurotic, cases that are most difficult to treat."[2] We are speaking here, of course, of the short term. In the long term almost all patients with depression except of the psychotic variety recover

1 E. A. Strecker and B. L. Keyes. 1922. Ovarian therapy in involutional melancholia. *NY Med J* 116: 30–4. The presence or absence of psychosis was inferred from the brief vignettes.

2 Alec Coppen in discussion. 1976. In B. I. Hoffbrand and G. F. B. Birdwood (eds) Biological aspects of clomipramine: Proceedings of a symposium held at Marbella, Spain, on March 12–15, 1976. *Postgrad Med J* 52(Suppl 3): 119.

spontaneously.[3] But the long term can be a long time in coming, and life is lived in the short term. The news that psychotic depressions recovered in the short term when treated properly was therefore very good news.

Convulsive therapy

This story of successful treatability started in 1935 with the advent of Ladislaus von Meduna's chemical convulsive therapy, and definitively so in 1938 when Ugo Cerletti began using electricity to induce the seizures. The real history of the treatment of delusional depression has been a tug-of-war between partisans of ineffective drugs that just happened to be under patent protection and were hyped by the pharmaceutical industry, and a handful of effective treatments from which no one was going to make a lot of money, but which actually worked.

It was thus convulsive therapy that began the modern era in the treatment of mood disorders. Ladislaus von Meduna, who originated convulsive therapy in 1935 in Budapest with pentylenetetrazol (marketed as Metrazol in the United States and as Cardiazol in Europe), envisioned the treatment for schizophrenia, and believed it most effective in catatonic syndromes. But when in 1938 Roman psychiatry professor Ugo Cerletti proposed electricity to initiate the seizures, almost from the beginning he realized that electroshock therapy, as he called it, was more effective in depression than in schizophrenia. As he wrote in the *Italian Journal of Psychiatry* in 1940, "In the treatment of manic-depressive illness we have obtained even more promising results than in schizophrenia, particularly in depressive episodes" (Cerletti, 1940).

Electroshock quickly established itself as a safe and effective treatment of the symptoms of both psychosis and depression. Indeed it was so

3 See S. J. Kantor and A. H. Glassman. 1977. Delusional depressions: Natural history and response to treatment. *Br J Psychiatry* 131: 351–60, to the effect that "[d]elusions were to be considered an ominous prognostic sign in patients with manic-depressive illness" (p. 352).

effective that the early electrotherapists believed that the great majority of patients would respond to the treatment. As New York psychiatrist Lothar Kalinowsky, the godfather of ECT in the United States, wrote in 1941, "Everyone who has seen depressive patients mute, stuporous and tube-fed for years, who after three or four convulsive treatments recover completely, will no more belittle the importance of these treatments. In this group, amazing recoveries are achieved in the majority of all treated cases" (Kalinowsky, 1941). Later ECT specialists adopted informally an "80 percent" rule: If fewer than 80 percent of your patients failed to recover, then you were doing something wrong.[4] (There is of course no pharmacotherapy of depression for which anything like 80 percent of the patients recover.) As a result of the remarkable effectiveness of ECT in endogenous depression, or melancholia, the psychotic form of the illness ceased to be singled out: ECT was equally effective in psychotic and nonpsychotic forms alike.

We are back in 1940. In October of that year Mr A. B., 40 and married, was admitted to Hillside Hospital in the New York borough of Queens, accompanied by his sister. "The patient states that he recently developed an obsession which he finds very peculiar. He claims that he was accused by a woman with whom he had lived for 4 years of having indulged in sexual perversions, although he had actually never done it. He claims that for the last 4 years this accusation has been bothering him and he feels that the accusation got around and became public knowledge." (So he has clearly been psychotic for some time, and there may or may not have been a stress trigger for this.) The story continues:

In September 1936, he met a woman to whom he became engaged. Shortly before the wedding, he became depressed, then following the ceremony he tipped into hypomania, bingeing on alcohol and gambling.

4 On the 80% rule, see J. D. Little et al. 2003. Right unilateral electroconvulsive therapy at six times the seizure threshold. *Aust NZ J Psychiatry* 37: 715–19: "As to patient selection, there is a body of evidence to suggest that a response rate above 80% . . . should now be routine. If the technique is unable to achieve this result, then either that technique or the patients selected, need to change" (p. 719).

After discovering that his new bride did not intend to pay his gambling debts, he became depressed again and stopped working – he had been a production employee at a newspaper – and now, at the time of admission, he had been fiercely biting his nails. As the chart noted, he "is dejected, apprehensive, mildly retarded, complains of loss of sleep and appetite and has severe guilt feelings about his debts and a fear of losing his job."

On the ward, he makes slow progress and continues to obsess about the idea that people think he is a sex pervert. A note in his chart of February 5, 1941, says that the woman he formerly lived with had

> kept bothering him to marry her. At one time he made her pregnant and she wanted to have the child. They were drinking in a saloon once when becoming angry with her for bothering him he called her a lousy c. and she called him a c. lapper. The bartender overheard this and told others and the rumors were spread around. He thinks that the patients here also think that he is a sex pervert. It was decided to try electric shock therapy.

On February 15, 1941, he began ECT and by March 25 had received eighteen treatments with ten major seizures. "There has been a marked improvement in his condition in the past few weeks," noted the chart. "He is now practically rid of his depression. He is bright, cheerful and active, and has spontaneously expressed his desire and readiness to resume life on the outside and has asked for his discharge." "Nothing of a psychotic nature remained," said the discharge note.[5]

ECT thus transformed the treatment of psychotic depression. Before, depression had been ineffectively treated with opium and, after 1900, with barbiturate sedatives. Agitated patients could be calmed with drugs but nothing existed in the pharmacopoeia to touch the underlying depression or the psychosis. ECT touched both. It is ironic, overturning the notion that "progress" is something that happens at the end of events not the beginning, that the best treatment of psychotic depression was the first to be discovered.

5 Hillside Hospital Archives, microfilm reel no. 14, case 1526.

Antimelancholic medication: Chlorpromazine

In 1952 the revolution in therapy that ECT had initiated spread to pharmacotherapy. This was really the beginning of biological psychiatry, an approach that emphasizes the brain rather than the mind as the seat of illness and endeavors to treat the brain with pharmacotherapy. Melancholia has always loomed at the center of biological psychiatry. As Gerry Klerman once said, "Melancholia is to biological psychiatry as neurosis was to psychoanalysis."[6] What one of us has called "antimelancholic medication" (AMM) (Swartz et al., 2001) would rush center stage.

It was in France that this revolution began. In 1952 French clinicians established the efficacy of chlorpromazine in psychosis, or "schizophrenia" as they called it, and the treatment of psychiatric illness with pharmaceuticals began to supplant talk therapy as the main instrument in the toolbox of psychiatry. Chlorpromazine was licensed in American psychiatry in 1954. The drug's success ended the belief that serious psychiatric illness was untreatable, essentially hopeless. A whole new era had begun.

The early psychopharmacologists quickly realized the effectiveness of chlorpromazine in psychotic and melancholic depression. In 1953, Paris psychiatrist Jean Sigwald described the use of chlorpromazine on an outpatient basis for a number of indications, including depression. "In general, treatment with chlorpromazine almost always affects the patient's mood and we have observed the disappearance of sadness and depression, as a certain euphoria takes their place" (Sigwald and Bouttier, 1953). Within 3 years' time Sigwald had successfully treated 150 patients with chlorpromazine, among them 23 with "psychoneurotic and psychotic depression" (Sigwald et al., 1956). Sigwald described

6 Gerald Klerman, discussion comment. Meeting of the APA Ad hoc advisory committee on melancholia, July 26, 1985, APA Archives, Williams Papers, Research, *DSM-III-R*, box 4, folder "Melancholia meeting."

chlorpromazine as "the insulin of the nervous" (Sigwald et al., 1956). (This, of course, is an oversimplification. Antipsychotics are really "thought simplifiers"; they decrease psychotic ideation by decreasing all ideation; they are like organizing a room by removing things from it until it is reasonably tidy. Today, antipsychotics would not necessarily be the treatment of choice, yet in an era where there was no pharmacotherapy for melancholia, they were a step forward.)

The positive results of these early French trialists were confirmed by other clinicians. In one of the earliest chlorpromazine trials outside of France, Paul Kielholz at the university psychiatric clinic in Basel, Switzerland, established the effectiveness of chlorpromazine in "endogenous depression"; he said that the drug clearly reduced "psychotic ideation" (Kielholz, 1954). At Baylor University in Houston, Texas, Vernon Kinross-Wright found chlorpromazine more effective in depression than in schizophrenia. In a study of ninety-five unselected patients admitted to the psychiatry service of a general hospital, 72 percent of the schizophrenics were much improved or better, 78 percent of the depressives (Kinross-Wright, 1955). At Manhattan State Hospital on Ward's Island in New York, Herman Denber tried several different treatments of "depressed psychotic patients" (meaning probably melancholia): placebo, chlorpromazine, the anti-Parkinsonian compound diethazine, and a combination of chlorpromazine and diethazine. Eight of the ten patients in the chlorpromazine-diethazine arm experienced a "complete remission" (Denber, 1957).

At nearby Hillside Hospital in the eastern part of Queens, in 1958–9 Max Fink and Donald Klein administered phenothiazine-type antipsychotic drugs to 120 patients without regard for diagnosis. The surprise finding was that the antipsychotics functioned as antidepressants, decreasing "agitated depression" in eight patients seen as having obsessive-compulsive states. "The depressive state was markedly alleviated," the authors found (Klein and Fink, 1962). When they reanalyzed these data in 1965, they put imipramine head-to-head against a chlorpromazine-procyclidine combo (procyclidine is anti-Parkinsonian).

The authors found chlorpromazine superior to imipramine in the treatment of agitated depression, imipramine superior in phobic anxiety states, and the drugs tied in treating retarded depressive syndromes (Fink et al., 1965).

Meanwhile Leo Hollister and John Overall were putting the antipsychotic drug thioridazine (Sandoz's Mellaril) head-to-head against imipramine in seventy-seven male patients who had depression as their major complaint at a number of Veterans Administration hospitals. "As a large proportion of the total sample of patients in the group were most responsive to thioridazine," they wrote, "the latter drug was slightly but not significantly better than imipramine in reducing total pathology in the total sample" (Hollister and Overall, 1965).

Thus did evidence build on behalf of chlorpromazine and the other phenothiazines as antidepressants in serious depression. By 1967 a report of the World Health Organization (WHO) on psychopharmacology concluded that chlorpromazine and imipramine were equally effective as antidepressants (WHO, 1967).

Antipsychotics became prescribed as adjuvants to ECT therapy for depression. In 1955 Douglas Goldman, a Cincinnati psychiatrist who helped pioneer the somatic therapies, reported a female patient, 31, with a long history of depressive illness, whom Goldman had been treating with low doses of chlorpromazine; she had been experiencing a bit of relief. "Apparently, however, some depressive affect had been building up for a short period and the patient's life was saved only by the skill of the driver of a tractor-trailer truck who was able to pull his outfit far enough to the side of the road so that the patient was able to strike only the rear wheel of his tractor with her car instead of hitting it head-on." She later told her husband that she had been planning her suicide at home but the opportunity afforded by the truck seemed just too good to pass up. Goldman put her on ECT, continued the chlorpromazine, and she did well thereafter. "The combination of chlorpromazine with electric shock treatment accelerated significantly her recovery from the depressive state," Goldman said (Goldman, 1955).

Then something happened that, generally speaking, is not supposed to occur in medicine with its emphasis upon progress and the building blocks of knowledge: the usefulness of chlorpromazine and the other phenothiazine antipsychotics in endogenous depression became forgotten. This did not happen accidentally. In 1966 the FDA, determined to cleanse the pharmacopoeia of useless traditional remedies, asked the National Academy of Sciences/National Research Council to conduct a comprehensive review of the efficacy of all drugs on the market. A psychiatry panel considered the psychiatry drugs, recommending, chiefly on the basis of personal opinion, that many of them be withdrawn as ineffective.[7] They said that chlorpromazine was definitely effective in psychosis and severe depression. The FDA on its own, however, in implementing the recommendations of the NAS/NRC review in a bureaucratic exercise called Drug Efficacy Study Implementation (DESI), decided to cut back the uses of the antipsychotics and limited the indications of chlorpromazine mainly to psychosis, omitting depression; in 1971 the FDA published a notice in the Federal Register to that effect. Despite Smith Kline's ongoing attempts during the 1970s to get the regulators to expand the indications for chlorpromazine, the Feds remained firm, willing to concede in the 1980s only a black-box warning on chlorpromazine for "non-psychotic anxiety."[8]

Thus, with the stroke of a bureaucrat's pen, chlorpromazine ceased to be advertised or detailed for depression. Other antipsychotics with fresher patents reached the market, and chlorpromazine started to be forgotten, despite remaining as effective as any antipsychotic ever marketed.[9] Given the general disadvantages of the antipsychotics – and the

7 Food and Drug Administration, archives, Drug Efficacy Study Implementation, NAS/NRC review nos. 1330, 1344.

8 On the largely unknown DESI story, see E. Shorter. 2002. Looking backwards: A possible new path for drug discovery in psychopharmacology. *Nat Rev Drug Discov* 1: 1003–5.

9 The entry for chlorpromazine in the Physicians' Desk Reference, 2003, is silent on depression as an indication, while admitting the management of mania and "severe behavioral problems in children," among other indications (p. 1651).

more recent availability of alternative agents – it is not clear that chlorpromazine today would be the remedy of choice in the management of psychotic depression. But aside from ECT, chlorpromazine was the first effective pharmacotherapy for severe depression.

The antipsychotics currently used in psychotic depression tend to be "atypicals" such as clozapine, not the classic antipsychotics of the chlorpromazine era. It is quite possible that they are less effective than chlorpromazine for this indication. We will probably never know. Trials are now funded mainly by industry, and it is inconceivable that a drug company would risk some precious new compound in a trial against a drug that is 40 years old! In any event, the point is not that chlorpromazine was a wonder drug for psychotic depression; it caused severe side effects, such as movement disorders and persistent psychosis. The point is, rather, that some of the past treatments that have proven clearly effective in psychotic depression have been forgotten today in favor of drugs that may be inferior, yet that have patent coverage.

Virtually all observers in the 1950s admitted that ECT was superior to any drug in the treatment of depression. So why bother with drugs? The search for pharmaceuticals in psychotic depression became necessary because the growing stigmatization of ECT in the 1960s and 1970s caused many patients to be fearful of electrotherapy. As well, many psychiatrists enamored of Freudian psychotherapy or psychopharmacology came to shun it as well. The result, in a society whose conception of ECT reflected what they had seen in the 1975 movie *One Flew Over the Cuckoo's Nest*, was that it became virtually impossible to prescribe ECT in many centers (even today it is unavailable in a third of United States metropolitan areas) (Hermann, 1995). Because of these fears, after the end of the 1950s drugs would have the main burden of treating psychotic depression. (ECT did not entirely go out of business, yet until its revival in the 1990s its use became greatly restricted and for most patients ceased to be a treatment option.)

There is one final point about this golden era of drug discovery in the 1950s and early 1960s, when it seemed as though a cornucopia had opened, pouring new compounds into the psychiatric marketplace whose uses were not well defined: There was probably too much too soon. "We have so many drugs whose effects we do not properly understand," Edinburgh psychiatrist Frank Fish told a meeting in 1959. "And we have sometimes very little idea of precisely what the condition is that we are trying to treat." Fish likened the situation "to what might have happened had somebody introduced simultaneously five powerful antibiotics in the middle of the eighteenth century." What diseases are these drugs actually good for? (Fish, 1964) There was not really time in the psychopharmacologic rush of the 1950s to undertake the careful clinical observation that might have differentiated the response profile of one drug from that of another. The companies all insisted that their products were useful for just about everything, and the trials contained vastly heterogeneous groups of patients, psychotic and nonpsychotic, depressed, tense and nervous alike. In careful hands, the drugs might have served as pharmacologic torches to chisel out new disease entities. In the pell-mell of marketing they became panaceas, good for everything and yet, somehow, superb for nothing.

Antimelancholic medication: The tricyclic antidepressants

In 1957 Swiss psychiatrist Roland Kuhn established the efficacy of imipramine, a Geigy compound closely related to chlorpromazine, in "vital," or endogenous, depression.[10] Imipramine was marketed as Tofranil later that year in Switzerland, and in 1959 in the United States. It was the first TCA, so-called because the two phenyl rings linked together by a chemical bridge have the appearance of a three-ringed structure. The TCAs quickly established themselves as effective in many forms of

10 For this story, see Thomas Ban et al. (eds) 2002. *From psychopharmacology to neuropsychopharmacology in the 1980s*. Budapest: Animula, pp. 282–353.

depressive illness, both endogenous and reactive, and the convention sprang up that drugs like chlorpromazine, called "antipsychotics," were mainly useful in the treatment of schizophrenia (the term schizophrenia in those years was virtually synonymous with psychosis). And that the TCAs and the monoamine oxidase enzyme inhibitors (MAOIs) were mainly useful in the treatment of depression.

Imipramine reached the United States in January 1957, as two psychiatrists in Saginaw, Michigan, received a supply, evidently directly from Geigy. They administered the drug to in- and outpatients with a wide variety of diagnoses. Of those with "psychotic depression," 42 percent were "markedly well," slightly smaller percentages of patients with involutional and neurotic depression. So the news from Saginaw was promising: "Patients frequently reported that delusional thoughts and hallucinations became more vague, 'like a bad dream that occurred a long time ago,' and they became less introspective and less ruminative" (Ruskin and Goldner, 1959).

In 1959 Geigy launched imipramine in the United States, followed by a slew of rival TCAs. The effectiveness of these drugs was at first unclear: So much serious depression was labeled "schizophrenia" by psychoanalytically oriented physicians who called schizophrenia everything they could not treat with psychotherapy. Much reactive depression was still concealed in the blanket label "nervousness"; the hospital depressions still seemed pretty much of a muchness.

It was, therefore, only in 1965 that Gerald Klerman, then at Harvard, and Jonathan Cole at the NIMH, achieved an overview of the twenty-three randomized clinical trials of imipramine in depression that compared the drug to placebo or a rival compound. Thirteen of the studies had been in hospital patients, and in seven of these imipramine had beaten placebo or the rival drug. Outpatient studies had found imipramine even more effective (Klerman and Cole, 1965). The Klerman-Cole paper represented the first definitive statement that the TCAs worked. In 2000, veteran psychopharmacologist Fridolin Sulser of Vanderbilt University looked back: "Though new drugs were discovered, in my opinion, there is not a single one that is more efficacious and faster acting than the original antidepressants discovered almost 40 years ago by serendipity."[11] Imipramine was one of psychiatry's historic drugs.

But early on psychiatrists realized, *pace* Saginaw, that imipramine was less effective in psychotic depression. The Germans and Swiss in these years were more immersed in psychopharmacologic research than the Americans, having a long tradition of drug discovery going back to the early days of the organic chemical industry in the 1850s. In June 1959, the department of psychiatry of Frankfurt University conducted a big imipramine symposium attended by many investigators who had received early samples of the drug from Geigy. As Hanns Hippius, then at Berlin and leader of the younger generation of German psychiatrists not contaminated by the Nazi experience, summarized the proceedings, the conference confirmed what Kuhn had already established: that imipramine worked best in vital depression. Yet Hippius also mentioned the consensus that imipramine was inappropriate in agitated or psychotic depression: "The more the psychopathologic picture is dominated by delusional symptoms and the more that inner unrest or agitation take the place of vital slowing, so much less are the prospects of a good treatment result with Tofranil" (Hippius and Jantz, 1959).

Several body blows to imipramine followed. In 1962 a team of VA psychiatrists led by psychologist John Overall and Palo Alto psychiatrist Leo Hollister conducted a large placebo-controlled trial of various possible antidepressants: One was a combo antidepressant-sedative marketed by Smith Kline called "Dexamyl" (it contained a mixture of amphetamine and barbiturate), another was imipramine, and the third the MAOI isocarboxazide (Roche's Marplan). The trialists looked at psychotic depression among other types. The news was crushing: Although at 3 weeks imipramine had a salutary impact on psychotic

11 Fridolin Sulser, interview. 2000. From the presynaptic neurone to the receptor to the nucleus. In David Healy (ed.) *The Psychopharmacologists*, vol. 3. London: Arnold, pp. 239–58, quote on p. 247.

depression, at 12 weeks none of the drugs beat placebo. (Here again, "psychotic" might have meant mainly severe; the authors are unclear; Overall et al., 1962.)

In these years there were a number of such studies of "psychotic" depression, difficult to evaluate because the investigators usually meant endogenous depression, in the belief that the delusional variant was not worth singling out.[12]

Then in 1975 Sandy Glassman at the New York State Psychiatric Institute entered the scene. His work is important because not only did he show that imipramine did poorly in actual psychotic depression, but as we saw in chapter 2, he also suggested that psychotic depression was probably a disease of its own, different from melancholia and from neurotic depression. Just hanging around the ward, he had noticed that most of the patients who were not improving on imipramine had psychotic thinking. He put them on ECT and they rapidly improved. This set Glassman pondering (Glassman et al., 1975).

Two years later, in 1977, Glassman and Shephard Kantor, in an article in the *British Journal of Psychiatry* (Kantor and Glassman, 1977), said that "the presence or absence of delusional thinking should be considered as a significant criterion in the classification of depressive disorders"; in other words, the disease's nonresponse to TCAs meant that it was probably a separate disease entity. This was a timely statement, given that the halls of the New York State Psychiatric Institute (PI) in those days were full of talk about the classification of illness, the third edition of the APA's *DSM*, edited by Glassman's colleague Bob Spitzer, being close to readiness.

Indeed, other nosology buffs at PI were quite unconvinced about the separate disease status of psychotic depression. Frederic Quitkin, Arthur Rifkin, and Donald Klein had diseases of their own in the mood area to propose; in an article in the *American Journal of Psychiatry* in

12 On this literature, see A. S. Friedman et al. 1966. Imipramine (tofranil) vs. placebo in hospitalized psychotic depressives. *J Psychiatr Res* 4: 13–36.

July 1978, they pooh-poohed Glassman's brainstorm as merely a more severe version of plain old depression (Quitkin et al., 1978). Goaded perhaps by this challenge, in 1981, Glassman and Steven Roose laid out the reasons why psychotic depression should be considered a separate disease: In addition to TCA unresponsiveness, these patients had "dramatically more psychomotor retardation," were less reactive to the environment, were unresponsive to placebo, and exhibited a different pattern of brain biochemistry (Glassman and Roose, 1981).

The controversy definitively fixed the unsuitability of TCAs in the treatment of psychotic depression. As the authors of one study explained rather casually, almost half of our melancholic patients are psychotic, and thus not candidates for TCAs (Nelson et al., 1981).

It was thus Glassman who showed that the classic distinction between "antidepressants" for depression and "antipsychotics" for schizophrenia was largely marketing baloney. Antidepressants were in fact of little use for a large chunk of depressive illness. Though Glassman had given his refractory patients ECT rather than chlorpromazine, people were aware that antipsychotics often suppressed symptoms substantially in depression. As far as psychotic depression is concerned, chlorpromazine seems to have been more effective than the TCAs. (The reverse is not true: antidepressants have a poor record as antipsychotics.) As the penny dropped that the TCAs were not the drugs of choice in delusional depression – although effective for nonpsychotic melancholia and for reactive depression – it started to make sense again to differentiate treatments for psychotic depression from those for the nonpsychotic variety.

One attempt to muddy the waters should be noted, however. After *DSM*-III came out in 1980, there was much agonizing about the "melancholia" qualifier. What was melancholia and how did it differ, except in terms of severity, from nonmelancholic depression? On July 26, 1985, Bob Spitzer and Mark Zimmerman, a pre-medical school research associate at the University of Iowa, convened an ad hoc committee to consider the role of melancholia in the forthcoming

DSM-III-R, planned for 1987. Zimmerman and Spitzer found, in the microstudies that cluttered the literature, relatively little support for separating the two conditions. Zimmerman and Spitzer pooh-poohed the idea that melancholia was more responsive to the "somatic therapies," such as antidepressant drugs and ECT, than nonmelancholia. In an article on the committee's work published in 1989 they claimed, "No study of antidepressant medication or ECT has supported *DSM*-III's suggestion that 'melancholics are particularly responsive to somatic therapy'" (Zimmerman and Spitzer, 1989). This was simply flat-out wrong. Melancholia's differential responsiveness to ECT in particular was a matter of fact, and constituted one of the reasons for insisting that melancholia and nonmelancholia were two separate illnesses.

When queried about the statement of Zimmerman and Spitzer, Max Fink said

> Neither Spitzer nor Zimmerman are 'clinicians' (Zimmerman was a student at the time) and so do not have a personal experience that patients with the most flagrant forms of melancholia do remarkably well with ECT and very poorly with psychotherapy and medications. We did know that the more severely ill, retarded, hopeless and suicidal patients did not respond well to TCAs or MAOIs and that they required ECT. On the other hand, ECT was so powerful an antidepressant that depressed patients who were not severely melancholic also responded well to it. (Max Fink, personal communication, 2005)

Yet the statement of Zimmerman and Spitzer reverberated across the literature, reinforcing skepticism about the notion of the two depressions (melancholic vs. reactive). Of course if there was no such thing as melancholic depression, then a psychotic cousin of it did not exist either as a separate entity.

Antimelancholia: new treatment possibilities

The rapid growth of interest in psychotic depression boosted the revival of ECT that Max Fink, then at the State University of New York's Stony

Brook campus, led in the 1970s and after. Fink and co-workers definitively established the effectiveness of ECT in this disorder. (In one trial, 95% of their patients with psychotic depression experienced a remission, as opposed to 83% of patients with nonpsychotic depression; Petrides et al., 2001.) Simultaneously, growing awareness of delusional depression triggered interest in other drug treatments.

Lithium was popular in the nineteenth century for psychiatric illness. In 1871 William A. Hammond, physician-in-chief to the New York State Hospital for Diseases of the Nervous System, described its use in various forms of what they were then calling "mania," one of which was psychotic depression ("acute melancholia").[13]

After 1949 lithium experienced a rebirth when Australian psychiatrist John Cade wrote his pioneering article on its use in the treatment of mania (Cade, 1949). In 1970, lithium was licensed by the FDA for use in the United States. Because lithium can be used to maintain depressed and manic patients between episodes, there was naturally curiosity about it in psychotic depression as well. Workaday psychiatrists in many places began giving it to their delusional depressed patients because its success in mania had been well documented, and so many serious depressions could, with the eye of faith, be considered manic-depressive illness. In France, lithium was used routinely in the treatment of such cases, many of them patients with long-standing psychoses. At a symposium on lithium in Marseille in 1972, Jean Broussolle, who ran a public psychiatric ward in Dijon, commented in the middle of an animated discussion of lithium use,

> Since we're talking about our collective experience, I myself have a hospital ward that in effect has the honor of receiving those whom the others don't want, and my friends have a private clinic which has a very very wealthy clientele with chronic manic-depressive psychoses that are extremely serious. When we compare our results [with lithium], mine aren't as good,

13 William A. Hammond. 1871. *A treatise on diseases of the nervous system.* New York: Appleton, p. 381; on acute melancholia, see pp. 362–6.

but theirs are without doubt excellent and that goes also for those extremely serious cases where it's really been a permanent family catastrophe.[14]

In Britain, senior psychiatrists had for years used the "Newcastle cocktail" in chronic depression, consisting of the MAOI phenelzine (Parke-Davis's Nardil), the amino acid tryptophan, and lithium. As Scottish psychiatrist Donald Eccleston remembered of this cocktail from the early 1970s in Edinburgh,

> George [Ashcroft] and I became more and more interested in clinical problems and people were beginning to send us patients who had resisted treatment. Very frequently, the answer was simple – you started lithium and they got better. But George had read an article . . . that said a combination of phenelzine and tryptophan was as good as electroconvulsive therapy, so we began trying that combination, but found that while patients might have a marvelous 6 weeks, it faded. We got the idea that, if we added lithium, the response might be perpetuated. And that was how the Newcastle cocktail, really the Edinburgh cocktail, evolved.

Yet they had no control group to demonstrate efficacy beyond the slightest doubt (as though penicillin had needed a control group); no academic journal would accept their work, and they never published.[15] (Pharmacologically the Newcastle cocktail did not make total sense, given that the logical amino acid would have been L-DOPA or tyrosine, related to dopamine and norepinephrine, rather than tryptophan, related to serotonin. But in any event, the effective ingredient was probably the lithium.)

Then lithium broke into academia. In 1981 Claude De Montigny at the University of Montreal gave lithium to eight patients with "major unipolar depression" who had been unresponsive to TCAs. All eight of them "experienced a marked alleviation of their depressive symptoms" within 48 hours (De Montigny et al., 1981). The study caused

14 [Jean] Broussolle, in discussion. 1973. Psychopharmacology supplement. *L'Encéphale* 62: quote on p. 60.

15 Donald Eccleston, interview. The receptor enters psychiatry (2). In David Healy (ed.) *The Psychopharmacologists*, vol. 3, pp. 201–12, quote on p. 208.

considerable interest. The following year at St. Hans Hospital in Roskilde, Denmark, a team of trialists found that lithium combined with L-tryptophan tied amitriptyline in the treatment of "endogenous depression" (Honoré et al., 1982).

Meanwhile, Yale University had become a beehive of research in psychotic depression. In 1983 Lawrence Price and J. Craig Nelson tried systematically administering lithium to these patients. Aware that delusional psychotics did not do well on TCAs – and with De Montigny's experience in mind – they gave lithium to six delusional patients who had not responded to combined antipsychotic-antidepressant therapy. Ms. A., for example, 55, had come into the university psychiatric hospital for her sixth episode of psychotic depression. "She thought she had driven away her children and ruined their lives, that she had cancer of the jaw, and that she would never be able to function or enjoy herself again." She had failed numerous trials of combined antipsychotic-antidepressants. They decided to give her ECT but initiated lithium while they prepared her for it. Forty-eight hours later she was substantially improved, with a "Hamilton scale" depression score of 4 (practically well). Five days after that she was discharged from the hospital, "marking the first time she had ever had successful treatment without ECT" (Price et al., 1983). The several other cases were similarly impressive. (Nelson gets full marks for lithium here, but one bears in mind that he opposed ECT, an even more effective treatment.[16])

Finally, the combination of an antipsychotic and an antidepressant had a certain record of success in psychotic depression. The combination was a natural concept, of course, and industry had for years offered such combo pills. In 1966, for example, Schering began marketing Etrafon, a combination of the antidepressant amitriptyline and the antipsychotic perphenazine, "for the emotionally distressed patient." A year later, in

16 One of the authors (CS) recalls that Craig Nelson discontinued use of ECT on the inpatient wards of Yale, where he was inpatient director. When asked face to face about ECT, Nelson replied that they were always able to avoid using it.

1967, Merck brought out the same combo as "Triavil," a "tranquilizer-antidepressant." Triavil was widely popular and became known as "the Certs for depression." The street rap: "It's for neurosis. It's for melancholia. It's for psychotic depression!" At some point, psychiatrists routinely began prescribing these combinations, without much of a sense of doing something highly innovative. "Triavil was the one pill to use when you have no idea what you're doing," it was said.

Then in 1978 Craig Nelson at Yale put the academic seal of approval on these combos for psychotic depression. As an antipsychotic they used perphenazine and as an antidepressant either imipramine or amitriptyline (Nelson and Bowers, Jr., 1978). Also in 1978 Donald Sweeney, Craig Nelson, and other colleagues at Yale offered in the *Lancet* an academic rationale for this kind of coprescribing, noting that changes in dopamine and noradrenaline might be involved in psychotic depression, and that antipsychotics regulated the metabolism of dopamine, antidepressants that of noradrenaline (Sweeney et al., 1978). (Subsequently this kind of thinking became known as molecular mythology.)

Under David Kupfer, the psychiatry department of the University of Pittsburgh became a power house of psychopharmacology research, and it was from this department that, in 1985, a team led by Duane Spiker conducted a randomized trial of an antipsychotic-antidepressant combo (amitriptyline and perphenazine), versus the two drugs alone (no placebo arm). The combo was so much more effective than each of the drugs on its own – the authors talked about "synergy" – that this trial became embedded in the literature as the gold standard. Seventy-eight percent of the patients on the combo therapy responded, about equal, they said, to ECT (and they recommended that henceforth ECT be used only on combo nonresponders) (Spiker et al., 1985a).

Yet, in retrospect the two-drug combination has not been shown more effective in psychotic depression than antipsychotic drugs alone in patients who already failed to respond to TCAs alone. The disadvantage of the combination is that patients get the extensive side effects of two risky drugs.

The antipsychotic-antidepressant combo reached a provisional crescendo in February 2004 when Eli Lilly marketed Symbyax, a combo of the company's antidepressant fluoxetine (Prozac) and its antipsychotic olanzapine (Zyprexa) for psychotic depression (see Chapter 7). It was an on-patent reincarnation of Triavil, yet painfully irrational because Prozac is not an antimelancholic agent and has no business being given to melancholics, catatonics, or psychotics. Worse, Prozac raises Zyprexa levels by about 50 percent, and the combination can cause a depressive-like syndrome of severe apathy (Nelson and Swartz, 2000).

There is an apparent basic inconsistency in administering a dopamine-blocking medication to patients who show impoverished thought content, akinesia, and motor retardation. Specifically, these are signs of Parkinson's disease, and they correspond to gross deficiency of dopamine in the basal ganglia. In contrast, the signs of too much dopamine include excessive and choreiform movements, hyperreactivity, and hypertalkativeness. Giving dopamine-blocking antipsychotic drugs to patients with psychotic melancholia seems to be as incomprehensible as infusing glucose into diabetic patients with hyperosmolar coma. That the antipsychotic drugs diminish the symptoms, sometimes substantially, is not logically attributable to dopamine blockade itself. Rather, it can be explained only by the thought simplification and the gross tranquilization provided by these drugs. This is not specific treatment but chemical restraint, obstruction of ordinary brain function, and obscuration of continuing active illness. It resembles covering a severe skin eruption only with skin anesthetics and cosmetics; underneath, the rash is still there, hopefully healing on its own but actually untreated.

Today, the distance created by 50 years of psychopharmacology is palpable. For a population shy of ECT, the treatment of psychotic depression has come to depend on drugs, and in these 50 years of drug therapy, treatment has come a long way. In 1958 Kuhn, who had discovered the clinical effectiveness of imipramine in depression the previous year, was invited to the annual congress of the APA in

San Francisco. Kuhn was a very austere, silent man. In San Francisco he found a somewhat hypomanic Nathan Kline, who had just come upon the psychiatric use of iproniazid (Marsilid), "strutting around," giving interviews to the press. "Kline told them that the Russians with their Sputnik were way ahead of the Americans in the Arms Race. Now it was important that America should get ahead of the Russians and they could only do it by increasing the psychic abilities of the American researchers. So he said that everybody should take Marsilid, in order to help with their psychic powers."

When Kuhn had announced his own discovery at a psychiatry congress in Zurich the previous year, there had been only a few people in the audience. There were no questions afterwards.

Kuhn was asked why the level of interest was so low.

"Because nobody believed that there could be a drug against depression," Kuhn said.[17] Several decades later, the terrible illness of psychotic depression is indeed being successfully treated with drugs.

17 Roland Kuhn, interview. From imipramine to levoprotiline: The discovery of antidepressants. In Healy (ed.) *The Psychopharmacologists*, vol. 2, pp. 93–119, quote on pp. 105–6.

6

Treatment: Pitfalls and Pathways

BEFORE THE ADVENT OF ANTIDEPRESSANT DRUGS AND ECT, patients with depression generally recovered spontaneously, excepting those with psychotic depression who often suffered chronically (Kantor and Glassman, 1977). This historical perspective continues to direct our concern about the fate of patients with undertreated psychotic depression.

With prompt treatment psychotic depression should generally remit, becoming an episode with a beginning and an end. In between episodes the patient should be able to pursue work, creative endeavors, and pleasure without impairment. Yet, many patients do not recover fully, and the alternative outcomes range from misery to disability, entailing years of quiet impairment. Delay in providing effective treatment risks the emergence of PTSD from the stigmatizing, debilitating, and often life-threatening experiences of psychotic depression, psychiatric confinement, tranquilizing drugs, and the reactions of others to the patient's vicissitudes. Moreover, PTSD itself is agonizing, impairing, and decidedly chronic. If psychotic depression is undertreated, one risks the chronicization of psychotic symptoms. Yet whether the cause is chronicization or PTSD, the longer the period between the onset of the first psychotic symptom and the treatment the worse the outcome, regardless of the actual diagnosis (Marshall et al., 2005).

Treatment of psychotic depression should match the exact type of the illness, as detailed in the diagnosis section (Chapter 8). Unfortunately, the literature on this subject has not considered the types of psychotic depression. Moreover, the descriptions of patients in reported studies are often not detailed enough to identify the type of psychotic depression involved. It is rare that treatment studies provide details of psychopathology beyond diagnosis itself. A few reports describe severe psychomotor slowing (e.g., Parker et al., 1997), a core sign of melancholia. However, these reports did not mention evaluation for catatonia, which also includes profound slowing. It is reasonable to expect many patients with melancholic and catatonic features in studies of psychotic depression. Yet, such a mixture confounds the results because melancholia often responds to TCAs or bupropion, and catatonia virtually never does. Moreover, the literature has not separated management from treatment.

Accordingly, studies of the treatment of psychotic depression blur together the types. Here, we shall try to interpret information on treatment outcome, however flawed or speculative, for the benefit of our patients. We will keep the shortcomings and the implications of previous writing on this subject in close view.

Generalizing from the prevalences we observe, in treatment studies of psychotic depression, about a third of patients each should have the melancholic type, the psychosis-dominant type, and the catatonic type, with other types less common. Although several studies have described a high incidence of melancholic symptoms in psychotic depression (e.g., Parker et al., 1997), the poverty of thought and psychomotor slowing of catatonic depression would overlap with and confound any rating of melancholic symptoms. Including patients with catatonic depression in studies of psychotic depression should explain much of the apparently lower medication effectiveness in psychotic than nonpsychotic depression. Few patients entering published treatment studies of psychotic depression were already taking antipsychotic drugs; accordingly, few should have had tardive-type psychotic depression.

Treatments of psychotic depression overlap substantially with treatments of nonpsychotic depression and other psychotic disorders, and sometimes even with anxiety disorders. This overlap occurs because there is an imperfect match between nonspecific psychopathology on the one hand and biogenic psychiatric illness on the other – especially when psychopathology involves subjective symptoms. Anxiety disorders can include the subjective symptoms of psychosis, and vice versa. According to *DSM* criteria, diagnosis is primarily according to subjective symptoms. As a result there are mismatches. For example, some instances of what is actually anxiety disorder meet the *DSM* criteria for psychotic depression. The simple and ordinary approach is to overlook such misfits as nonresponders; however, this approach puts *DSM* ahead of patients. The patient-centered approach is to describe how well actual patients match – and do not match – the diagnostic criteria. This means evaluating and treating patients according to their complexities, not merely by the simplifications and subjectivities of *DSM*. This is our philosophy of treatment according to diagnosis subtype.

The benchmark for success in long-term treatment of psychotic depression seems ready to be set rather low. Of thirty-two patients located 8 years after discharge from treatment for psychotic depression at a rural major university hospital, the University of Iowa, only 44 percent were free from psychosis (Tsuang and Coryell, 1993). While this is far better than the zero percent of patients with schizophrenia who remained free of psychosis, it leaves enormous room for improvement.

Different treatment philosophies produce different outcomes; for example, readiness to use ECT. That particular university hospital receives resistant patients, ECT patients, and uninsured patients referred by psychiatrists around the state. After being discharged from the hospital, most patients were probably treated at mental health centers where ECT is not locally available. Yet, at the university hospital at Iowa, clinicians did administer ECT. Scored 6 months after hospital discharge, patients with unipolar psychotic depression were more frequently back to their normal selves than patients with nonpsychotic major depression (Coryell et al., 1986). Presumably these psychotic depressives had more frequently received ECT. The apparent explanation of widely varying outcomes such as these is that the outcome of treating psychotic depression depends strongly on physician practice philosophy and availability of treatment resources.

Treatment versus management

For the sake of discussion, we could say that one way to terminate all hallucinations, delusions, insomnia, and complaints of low mood and loss of interest would be to anesthetize the patient to unconsciousness. Depression scores such as the Hamilton Depression (HAM-D) rating would show a large reduction. Yet this would be symptom management, not treatment, scarcely a desirable or sensitive form of practice. More feasible than complete anesthesia are drugs that only partly inhibit the brain from operating and superficially appear to leave the patient conscious. This is tranquilization. Physiologically, benzodiazepine and barbiturate tranquilizers are called "depressants" because they diminish brain functions. In low to moderate doses they inhibit learning, recall, coordination, awareness of complexity, problem solving, willpower, and attention. In larger doses they are general anesthetics and can cause unconsciousness; in overdose, diazepam can produce unconsciousness for several days.

Antipsychotic tranquilizers inhibit the functioning of only some parts of the brain: those related to new thoughts, novel problem solving, social complexity, initiative, and motivation. These functions are housed in the prefrontal section of the brain. This sounds like a small fraction of the brain but in humans the prefrontal region is almost half the brain cortex. Its functions represent the essential differences in psychological performance between humans and animals, and also between human adults and children. Antipsychotic drugs suppress these differences by inhibiting prefrontal cortex function or neural outflow from the prefrontal cortex (Swartz, 2003a; 2003b).

The deficits in psychological performance caused by antipsychotic drugs mentioned here occur similarly in patients with Parkinson's disease. Parkinson's disease essentially represents what happens physically and psychologically when certain crucial dopaminergic brain cells are lost, cells located in the deep brain region called the pars compacta of the substantia nigra. Both with antipsychotic drugs and Parkinson's disease, the function of dopaminergic brain cells is deficient. Patients who take antipsychotic drugs often show the same physical signs as patients with Parkinson's disease because of this dopamine deficiency, including muscle rigidity, tremor, tendency to fall, and akinesia (generally decreased movements). Both groups also show impairments in problem-solving abilities, planning, initiative taking, and dealing with complexity (Bassett, 2005). These are called "executive" cognitive functions and are generally associated with the dorsolateral prefrontal cortex.

The behavioral results of this removal of participation in thinking by the prefrontal cortex vary with the particular antipsychotic drug. Dopamine-blocking antipsychotic drugs, such as haloperidol, perphenazine, and risperidone, decrease motivation to speak, together with lessening complexity and amount of thought. Some of the more recently introduced antipsychotics (e.g., olanzapine, clozapine, quetiapine) decrease thought complexity more than motivation to speak, and because the patient speaks abundantly the thought simplicity is easier to notice. Decreases in self-discipline and organization contribute to the weight gain patients experience from olanzapine, clozapine, and quetiapine. Olanzapine and clozapine also obstruct the function of the medial prefrontal cortex, which causes apathy, somnolence, and generalized weakness (Nelson and Swartz, 2000). Anesthetizing brain function is surely a last resort. It is management, not treatment.

The goals of treating and managing are also different. Treatment aims for remission of symptoms and return of the patient to preillness function and abilities. Management aims to stop complaints and behavior that causes complaints. Treating requires diagnosing the disease that causes the problematic behavior and acting against this disease. Managing focuses on diminishing symptoms such as problem behaviors and complaints; an accurate and specific diagnosis is not needed. These distinctions are important in treating psychotic depression because treatments and managements alike are available, commonly used, and mistaken for each other.

Nevertheless, when treatment is not available or not tolerated by the patient, or unsuccessful, thoughtful management is important to relieve suffering. This applies to the relief of psychotic depression symptoms just as to relief of pain from joint deterioration or cancer. Surely, management is better than nothing, but let us avoid mistaking management for treatment. In some instances, time is the healer, and treating psychopathology with temporary tranquilizers to buy time will produce a good result in several months, if the tranquilizer is indeed eventually tapered out.

Even an express tour through the psychiatric literature reveals that virtually anything is claimed to help depression. As a sampling there are exercise, acupuncture, pet therapy, computer use, aromatherapy, chocolate, group therapy, talk therapy, art therapy, dance therapy, bright light, sleep deprivation, herbs such as St. Johns Wort, natural amino acids such as S-adenosyl methionine (SAMe), natural sugars such as inositol, natural fats such as omega-3 oils, natural androgenic steroids such as DHEA and testosterone, SSRIs such as fluoxetine (Prozac), tricyclics such as imipramine (Tofranil), antipsychotic drugs, amphetamines which are the opposite of antipsychotics, benzodiazepines, lithium, ECT, vagal nerve electrode implantation and stimulation, magnetic brain stimulation, deep brain electrode implantation and stimulation, brain surgery (e.g., cingulotomy), and even placebo, which for a biological illness means the passage of time. Some people find that list making improves mood. Combination therapies use two or more treatments together, and the number of possible combinations is unruly.

This broad range of treatments is made possible by nonspecificity – indeed formlessness – in diagnosing depression. Some treatments noted earlier equal placebo and most equal placebo when treating psychotic depression. Psychotic depression simply does not respond to placebo. It is improper to prescribe talk therapy, chocolate, or placebo as primary treatment for pneumonia, and likewise for psychotic depression. It is not appropriate to treat psychotic depression as if it were not psychotic, or not depressive, or if it were two separate conditions of psychosis and depression.

A good and prompt result is essential, so we will consider what this means and how to get it. Remission, which means full restoration, is the routine good result of treating psychotic depression. Remission, of course, avoids injury to self or others as well as suicide; it also averts lingering impairment from treatment or remaining illness. Three months to achieve remission is good timeliness, four months is fair, and more than that is slow. Two months is very good, and one month is excellent. These are realistic goals and, as always, excellent is what everybody wants most.

In other words, remission is resumption of the patient's abilities and performance at preillness levels. Understanding the meaning of "without impairment" requires recognizing what can be impaired and how. Unfortunately, descriptions of the psychological impairments caused by antipsychotic tranquilizers and benzodiazepines are omitted or glossed over by textbooks of psychiatry and by other information provided to physicians, such as the Physicians' Desk Reference (PDR).

Common pitfalls in studying treatment

The concepts and plans in this book are related to the results of studies. However, obtaining data is one thing and interpreting it properly is another, as stock market investors can attest. This means that we must identify the strengths and weaknesses in the study methods to understand the implications of the results. Weaknesses in method produce misleading results, and there are several common weaknesses in studies of psychotic depression. Understanding the results of the study requires knowing the weaknesses along with the results themselves.

Treatment of psychotic depression requires proper diagnosis, made on the basis of evidence. In psychiatry, evidence is no less useful and valid than in a courtroom. Evidence might be incomplete or imperfect, but professionalism demands that the available evidence be identified and accounted for. This involves systematic collection of evidence, its inventory, and assessment of its quality and specificity.

In contrast, the primary purpose of the *DSM* is to serve the needs of psychiatrists in making a living, that is, for reimbursement. *DSM* makes diagnosis easy to assign by making evidence optional and omitting any standard for evidence. Someone's subjective opinion can substitute for any evidence. This is emphatically true for the diagnoses of mood disorders such as depression, and indeed psychotic depression. A commonly printed and spoken rationalization for the *DSM* is that it is better than the alternative. The implied alternative is that psychiatry fails as a profession. This oversimplistic rationalization coerces conformity to the criteria of *DSM*.

There are high stakes here. What most psychiatrists do overall is worthwhile, and it is proper and important that the profession and business of psychiatry succeed. But the suitability of *DSM* for psychiatry's business needs has nothing to do with its scientific validity, as shown by the Manual's elective use – and frequent disregard – of available evidence. The *DSM* is thoroughly unsuitable for scientific work, impartial study, evidence gathering, or evidence-based clinical practice. Sadly, studies of psychotic depression where diagnosis was made according to *DSM* without further detail can have little evidence-based or scientific meaning. These studies cannot and should not bind us in clinical practice, although they might give us some impressions and expectations that turn out clinically useful.

The veracity of the diagnosis is only the deepest of many pitfalls in studies of psychotic depression. A related problem is that the types of psychotic depression included in a study make a huge difference. Simply, the relative number of patients with each type strongly affects the outcome. Because studies of psychotic depression have not separated them with reference to type, there is no clear interpretation of the results.

Finally, some studies of psychotic depression have silently toppled into statistical pitfalls and have become traps themselves. The sample size might be too small (in statistical terminology, "underpowered") to detect a difference that actually exists. Published results are often statistically significant but not large enough to be clinically significant, especially when the sample size is very large. Commonly, Pearson's *r* ("product-moment" correlation coefficient) is used on data that includes outliers, which is not proper. But this is not a statistics textbook. Interested readers will want to know merely that the pits are there for the unwary.

Unaccounted drug effects

The types of psychotic depression have greatly different responses to specific medications. One problem is the presence of undiagnosed catatonia patients. Catatonia but not melancholia is usually temporarily mitigated by benzodiazepines, sometimes markedly. Even 2 mg/day lorazepam can have a large effect on some catatonic patients. If, in a study, you give undiagnosed catatonics benzodiazepines alongside the treatment drug, the patient will respond well. The problem is that benzodiazepines are commonly given to patients taking part in depression studies to calm uncomfortable tension or insomnia. With drugs like lorazepam, patients are less irritable and more cooperative, and so less likely to withdraw consent to undergo the study. This same consideration applies when restless tension (akathisia) or insomnia is caused by the study drugs themselves, as many SSRIs and antipsychotic drugs do. When patients with catatonic psychotic depression are included in a study of psychotic depression, the use of benzodiazepines in all treatment groups will raise the apparent effectiveness of the study drug across the board. Unless the investigators have expressly excluded patients with catatonic features, the presence of catatonia may be counted on because catatonia is present in a large fraction of patients with psychotic depression. Essentially, no reports of studies of psychotic depression mention efforts to identify catatonia, account for its effects, or exclude it; this is a major shortcoming.

While benzodiazepines can covertly diminish catatonia-related symptoms in some patients, they often cause delirium in elderly patients. Accordingly, in studies that include elderly patients, benzodiazepines can decrease treatment effectiveness. Whenever benzodiazepines are given in studies of psychotic, melancholic, or catatonic depression, assessing and accounting for their effects is a basic necessity, and yet rarely done.

Another problem is with regard to antipsychotic tranquilizers (i.e., "antipsychotics") in studies. These drugs have many effects on patients with psychotic depression besides possible improvement in depression or psychosis. Antipsychotics can exacerbate catatonia, sometimes suddenly and severely, producing a clinical picture similar to neuroleptic malignant syndrome. Yet, in other patients antipsychotic drugs lessen catatonia, even in the absence of hallucinations or delusions. We cannot predict which patients will improve on antipsychotics and which will worsen. It is a troubling gamble we cannot recommend because of the Hippocratic promise to "above all do no harm."

The common antipsychotic drugs olanzapine and clozapine induce apathy that some psychiatrists mistake for melancholia (Swartz, 2002). Other antipsychotic drugs often cause restlessness (called akathisia), provoking patients to pace or show other signs of agitation and thereby appear worse. Elderly patients are at high risk for rigidity, akinesia (loss of spontaneous movement), and other extrapyramidal symptoms from antipsychotics. These extrapyramidal symptoms can be mistaken for melancholic major depression because they involve motor retardation, impoverished thought and speech, and general slowing. All these side effects can confound ratings of depression, as used in studies of depression.

A key idea about the effect of antipsychotic drugs in tardive psychosis is that tardive psychosis is caused by antipsychotic drugs (Swartz, 1995). Continuing the antipsychotic drug makes it gradually worse, even if it controls the condition acutely. A core symptom of tardive psychosis is that patients are extremely sensitive to small adjustments in dose. A small increase in a large dose brings a huge improvement. A small decrease brings a huge worsening. Cutting it out altogether and giving lithium, or perhaps carvedilol, can bring remission (see Chapter 8). The picture resembles giving alcohol to an alcoholic who has the shakes. It will calm him down, but fundamentally it was the cause of his sickness, and if he continues drinking it will make everything worse. Giving alcohol calms the patient. Cutting the daily alcohol dose down makes him more tremulous and nervous. Cutting out alcohol altogether and treating the associated nutritional deficiencies and health problems can bring remission.

Analogies between tardive psychosis and alcohol withdrawal are infrequent in the literature. The analogy is startling and disturbing in its fidelity: Alcohol withdrawal syndrome does not occur in young alcoholics regardless of how much they drink. They can drink a gallon of hard liquor a day for a year and then stop suddenly, and typically have no withdrawal symptoms. Only the long-term alcoholics experience symptoms of alcohol withdrawal, and only the longest and most severe of these have delirium tremens (DTs). Tardive psychosis is just as real and palpable as alcohol dependence and withdrawal; it is antipsychotic dependence and withdrawal. Alcoholics behave as if withdrawal and DTs will not happen to them, as they continue to take alcohol. Just as patients with substantial alcohol intake cannot properly be included in studies of psychotic depression (except alcohol-related studies), neither can patients with substantial antipsychotic drug intake for longer than about 4 months, which is about how soon tardive psychosis can start developing. Accordingly, patients with possible tardive psychosis should not be grouped together with other patients in treatment studies (as in Margolese et al., 2002).

The simplest mechanism of the peculiar dose relationship between antipsychotics and tardive psychosis is explained in terms of neurotransmitter receptors and the principle of homeostasis. Homeostasis means that the body tries to maintain its ordinary balance of processes, and that attempts to change body processes are resisted by the body. Giving a dopamine blocker (such as haloperidol) causes the body to try to compensate for the lack of dopamine effects, that is, to overcome the dopamine block. The dopamine receptors become hypersensitive to dopamine, and they increase in number. As time goes by, higher doses of haloperidol are needed to block the dopamine receptors because there are more of them and they are more sensitive. (This is called "upregulation.") In this situation small gradual increases in haloperidol will block the growing dopamine "supersensitivity," and small increases in dose can bring large decreases in symptoms. Conversely, with supersensitivity present, small decreases in the dose of haloperidol can lead to severe worsening. The simplest explanation of tardive psychosis is as "dopamine supersensitivity psychosis" (Chouinard and Steinberg, 1984).

This simplest mechanism is not complete. It does not explain some accompanying irreversible effects, such as tardive dyskinesia and tardive psychosis that persist despite high doses of antipsychotic drugs or discontinuation of the antipsychotic drugs. These effects presumably involve the neurons that change in response to absence of dopaminergic neurotransmission. Generally, irreversible neurological changes such as tardive dyskinesia correspond to brain deterioration, and long-standing blockade of dopamine receptors in the basal ganglia kills neurons within them (Naidu and Kulkarni, 2001; Andreassen et al., 2003). This brain deterioration further resembles alcohol dependency. These changes are an end-run around the dopamine blocker–dopamine receptor standoff. The patient becomes psychotic despite the dopamine-blocking antipsychotic drug – and because of it. The only way to stop losing this game is to stop playing it, that is, to stop the "antipsychotic" drug. Again, this is analogous to symptoms of alcohol dependency and alcohol-induced brain deterioration; the only way out is to stop alcohol.

How about anxiety? A severe artifact in depression studies is that anxiety symptoms are calmed by drugs that do not treat depression. But as the anxiety improves, it appears that the drugs are acting as "antidepressants." One must be on guard for this. Specifically, sympatholytic antipsychotic drugs such as thioridazine and olanzapine cut somatic tension anxiety symptoms; as well, antipsychotic drugs with serotonin-1 agonism such as ziprasidone diminish worry. At least one-third of patients with psychotic depression have a concurrent anxiety disorder. The longer and more intensely that patients suffer from serious depression, bipolar disorder, or medical illnesses, the more severe the anxiety disorder.

Anxiety can also make the depression appear worse. As with any psychiatric disorder, anxiety disorders make patients unhappy, and unhappiness raises scores on depression rating scales such as the HAM-D and Montgomery-Asberg (MADRS). Somatic tension anxiety symptoms such as agitation, hyperreactivity, irritability, threatening behavior, strident voice, and rapid speech are generally calmed by some antipsychotic drugs (e.g., quetiapine, thioridazine, ziprasidone) and are largely unaffected by low to medium doses of others (e.g., perphenazine, loxapine, haloperidol) if not worsened.

The bottom line is that psychological anxiety symptoms such as dissatisfaction, worry, and obsessions are decreased by antipsychotic drugs that activate the serotonin-1A receptor, such as ziprasidone. Such drug-induced changes in symptoms of concurrent anxiety disorders profoundly influence depression rating scale results.

This antianxiety effect of antipsychotics is so intense that it accounts for much of the usefulness of antipsychotic drugs. In other words, most antipsychotic drug use is for conditions that are not psychotic (Weiss et al., 2000; Glick et al., 2001); they are being used to tranquilize anxiety. Moreover, drug companies have been seeking FDA approval for antipsychotic drug use in conditions that are not psychotic, specifically depression. The Eli Lilly Company received approval to use the antipsychotic olanzapine (in "Symbyax") for depression that is not psychotic. Numerous medical publications claim antipsychotic drugs work in nonpsychotic depression anxiety disorders and other conditions (e.g., Calabrese et al., 2005).

You might suppose that an antipsychotic that decreases anxiety is better than one that does not, but these drugs are not appropriate for treating anxiety disorders or depression except as a truly last resort. This is because these drugs are noxious when taken long term. Unfortunately study publications usually emphasize the desirable results and understate the undesirable effects. There is a "conflict of interest" built into the system that encourages physician-investigators to seek and emphasize positive findings and overlook quiet undesirable effects. Success of the treatment paves the career path, especially when the success can be stated in a simple and straightforward manner. Imagine a study that compares a TCA against the combination of this same antidepressant given with an antipsychotic drug. Patients in the combination group might well show more improvement on depression ratings because the antipsychotic decreased anxiety symptoms. Anxiety disorder and psychotic depression must be specifically assessed and rated separately from each other. However, this has never been done. Rather, the opposite has been embraced, that is, concurrent anxiety disorder is overlooked and all psychopathology is simplistically attributed to psychotic depression.

Overall, identifying the antidepressant effects of antipsychotic drugs in depressed patients requires systematic impartial assessments for anxiety disorders, catatonia, apathy, extrapyramidal symptoms, and tardive psychosis. Of these, only extrapyramidal symptoms have been assessed.

Rating scale shortcomings

Another crucial problem is distinguishing between relieving depression symptoms and recovering from depression. Unfortunately, depression rating scales do not make this distinction. The most common scales are the HAM-D and the MADRS. These scales were never intended to be sensitive to the presence of depression, only to the severity of symptoms that occur in depression. Even when high ratings occur on these scales, they do not indicate the existence of depression – the scales are just not specific. Patients with borderline personality disorder, alcohol or abusive substance withdrawal, PTSD, or GAD typically have high ratings on these scales from these conditions themselves. Depression rating scales are appropriate only when there is a separate determination that major depression is present.

There are two opposite types of problems with depression rating scales, and both are common. First, depression can remit while the rating stays high, and second, depression can continue while the rating drops.

These problems with depression rating scales are analogous to temperature in patients treated for pneumonia. First, let us suppose a patient with pneumonia and a 104°F fever. With treatment the temperature drops to 99°F. The patient is improved, but is the pneumonia gone? Not necessarily; the bacteria might be evolving for a comeback. What if the temperature drops to 100.5°F but the patient has a concurrent condition that can cause fever, such as leukemia or chronic malaria? The pneumonia might be gone, but the judgment of how well the antibiotic worked depends on the physician's examination of diagnostic signs, not the temperature.

This translates strongly to the interpretation of HAM-D and MADRS depression rating scales in patients who were depressed. This is because anxiety disorders by themselves raise HAM-D and MADRS ratings. A patient's HAM-D might fall from 30 before treatment to 14 on treatment. This is analogous to a fever of 100.5°F. The temperature has not regained normality, but you should be able to take care of your daily needs outside a hospital.

On the opposite side of the coin, if aspirin were given to the patient the fever might disappear although the bacteria continue to flourish. Without fever, the patient usually looks better and feels better. The response to aspirin is misleading. If the patient were taking both an antibiotic and aspirin, attributing loss of fever to the antibiotic is not proper without additional examination. An afebrile patient might go home with aspirin and an ineffective antibiotic and die quietly and peacefully in his sleep. Despite peace of mind, his illness was not appropriately treated.

Tranquilizing drugs are psychiatry's aspirin. They leave patients calm and quiet so they do not feel like complaining. While taking tranquilizers the thought processes of patients become simpler, new thoughts become rare, and complex thoughts are diminished. Patients lose abilities and skills, and they are not upset by this loss. Indeed, they are usually not even concerned or aware of the loss. This should be no surprise because this is what tranquilization means. Giving tranquilizing drugs makes psychiatric symptoms of all types decrease, as aspirin does to a fever. Let us not believe or pretend that tranquilizers cure psychotic depression. The depressive illness and its risks remain.

Look, for example, at the problem of treating mania with antipsychotics. For many years, the standard of efficacy in the treatment of a manic episode (i.e., mania) was chlorpromazine (Thorazine). But wait: Lithium is famously effective for treating mania. The puzzling aspect of lithium treatment was that, although lithium's reputation is well deserved, mania severity ratings of patients treated with lithium show scores no lower than for patients treated with chlorpromazine. Yet, virtually no manic patients treated with chlorpromazine are well, they are all still somewhat manic. Even when the hyperactivity of mania fades, its thought disorder continues, with grandiosity, distractibility, delusions, or paranoia. But now the patient can hide it from a superficial inquiry. Moreover, reasoning and problem-solving abilities are impaired by the tranquilizing effects of chlorpromazine. This is not necessarily true of lithium.

The same considerations apply to psychotic depression. Antipsychotic tranquilizers make the patients somewhat better without really curing them – and drag a boat load of disadvantages in their wake. To illustrate, one group of sixteen depressed patients receiving the antipsychotic tranquilizer perphenazine (64 mg/day) included two patients who plainly remained delusional although their HAM-D ratings fell to "normal" scores of 7 and 4.5 (Spiker et al., 1985b). This is a serious and dangerous shortcoming and it understates the problem of less obvious thought disorders remaining with antipsychotic drugs. It indicates that the effectiveness of antipsychotic drugs in psychotic depression is overstated by the HAM-D scale and similar scales such as the MADRS. In a retrospective study, seven of ten patients receiving haloperidol and amitriptyline for psychotic depression were rated as responders, but all ten continued to experience at least mild psychotic depression – there was no remission (Grunze et al., 2002).

Moreover, these depression rating scales fail to examine for the adverse cognitive, behavioral, and problem-solving psychological effects of antipsychotic tranquilizers. This is analogous to looking only at the temperatures of patients with pneumonia in order to rate treatment outcome.

These problems are relatively basic. Their resolution should be straightforward. Diagnostic evidence must be systematically gathered and accounted for. Concurrent psychiatric illnesses including anxiety disorders must be diagnosed and accounted for before and after treatment. The presence of psychotic depression and its subtypes must be examined for before and after treatment regardless of any rating scale results. The extent of side effects from benzodiazepines and antipsychotic drugs must be measured. Any shortcutting of these procedures obscures data interpretation and facilitates unjustified conclusions and clinical recommendations – it makes the study misleading. Unfortunately, these are not done and the associated shortcomings have not been discussed by the research study reports.

Then there is the question of placebo responsiveness, which does not exist in psychotic depression. If you were a drugmaker, you could not get your psychiatric drug approved by the U.S. FDA without including a study of a placebo comparison group, called a control group. When a placebo group is included, its outcome can help us interpret the sensitivity of the study. Yet, in some treatment studies it may be legitimate to omit placebo controls because some psychiatric diseases are so distinctly observable and unresponsive to placebo that placebo control is not always needed. Psychotic depression is one of these.

Both acute euphoric mania and psychotic depression are severe conditions with low spontaneous remission rates (i.e., when untreated). It would be unusual in a study of psychotic depression for placebo patients to show a remission rate substantially above 2.5 percent per week of study. If the placebo response was higher than this, what was studied was probably not psychotic depression. This is because average episode duration is about 9 months after diagnosis; accordingly, the rate of spontaneous remission is about 2.5 percent per week after entry into the study. This rate is a benchmark to interpret study results against. This is mathematical logic. The whole placebo question is a distraction in treatment studies of psychotic depression.

Then there is the issue of misdiagnosis in treatment studies. Studies tell us that the SSRIs do not perform well in the treatment of psychotic depression. Even in treating anxiety disorders and atypical major depression, well-designed placebo-controlled studies indicate that SSRIs have a remission rate only minimally higher than placebo. Of course, studies that do not reach that minimum are not published, which means that the published literature does not provide a balanced picture. In patients who have major depression without psychotic, melancholic, or catatonic symptoms, about 25 percent respond to placebo in 6 weeks, while 35 percent respond to an SSRI (e.g., Schneider et al., 2003). Any

SSRI study with response rates much higher than this (and there are several, all from Milan, Italy, e.g., Zanardi et al., 2000) was studying something other than depression, and surely not psychotic depression.

Giving ECT while stopping medications will have a strong effect on all types of psychotic depression. ECT reliably treats melancholia, catatonia, mixed manic-depressive episode, and acute psychoses other types. There will be other benefits from ECT treatment as well. ECT is anticonvulsant and should diminish seizure effects. Likewise, in tardive psychosis or drug-dependent psychosis, ECT should buy time while the adverse effects of drug and drug discontinuation wear off. In other words, ECT provides a temporary antipsychotic effect while drug-induced psychosis and drug-discontinuation-induced psychosis diminish. Besides these effects, in many patients, ECT also has a temporary antianxiety or euphoric action, and patients with anxiety disorder and or pseudopsychosis will tell of feeling calmer and happier for a few weeks. Still, ECT has no clear record of persisting benefit for anxiety disorders and our recommendations for its use are elsewhere.

Places for treatment and ECT

This topic is important because in the United States many people with psychotic depression receive evaluation and treatment at state hospitals, public mental health centers, or clinics for the uninsured or indigent. For proper treatment, all patients with psychotic depression need to be treated at facilities where all effective and safe treatments are available. Sometimes when a treatment is not available at a facility, the staff will routinely discourage if not disparage that treatment. Discouragement might be primarily passive, that is, by ignoring it. Surely, some treatments that are not widely available do not seem reasonably effective for psychotic depression, such as vagal nerve stimulation (VNS) and transcranial magnetic stimulation (TMS). Psychotherapy by itself is also inappropriate. However, modern ECT is safe and particularly effective, but available in only a minority of facilities. Very few state hospitals provide ECT. Some hospitals that do not provide ECT claim to arrange it when needed at other hospitals, and transfer patients accordingly. Yet they arrange for ECT only so rarely that their claim of providing it when appropriate is deceptive. When they say appropriate they mean unavoidable.

As shown by several generations of official APA Task Force reports, no controversy remains about ECT's acute efficacy and general safety. There is no room for doubt about the restorative effects of ECT as patients with painfully obvious debilitation from psychotic depression routinely return to appearing normal within a few days. ECT has been in wide use for over 60 years around the United States and the world. Nearly all patients who receive ECT are white, middle class, and insured (Kramer, 1999). African American patients are more likely than Causasians to be diagnosed as having schizophrenia instead of psychotic depression, and clinician deviation from DSM criteria contributes to this (Strakowski et al., 1996). Timely delivery of ECT treatment to suitable patients is good psychiatric practice, regardless of race or ethnic group.

Lack of ECT availability in state hospitals has political causes. From about 1945 until 1952, ECT was widely provided at state hospitals, but both the method and patient selection were crude. Before the first antipsychotic tranquilizer chlorpromazine (Thorazine) was commercially introduced in 1954, ECT was the best means of calming dangerously agitated psychotic patients, regardless of diagnosis. Although no anesthesia was used, ECT was safe and effective, much more so than the alternatives. (Also, ECT is not painful; the patient is instantly unconscious. Anesthesia is used only to remove the worrisome awareness of paralysis by succinylcholine. Anesthesia is not needed for ECT itself.) ECT is still used primarily without anesthesia in Russia and most Asian countries. Surely ECT receives low priority within U.S. state hospital systems because administrators are simply not familiar with ECT – they were hired on the basis of management experience. Because of politics, the tenure of a physician administrator and team averages under 2 years; this instability hinders development of ECT services. An ECT program can be cheaply deconstructed but rebuilding it takes time and work – and who will do it?

In the face of obstructions, state hospital psychiatrists become acclimated to the practical unavailability of ECT and eventually stop considering it. A system of transferring ECT patients elsewhere for treatment and inpatient care gives a tacit suggestion of clinical failure with every transfer, with lower stature and morale. Of course, this inhibits ECT use.

Financially speaking, ECT costs are typically less for a patient than a couple of days in the hospital, and are paid by fee-for-service insurance, Medicare, and Medicaid. ECT costs are also less than a few months' supply of patented antipsychotic tranquilizers, such as Zyprexa, Symbyax, and Risperdal. Moreover, in treating psychotic depression, prompt ECT use reduces hospital stay and hospital costs to well below those accompanying medication use (Markowitz et al., 1987; Olfson et al., 1998). Even if there were no reimbursement, ECT operations should cost less than 0.1 percent of hospital operation, so that is not a real reason for state hospitals not giving ECT. It is not clear how proper psychiatric evaluation or treatment can be provided in state hospitals when ECT is difficult to obtain and usual patient handling is tranquilization. Between state hospitals where ECT is not given, and hospitals where ECT is available, there are two sharply different standards of care.

If the hospital administrator says his hospital is not able to administer ECT safely, that hospital is probably not able to reliably provide safe and effective treatment for seriously ill patients through any means. Patients in state hospitals are commonly exposed to harmful experiences (Frueh et al., 2005). About twelve patient deaths occur yearly in U.S. hospitals from involuntary restraints (Masters and Wandless, 2005). If a patient with psychotic depression is in restraints for more than a few hours during the first day or two, medications are not adequate and ECT should be urgently considered.

When ECT is discussed, administrators of state hospitals might claim uncomfortable feelings on the subject. In doing so they imply that their impressions are more valid than data about ECT effectiveness. This makes the decision personal, not professional. To improve ECT resources, the psychiatrist has to change the personal opinions of state hospital administrators and perhaps government officials. Changing personal opinions is a challenge. It can involve overcoming biases against biological psychiatry and ECT propagated by people looking to sell movies, books, newspapers, politics, or sci-fi religions to the public.

The image of ECT outside psychiatry has been influenced by several movies reprising its overuse in state hospitals 50–60 years ago, recently summarized by Banken (2002). Many effective and useful medical treatments have been overused, from cardiac bypass surgery and hysterectomy to penicillin and benzodiazepines. Perhaps overuse reflects effectiveness when used appropriately. Past overuse is no reason to obstruct proper use in suitable patients. However, polemical statements about inappropriate use in the past can incite undiscriminating people. Reality is the suffering, debilitation, and stigmatization of patients with illness that is undertreated or not treated appropriately. In our society who is familiar with severely ill psychiatric patients? These patients are separated from the community and placed in hospitals and nursing homes, and sometimes in prisons. Until you enter such places you might never see the misery of severe psychiatric illness, including psychotic depression and the conditions it becomes when not promptly, thoroughly, and appropriately evaluated and treated. People who do not work with mentally ill patients should not meddlesomely and uninformedly limit the access of these patients to treatment, including ECT.

In Texas, antipsychiatry groups persuaded the state legislature to severely inhibit ECT access. Recently the state of Texas executed mentally ill patients. Proper and compassionate treatment of the mentally ill has always been a matter of civilization and character. Nota bene, residents of Texas.

That some government hospitals provide ECT stands as a challenge to those that do not. Moreover, psychiatrists at government hospitals have notably advanced the practice of ECT and of a psychiatry that incorporates ECT. Many but not all hospitals operated by the U.S. Department of Veterans Affairs provide ECT. Generally it is those in the same city as a medical school and affiliated with it that maintain an ECT unit. Conversely, some private psychiatric hospitals and community hospitals with psychiatric beds do not provide ECT; obviously their quality is more variable than hospitals that provide ECT. Surely, psychiatrists with extensive ECT experience have observed more about when and how to use it and when not to.

A common path to treatment

Treatment starts after assembling the details of history, interview, examination, and identifying the type of psychotic depression. It does not help to prescribe antipsychotics for every patient who could receive a diagnosis of psychotic depression or schizo-something. We will do better, starting with efficiently assessing the possible patient response to treatment. Treatment begins with planning.

There are two separate ways to judge treatment results. These are observable illness and patient satisfaction, the former objective and the latter subjective. The first step in treating is identifying the signs you and your staff can see that indicate the patient is ill. Second is identifying the patient's subjective dissatisfactions and worries. Third is clearly separating evidence you can see from subjective dissatisfaction; this step is crucial.

Fourth is being aware of how the observable illness might change as the patient improves, regardless of satisfactions and dissatisfactions. With this, you should include a time frame for improvement, meaning when you might recommend ECT to a patient if an initial drug trial does not succeed within that time frame. It should help the patient and family accept ECT if you mention the ECT plan when the drug trial starts. Because psychotic depression is not psychological, the patient's improvement from this drug trial is not affected by psychological expectation or pressure. Rather, mentioning ECT before the drug trial gives the patient and family a sense of depth in your experience and a feeling of participation in selecting ECT if it becomes needed. Remission and patient satisfaction are two separate goals. We need both, but this might take two separate plans.

Fifth is deciding how quickly response is needed and how resistant the patient has been to treatment already received. Urgency typically corresponds to suicidality, somatic tension, inanition, or hypoactivity. If the patient wants to die and is not convincingly against suicide, quick response is needed. Strong somatic tension means that the patient looks or sounds markedly agitated, irritable, or hyperreactive; patients with it urgently seek relief, sometimes by self-destruction. Some underweight depressed patients decline food and lose weight despite denying any death wish; this is de facto suicidal behavior and it can and does produce sudden cardiac death. Low serum albumin, low or unstable pulse or blood pressure, or electrolyte abnormalities are signs of special urgency in patients after weight loss. The hypoactivity of undertreated catatonic depression is presumably responsible for their excess death from lung and cardiac causes, such as pneumonia, myocardial infarction, arrhythmia, and emboli (Swartz and Galang, 2001; Swartz et al., 2001).

Usual treatment resistance means that the patient received a full-dose course of TCA or bupropion yet remains psychotically depressed, not just dissatisfied or worried. These meanings of urgent and resistant are perhaps unrealistically clear cut. Most patients have their own complex blend of urgency and resistance additionally related to psychosis-driven behavior, other disordered behavior, personal expectations, financial pressures, living conditions, or concurrent medical conditions. With elderly patients who are psychotically depressed, serious concurrent medical conditions are ubiquitous. Moreover, the medical conditions and the depression become an enmeshed complex in which both must be treated collaboratively to obtain improvement. Patients with weakness or apathy from depression cannot recover from respiratory failure (as from pneumonia) until they regain strength and willpower to deliver effort. The same is true of patients in physical rehabilitation. Not effectively treated, they may die of pneumonia.

In the following two chapters, we see how to treat such patients, and others.

7

Treatment: ECT, Medications, and More

THE ENORMOUS PERSONAL improvements we have seen in patients who receive ECT and AMMs, and the suffering and incapacitation these patients escape, are beyond the ability of language to convey. We can spell out how to provide these treatments, and do so here. The information provided in this chapter is primarily for physicians, yet patients and their families can have a front row seat as they see how this fearful illness must properly be treated.

Electroconvulsive therapy

Catatonia, suicidal intent or activity, dangerous or unpredictable agitation, weight loss, inability to swallow medication, and severe impairment of self-care are reasons to begin ECT urgently in patients with an ECT-responsive type of psychotic depression. Failure of a previous medication trial, need for inpatient confinement, need for a prompt or reliable response (i.e., cannot wait), medication intolerance (because of age or medical problems), or patient preference are compelling reasons to choose ECT as the next treatment. Of course, patient preference is influenced by what the physician chooses to say (or omit) about the up- and downsides of treatment alternatives, and how this meshes with patients' desires for reliability, promptness, comfort, and avoidance of impairment or disempowerment.

A meta-analysis of forty-four treatment studies of psychotic depression concluded that ECT tends to be superior to the antipsychotic-TCA combination and is distinctly superior to tricyclics alone (Parker et al., 1992). Those studies primarily focused on changes in symptom severity according to the HAM-D and similar scales, not on completeness of remission or psychological impairments from antipsychotic drugs. Accordingly, their results represent only average suppression of symptoms, not the regaining of preillness good health and performance abilities. Their method somewhat overstates the effectiveness of antipsychotic tranquilizers, as detailed in the "pitfalls" section of the last chapter. In a simpler report of summation of seventeen studies, 82 percent of psychotic depression patients responded to ECT versus 77 percent with the antipsychotic-tricyclic combination (Spiker et al., 1985b).

ECT is effective in removing suicidality in psychotic depression. Of thirty-five patients with active suicidal thoughts or behavior, after ECT, thirty patients had no further thoughts of death or feelings that life is not worth living (Kellner et al., 2005). The median total number of sessions of bilateral ECT given in treating psychotic depression is 7.0, the same as in nonpsychotic depression (Petrides et al., 2001).

Several studies have reported that ECT is more effective in psychotic depression than the combination of antipsychotics and antidepressants. In a retrospective study, good response occurred in 86 percent of ECT patients and 42 percent of antipsychotic-antimelancholic drug patients; improvement occurred in all ECT patients and 50 percent of the drug patients (Perry et al., 1982).

ECT has been reported to produce a larger response in psychotic depression than in nonpsychotic depression, 92 percent versus 55 percent (Birkenhager et al., 2003). Similarly, with ECT 83 percent of 77 psychotic depression patients achieved remission, as did 71 percent of 176 nonpsychotic depression patients (Petrides et al., 2001). Excluding the 14 percent of patients who stopped ECT treatment prematurely, the remission rates were 95 percent and 87 percent, respectively. This makes sense because nonpsychotic depression is sometimes primarily an anxiety disorder or a psychological reaction rather than a biological illness. Specifically, atypical depression (which is never psychotic) is difficult to differentiate from anxiety disorders, and *DSM* confuses rather than clarifies the distinction. Some patients with atypical depression or primary anxiety disorder who have been diagnosed as having major depression receive ECT because of medication resistance or suicidality; this lowers the overall ECT response rate in nonpsychotic depression. In psychotic depression, by contrast, the psychomotor slowing, sickly appearance, and blunted affect do not overlap with symptoms of anxiety disorders. Of course clinicians who avoid giving ECT to patients with atypical depression obtain higher ECT response rates. Greater use of ECT in nonpsychotic depression or less selective diagnosis of psychotic depression can explain reports that response to ECT is about the same in psychotic and nonpsychotic depression (Solan et al., 1988; Black and Winokur, 1989).

Over 80 percent of patients with psychotic depression who fail to respond to a TCA respond to ECT (Glassman et al., 1975; Avery and Lubrano, 1979; Lykouras et al., 1986a, 1986b; Spiker et al., 1986). In treating corticosteroid-induced major depression, whether psychotic or not, ECT was effective but tricyclics were not (Brown et al., 1982; Lewis and Smith, 1983). ECT was effective in nine of fifteen patients who failed to respond to the combination of antipsychotic and AMMs (Nelson and Mazure, 1986), a result not significantly different from 80 percent. ECT was more effective than the combination of amitriptyline and the MAOI phenelzine (Davidson at al., 1978).

ECT: The procedure

ECT treatment is painless, and after the treatment most patients are surprised to hear that it has occurred. MRI studies in humans, post-mortem studies, and animal studies have found that it does not injure the brain. Moreover, if injury occurred from ECT, patients would show the same physical problems that occur after stroke, such as paralysis, and this does not happen. Physical risks from ECT are about the same size as risks from brief anesthesia alone. The risk of death from ECT is about 1 in 22,000; this is less than the lifetime risk of death from taking a bath, 1 in 10,000 (Seach, 2005). It is also less than the risk of dying in a car accident over the next year. Still, for safety you need to know how to drive a car. Similarly, you need to know some things about the ECT procedure.

The ECT procedure consists of inducing a controlled brain seizure for therapeutic purposes, by applying a measured dose of electricity. There is a well-developed technology to do this. The patient is given anesthesia as for surgery and is asleep during the entire treatment. There is little muscle movement during the treatment because of the anesthesia. The most effective electrical stimulus is a series of pulses, each 1/2,000 second wide, applied at a rate between 60 and 140 pulses per second, for several seconds (Swartz and Manly, 2000). The amount of electrical energy entering the brain at the largest electrical dose used is not enough to raise brain temperature by 0.10 of a degree (Swartz, 1989). The brain seizure typically lasts between 25 and 50 seconds. Patients ordinarily awaken 5–10 minutes after the seizure.

The ECT procedure begins with obtaining written informed consent from the patient and at least tolerance from close family members. Educational pamphlets and videotapes for patient and family can help, and so can advocacy by former patients who recovered their health with ECT (Parvin et al., 2004). It also begins with the plan of medical evaluation to determine what special precautions are needed during ECT anesthesia, if any. This usually includes physical examination including mouth inspection for loose teeth, electrocardiogram

(ECG), serum potassium, blood hemoglobin and hematocrit, and anesthesiology consultation. Spine x-ray films are not routinely needed. Possible or actual illnesses such as diabetes can require additional tests.

There are two different moments for assessing the response of depression to ECT. One is immediately after completing the series of ECT sessions. The other is 3–6 weeks later. Much more time and effort is needed to assess patients after they are discharged from the hospital. This is why few studies assess patients more than 4 days after ECT. Relapse that occurs 6 weeks or more after the completion of ECT is attributable to ineffective prevention of recurrence, not to ECT. Relapse 4–6 weeks after ECT is still probably from weak prevention. However, relapse within the first 4 weeks usually indicates treatment ineffectiveness or unsuitability, or an untreated separate problem such as an anxiety disorder.

There are several different methods of ECT, largely consisting of varying electrode placements, electrical doses, and anesthetic medications. The four common electrode placements are traditional bilateral, bifrontal bilateral, LART bilateral, and (right-sided) unilateral. Traditional bilateral is also called bifrontotemporal or bitemporal. LART represents left-anterior right-temporal bilateral placement. The different methods of ECT represent different balances between effectiveness and temporary side effects.

Usually ECT is selected to treat psychotic depression because there is urgency for response or resistance to antidepressant medication. If the patient has had many episodes, is seriously suicidal, is in a long episode, has unstable vital signs, or shows behavior affected by hallucinations or delusions, the ECT method should be weighted more to assure efficacy rather than to minimize side effects. Unstable vital signs mean a fever, a rapid or rapidly varying heart rate, peculiar excessive sweating (hyperhydrosis), rapidly varying blood pressure, or high blood pressure that began during the episode of depression. These circumstances warrant giving effectiveness a higher priority and using one of the three bilateral placements. LART and bifrontal placements have fewer side effects than traditional bilateral ECT with comparable efficacy. There are several rationales by which LART should have fewer side effects than bifrontal but these have not been tested (Swartz and Nelson, 2005). Particularly in elderly patients, traditional bilateral ECT causes more disorientation and need for supervision than the other placements do. Nevertheless, while there is emergency and not mere urgency, the long usage of traditional bilateral ECT makes it desirable.

Treatment ineffectiveness of unilateral ECT is seen in the much higher rate of early relapse after unilateral than traditional bilateral ECT (Sackeim et al., 1993). The overall effectiveness of unilateral ECT can be increased by using higher electrical stimulus doses, but this increases side effects.

Other remediable causes of incomplete success with ECT treatment include low electrical stimulus dose, weak ECT seizure, use of interfering medications (such as benzodiazepines, anticonvulsants, or high-dose anesthesia), or an insufficient number of ECT sessions. Six good quality ECT sessions is the usual minimum, five is an absolute and rarely used minimum, and seven to eight sessions is a good median number. It is unusual for a treatment course to exceed twelve sessions. Effectiveness is surely lower if several problems of method happen to be present simultaneously.

A few patients with conditions suitable for ECT may relapse quickly despite receiving long courses of high-dose medication-free vigorous bilateral ECT. Generally these patients have been severely and continuously ill for at least 2 years. However, the studies of relapse have not distinguished between true relapse of psychotic depression and the emergence of unhappiness from underlying anxiety disorders or adjustment disorders, themselves resulting from the threatening stresses of experiencing severe and long-standing illness.

The most common reasons for apparent ineffectiveness of ECT are an underlying anxiety disorder, personality disorder, alcohol problem, substance abuse disorder, or an undiagnosed or undertreated medical illness. Typically these patients will appear dissatisfied or tense but not slowed in movements, thought production, or emotional expression.

A crucially important part of the ECT procedure is avoiding unnecessary medications along the ECT course. The only medications known to speed response to ECT increase the intensity of the ECT seizure. These are stimulants, such as theophylline and caffeine; they should be given only if the patient shows weak ECT seizures or if medically unavoidable (as in some asthma cases). Conversely, ECT response is decreased by medications that act opposite to stimulants, such as lorazepam and other benzodiazepines. Antipsychotic medication can interfere with swallowing and increase risk of aspiration during or after ECT, especially when anesthesia is given with propofol, the patient is elderly, or no pretreatment atropinic agent is given. If an ECT patient needs night-time sedation, promethazine should work without interfering with ECT; elderly patients would receive 12.5–25 mg, and adults 25–50 mg orally or intramuscularly, or half these doses intravenously. Nevertheless, if possible all medication should be avoided.

During each ECT treatment the physiological effects of the ECT seizure should be examined for weakness. A weak seizure generally indicates a suboptimal treatment, although sometimes it reflects aging or illness in the patient. The physiological effects to know about include duration of the tonic phase of the motor seizure, peak heart rate, EEG waveform, EEG amplitude, and postictal suppression. Specific details and suggestions are available in a clinical textbook (Abrams, 2002) and for further development (Swartz, 2000).

ECT: Mechanisms

A basic mechanism of how ECT works in treating psychotic depression has not been proven, but there have been many hypotheses. Some psychiatrists have postulated that ECT causes production of specific therapeutic substances such as hormones or neurotransmitters (Fink,

1979); their identity remains unknown. We will review a structural mechanism of ECT previously published by one of us (Swartz, 1984). It does not require mentioning specific hormones or neurotransmitters and it provides a simple way to understand how ECT works in several different psychiatric disorders.

A realistic ECT mechanism must account for the facts that ECT works by inducing a generalized seizure, and that the quality of this seizure generally determines the extent of therapeutic benefits. Seizure quality refers to its intensity and generalization; that is, a seizure that spreads only weakly before stopping has low effectiveness. Our structural mechanism has two parts, both related to seizure effects. First, the ECT seizure depletes brain neurotransmitters. Second, this depletion is followed by neurotransmitter replenishment according to the genes.

It was the pretreatment pattern of neurotransmitters that mediated psychiatric illness, as in psychotic depression. This neurotransmitter pattern of illness resulted from the interaction between the patient's genes and his environment, presumably experiences that affected body physiology. As an ECT seizure depletes the neurotransmitters, the pretreatment patterns mediating the illness are disrupted. In the process of neurotransmitter replenishment, gene DNA is transcribed, leading to the production of enzyme proteins and their catalysis of new production of neurotransmitters. This healthy pattern differs from the previous pattern that had become maleficent because the pattern of newly replenished neurotransmitters reflects only the genes, not the environment or its interaction with the genes. Accordingly, the new pattern differs from the pathological pattern that was present before ECT. With each ECT treatment, the pattern of illness is disrupted further. Eventually the pattern is sufficiently erased to stop the psychiatric disease.

Here is an analogy. Write "psychotic depression" on a chalkboard; this represents the pretreatment pattern of illness. Then erase several letters and write the letter "h" underneath to start spelling the word "health"; this represents an ECT treatment. Each additional ECT is reflected by erasing several more letters from "psychotic depression" (as depletion of illness pattern) and adding another letter to "health" (as replenishment according to the genes).

This mechanism is consistent with ECT providing therapeutic benefits in several different conditions, including mania, catatonic depression, melancholic depression, and other types of psychotic depression. The benefit of resetting the pattern of brain neurotransmitters should persist if the environmental effects do not overcome it. Presumably lithium decreases the effects of the environment on neurotransmitter patterns; this is consistent with lithium pharmacology of diminishing second messenger effects at neurotransmitter receptors. In this mechanism, ECT restores brain neurotransmitter function to normal preillness state. This restorative mechanism delineates a clear distinction between ECT and medical interventions that obstruct parts of brain function, interventions such as ablative brain surgery, deep brain stimulation, and antipsychotic tranquilizers.

In this mechanism, psychotic depression resembles errors accumulating in the operation of a computer program, eventually leading to generalized computer malfunction. ECT is then analogous to clearing the program from the computer and reloading a fresh copy of the program. Most old memory is stored in physical brain structure, not in neurotransmitters. Very recent memory is stored in neurotransmitters. The older and better learned the memory, the more it resides in the brain structure. Neurotransmitter memory is analogous to random-access memory (RAM) in semiconductor chips. Structural memory is analogous to hard disk storage. ECT is analogous to clearing RAM but not hard disk storage. This analogy illustrates how ECT can provide therapeutic benefits without impairing brain function or psychological performance.

ECT surely causes other neurochemical changes besides depleting neurotransmitters, such as generating anticonvulsant activity and briefly releasing hormones from anterior and posterior pituitary. ECT's anticonvulsant benefits may help relieve psychotic depression resulting from seizure disorders. Because several anticonvulsant medications treat mania or diminish somatic tension anxiety, the anticonvulsant effects of

ECT might do likewise. However, ECT's anticonvulsant effects persist for only several weeks, so are unlikely to produce the persistent benefits in psychotic depression that are regularly reported.

Prevention of recurrence after ECT

In the absence of continuing therapy, patients who benefit from ECT can quickly relapse (within 2–4 months) or experience recurrence (after 2–4 months). Early relapse suggests incomplete treatment, while later recurrence suggests incomplete maintenance. How should treatment be continued? Of patients over age 60 who achieved remission from psychotic depression with ECT and were maintained on TCAs alone, 10 percent relapsed within 4 months and 36 percent had recurrence after 4–24 months (Flint and Rifat, 1998b). This is a fairly good outcome, but recurrence should be even lower with maintenance on lithium or a combination of lithium and nortriptyline. In patients with nonpsychotic depression, after remission with ECT, relapse occurred in 4 percent and recurrence in 10 percent.

Maintenance with TCAs alone brings only moderate success. One study of psychotic depression after ECT remission found that, when checked on average 3.5 years later, 78 percent of patients had relapsed. All twenty-three patients had failed to respond to tricyclics prior to starting ECT (Aronson et al., 1987). Another study reported 50 percent relapse of psychotic depression within 1 year of ECT remission (Spiker et al., 1985a). Again, most patients had been discharged on a TCA alone.

Of patients over age 50 (average age 72 years) who responded to ECT for delusional depression, 33 percent of those maintained on nortriptyline (average 55 mg/day) and perphenazine (average 10 mg/day) relapsed within 6 months. Although only 15 percent maintained on nortriptyline alone (average 70 mg/day) relapsed, the difference was not statistically significant. Nevertheless, it does suggest that the combination is not superior to tricyclic alone in post-ECT maintenance.

Combination subjects experienced more falls to the floor and more troublesome extrapyramidal symptoms and tardive dyskinesia, despite the low perphenazine doses. Only one patient relapsed into psychotic depression; the other six relapses were nonpsychotic (Meyers et al., 2001).

This distinction is a revelation, and no other study of relapse has described it. This nonpsychotic "relapse" might well have been an exacerbation of an underlying anxiety disorder such as PTSD, or adjustment disorder reaction. This would not be a true relapse of psychotic depression. It might be somewhat analogous to the high occurrence of factitious seizures (pseudoseizures) in patients with a genuine seizure disorder; some patients seek help for life frustrations by assuming the sick role. Older patients with psychotic depression have a lower relapse rate, which suggests that greater relapse in younger patients might be due to more anxiety and adjustment disorder in this age group. After elderly patients recover from psychotic depression, outpatient maintenance ECT is recommended for them as effective and economical (Rabheru and Persad, 1997).

In two studies carbamazepine was found superior to lithium in preventing recurrence of psychotic depression (Placidi et al., 1986; Kostiukova, 1989). Another study found suggestive data that oxcarbazepine is effective (and more effective than valproic acid) in treating psychotic depression (Raja and Azzoni, 2003). Several reports have described good effectiveness of valproic acid in treating psychotic mania and manic schizoaffective disorder, but no reports of success with it in treating psychotic depression were found. Carbamazepine and its metabolite oxcarbazepine might be a little less effective than valproic acid in treating mania, but they appear more effective in depression.

ECT versus medications

Suitable ECT patients are common on psychiatric wards. Before receiving ECT they have palpably serious illness – they appear ill, cannot manage their lives independently, and often have deficient self-care. Inhibiting their access to ECT prolongs this suffering and debilitation, and so risks loss of job, family, property, and financial independence, and with these the respect of others and self. Undertreatment of psychotic depression increases hospital and physician liabilities if a patient commits suicide. Delaying ECT for catatonic psychotic depression predisposes to life-threatening cardiopulmonary events (Swartz and Galang, 2001; Swartz et al., 2001). The suffering and stigmatization of undertreated psychiatric illness is a stress of traumatic proportions, itself harmful. Moreover, allowing psychosis or catatonia to continue uninterrupted predisposes to it becoming chronic.

Becoming chronic seems to be the essential difference between schizophrenia and psychotic depression. It is the simplest explanation of the nearly complete overlap in family occurrence of schizophrenia and mood disorders, including among identical twins (Taylor et al., 1993). Because psychotic mood disorders and schizophrenia seem to share the same genotypes and biological abnormalities, clinical differences between them apparently derive from the patient's experience. Not everybody will agree with this, but we suggest it anyway because it is patient centered: A treatment that effectively interrupts psychosis and catatonia may diminish the chance of psychosis becoming chronic, that is, turning into schizophrenia. A couple of years ago we were delighted to hear of an ongoing study of this concept, using ECT to prevent chronic psychosis, although it was overseas; publication is several years distant.

What limits the use of ECT in treating psychotic depression? The all-inclusive judgments some psychiatrists have openly published in peer-reviewed medical journals that aspire to scholarship suggest that personal opinions are involved. The citations here were taken solely from articles focusing on psychotic depression, in which ECT efficacy is not in doubt. This collection is illustrative, not comprehensive. We will start with dismissive comments that do not enforce a personal boundary between patient and doctor, "ECT does not provide ... for the large numbers of patients who prefer pharmacologic treatment" and "patients don't like

ECT." As one group declared dramatically, "[by] its very nature, the induction of an epileptic seizure, can seem barbaric, and overtones of social control remain . . . its use is complicated by the . . . need to starve the patient." A psychiatrist wrote, "the availability, cost, stigma, and side effects associated with ECT have limited its use as a first-line treatment." We ask our readers to reconsider each of these statements with the word "surgery" in place of ECT. The statements about surgery will be quite accurate. However, this word-substitution exercise reveals the distortion in the statements about ECT. All these "reasons" are only personal opinions. They are factually incorrect or self-fulfilling, as detailed below.

Does ECT smack of barbarism, social control, and starvation? Incomparably more cruel is allowing the patient to remain ill rather than regaining his health and persona. Continuing illness or tranquilization with antipsychotic drugs controls patients profoundly and directly. In contrast, ECT is painless, does not control anyone, and avoids leaving patients tranquilized or partially ill. It enables life, liberty, and the pursuit of happiness, while tranquilizers risk or impair these. Regarding the word starvation, it is out of proportion with postponing breakfast until 9 AM. The use of the word "starve" suggests that those authors are not acquainted with the ECT procedures they criticize.

Patient and family preferences are overwhelmingly influenced by the knowledge, sensitivity, and relevance of the psychiatrist's explanation. Patients and families do not know what to think about ECT. Most realize that what they have seen in the movies and on television might be medically inaccurate or out of date, and they depend on the doctor to educate them. Here is a simple and realistic explanation we suggest you adopt to help patients understand the value of ECT. It starts with "other people easily see that you are ill. You look ill, as if you have the flu." Then you describe to the patient the signs of illness that other people see, such as: "you look severely exhausted and worn out, you hardly move, you hardly speak, your voice sounds weak, your face looks stiff and wooden like a mask, you are drawn in to yourself and don't notice other people or try to help them." Then continue, "when other people see your movements and hear your speech they see that you are ill. They know your private business. There is a treatment that usually brings people back to looking normal and healthy, so that your health can be your private business again. This treatment is modern ECT."

Your patients may come in believing that drugs such as antidepressants, mood stabilizers, and antipsychotics are equivalent substitutes, but they are not. Antidepressants and mood stabilizers work well but only for a third to half of patients, and the recurrence rate is not lower than after ECT. The regular use of ECT in academic medical centers and nearby hospitals (Hermann et al., 1995) illustrates the absence of equivalent substitutes in places where scholarship is prominent. We fervently wish that pills were available to make surgery unnecessary, but we know that no pill can properly fix a hernia, a ruptured spleen, or a brain tumor. Surely we wish that medications worked as well as ECT, but they do not, and pretending they do is harmful to patients.

Safety of ECT versus antipsychotic drugs

Treating psychotically depressed patients with ECT rather than antidepressant drugs may substantially reduce the harm that awaits many of these patients down the road. So many patients continue to suffer when they could be well, are driven to suicide, and die prematurely from heart and lung diseases associated with hypoactivity and abulia such as pneumonia. As an example, 40 percent of patients treated for psychotic depression without ECT at Yale University Hospital died within 15 years (Vythilingam et al., 2003), a markedly excessive rate. About 90 percent of deaths were from medical causes, not suicide. A recent Scandinavian study found that after hospital discharge ECT patients had a substantially lower death rate from lung diseases such as pneumonia than discharged psychiatric patients who did not receive ECT. Moreover, patients who have asthma and received antipsychotic drugs in the previous year had a 3–6-fold greater risk of death or near-death from asthma

(Joseph et al., 1996). Likewise, aspiration pneumonia was associated with antipsychotic drugs in ambulatory elderly patients with Alzheimer's disease (Wada et al., 2001). In a study of over 500 depressed inpatients, ECT recipients had a significantly lower death rate than patients who received low dose antidepressant and those who received neither ECT nor antidepressants (Avery and Winokur, 1976). This was particularly true for nonsuicide deaths.

There are two quite separate reasons for higher death rates from medical causes when psychotic depression is treated with antipsychotic tranquilizers instead of ECT. These are continuing depressive illness and antipsychotic drug side effects, and they apply whether or not the antipsychotic drug is given together with an antidepressant. First, medications are inferior to ECT in rate of remission, completeness of response, and speed of response. Because more patients remain ill and partially ill with medications than ECT, they are more likely to experience heart and lung diseases associated with the hypoactivity of continuing depressive symptoms, diseases such as pneumonia and pulmonary embolus.

Second, the antipsychotic drugs commonly used in treating psychotic depression cause behavioral problems with medical risks as well as risky medical conditions. The behavioral problems include hypoactivity, diminished initiative, and weakened willpower; these provoke pneumonia and pulmonary emboli. They also inhibit the patient from requesting help when illness starts. Adverse medical conditions caused by antipsychotic drugs induce cancer (Swartz, 2004b) and weight gain. In turn, weight gain increases risks of high blood pressure, atherosclerotic coronary vascular disease, diabetes, strokes, myocardial infarctions, and further hypoactivity. The lethal medical risks of antipsychotic drugs are illustrated by the observed 50 percent higher death rate within 12 weeks of starting antipsychotic drugs (3.5%) compared to placebo (2.3%) in randomized studies of over 5,000 elderly patients with dementia (Schneider et al. 2005). These data concern patients taking only the recently introduced costly antipsychotic drugs olanzapine, risperidone, ziprasidone, aripiprazole, quetiapine, and clozapine. Individual drugs, severity of illness, and type of dementia did not influence the death rate. The excess rate of brain stroke from these drugs led the FDA to require a "black box warning" in the printed information included with these drugs, similar to the warning on cigarette packs.

Antimelancholic drugs alone

AMMs (an abbreviation that one of us coined in an earlier publication) (Swartz et al., 2001) refers to effective treatments of melancholic depression. This includes tricyclics, MAOIs, bupropion, and high-dose venlafaxine. It does not include SSRIs such as fluoxetine and escitalopram, which can treat atypical major depression, by definition a nonmelancholic disorder. Because SSRIs are widely referred to as antidepressants, to prevent confusion we will avoid this term whenever this drug class is under discussion, because the SSRIs do not, in fact, treat successfully the kinds of depression considered here.

The distinction between psychotic and nonpsychotic depression corresponds to a large difference in response to antimelancholic drugs. With a high dose of TCA alone, only one-third of patients with psychotic depression achieve remission, compared to two-thirds of those with nonpsychotic melancholia (Avery and Lubrano, 1979; Coryell and Tsuang, 1982; Kroessler, 1985; Coryell et al., 1986; Spiker et al., 1986; Chan et al., 1987; Parker et al., 1991a). The distinction between the patient feeling as if he is condemned and believing that he is can be subtle, but it corresponds to a huge difference in success rate with this treatment. The lower rate of drug response in psychotic depression decreases expected drug benefits, increases expected costs and risks because of longer average episode duration, and should influence patient and family preferences among treatments.

Severity difference might explain the difference in outcome between psychotic depression and nonpsychotic melancholia. Severely depressed nonpsychotic patients respond to tricyclics at about the same (one-third) rate as those with psychotic depression (Kocsis et al., 1990). Another possible explanation is that many patients with psychotic depression have a tricyclic-nonresponsive type of depression, such as catatonic or tardive (see Chapter 8).

Concurrent anxiety disorder can also affect outcome and might be worse in patients with more severe and long-lasting depressions, that is, psychotic rather than nonpsychotic. As for depressed patients who are also anxious, the practical clinical approach remains to evaluate and treat underlying anxiety disorders before concluding acute treatment, and to expect 33–50 percent remission rate to high doses of AMMs in all severe depressions including psychotic depressions. This perspective includes adding lithium or triiodothyronine when possible and placing a short time limit for initial improvement from antidepressants before switching to ECT, such as 1 week.

Antimelancholic blood levels can influence outcome in psychotic depression. With amitriptyline, a blood total tricyclic level above 250 ng/ml is associated with greater response (Spiker et al., 1986); imipramine should be similar. Patients commonly vary ten-fold in the blood levels obtained from a particular tricyclic dose, but an amitriptyline blood level above 250 ng/ml usually requires a daily dose of 200 mg or more. The usual target for serum nortriptyline level of 50–150 ng/ml came from one small study that was not restricted to psychotic depression. There is an internal inconsistency between aiming above 250 ng/ml (for total amitripyline and nortriptyline) when prescribing amitriptyline but below 150 ng/ml when using nortriptyline. Accordingly, there is no established error in exceeding 150 ng/ml with nortriptyline in psychotic depression.

No differences in age, sex, or duration of illness were found between patients with psychotic depression who responded to a TCA alone and those who did not (Spiker et al., 1986). Some studies with small numbers of patients reported low rates of response to tricyclics, but because of underpowering they were not significantly different from one-third (e.g., 17% response, Brown et al., 1982).

Antidepressant-induced mania

In exceptionally high doses, TCAs can induce a manic episode in susceptible patients (Jain and Swartz, 2002); so can bupropion (Goren and Levin, 2000). Patients with types of psychotic depression that occur in bipolar disorder are susceptible. At ordinary doses, antidepressant-associated mania is mild and brief, as compared to endogenous mania (Stoll et al., 1994). This study was conducted soon after SSRIs were introduced and fluoxetine was the only SSRI widely used. Antidepressant-associated mania occurred in nineteen patients taking tricyclics, thirteen taking fluoxetine, six on bupropion, and thirteen on MAOIs. Because fluoxetine is equivalent to placebo in treating psychotic depression, it is logically equivalent to placebo in inducing mania. These numbers suggest that the mania induced by tricyclics and bupropion is less frequent as well as milder than naturally occurring mania. In contrast, with these numbers the relative rarity of MAOI use suggests that it readily induces mild mania.

Because the depressive episodes linked to bipolar I disorder are of the psychotic, melancholic, or catatonic type, but not atypical type, it is essential that studies of switching exclude atypical depressions. Atypical depression outnumbers the other types of depression put together, and if atypical depression is included, patient selection will not be proper. The information needed is how much switching from depression into mania occurs with patients who have psychotic, melancholic, or catatonic depression, not atypical depression. Unfortunately, rather than excluding atypical depression we have the opposite. Apparently to increase the numbers of patients and the apparent noteworthiness of the results, recent switching studies specifically include atypical depressions and bipolar II patients. This makes the switching results uninterpretable.

The numerator, the number of mania cases, can also be artificially inflated: This happens when the occurrence of hypomania is scored as equal to switching into mania. However, hypomania is not mania of mild severity but often represents an anxiety disorder (Swartz, 2003c). On followup 1–2 years after a first hospitalization for psychotic depression, 13 percent of patients were said to have developed "mania or hypomania" (DelBello et al., 2003). This followup period is appropriate because 1–2 years of wellness is as long as a patient would be maintained on an antidepressant after remission from a first episode of depression. However, 13 percent is an overestimate of switching because it includes hypomania. In the United States the incidence of diagnosable anxiety disorders in bipolar I patients is about 35 percent and in bipolar II patients essentially 100 percent. Anxiety is high in bipolar I because the illness causes anxiety; it is universal in bipolar II because hypomania in bipolar II is equivalent to anxiety disorder with only rare exceptions.

The rapid cycling and premature episodes of mania attributed to tricyclics can also be accounted for by bipolar disorder worsening with time. The only way to identify tricyclic-induced mania would be to find a difference from another antidepressant treatment, randomizing patients between the two methods. Patients who enter such a study should have just recovered from an episode of psychotic depression and must continue with treatment to avoid rapid relapse. In such a study the comparison treatment should not have an antimania effect, as lithium and ECT do, because it would bias the result. It should not obscure the symptoms of mania, as antipsychotic drugs do.

This whittles down proper drugs to compare against tricyclics to bupropion, high-dose venlafaxine, and MAOIs. There are a few single-case studies of venlafaxine treating psychotic depression, but no studies of patient groups. Several psychiatrists have reported single cases of mania apparently associated with venlafaxine. Still, we can draw conclusions from studies that used medication equivalent to placebo for psychotic depression as a comparison group, specifically SSRIs. Indeed, SSRIs do not induce mania (e.g., Amsterdam and Shults, 2005). No difference was found between bupropion and SSRIs regarding onset of mania or rapid cycling, and both were rare (Joffe et al., 2002).

The conclusion is that if unusually high doses of bupropion, tricyclics, or venlafaxine are avoided, the incidence of drug-induced mania is negligible. This applies as well to depressed patients who are at risk for bipolar episodes, but these patients generally need to also take an antimanic drug, for example, lithium, valproic acid. Because lithium also prevents recurrence of depression and valproic acid does not, all else equal lithium is preferable.

Tricyclics with triiodothyronine in females

Triiodothyronine (T3, liothyronine, brand Cytomel) is one of the two principal thyroid hormones in the body; the other is thyroxine (T4, brands Synthroid, Levo). When T3 is given together with a TCA to female patients who have melancholic psychotic (or nonpsychotic) depression, full remissions are often obtained in 3 or 4 days, sometimes in just 1 or 2 days. This is usually faster than the usual 3–4 weeks for response to tricyclics alone. Moreover, this method allows faster determination of nonresponse to tricyclics, so you can move more promptly to another treatment. Mysteriously, T3 potentiation does not have such large effects in males (Wheatley, 1972). Patients who do not respond to tricyclics alone can respond when T3 is added, although this is not specifically in psychotic depression (Goodwin et al., 1982).

By itself no thyroid hormone treats psychotic depression or any other depression. Indeed, supraphysiologic doses of any thyroid hormone cause hyperthyroidism, which has several unpleasant body tension anxiety symptoms such as agitation, tremulousness, and hyperreactivity. In treating depression, triiodothyronine is used only to supplement TCAs. The standard T3 dose is 25 μg (equals 0.025 mg) once daily, and it is started at the same time as the TCA. Before the first T3 dose, patients should have a recent serum T4 or TSH level, to screen for thyroid hormone abnormalities.

Continuing this dose of T3 for as long as the TCA is given should prevent the rapid relapses seen when T3 was withdrawn soon after remission (Swartz, 1982). The relapse risk from premature T3 discontinuation outweighs the presumably negligible benefit.

The daily T3 dose is about one-seventh of the 150–200 μg of thyroxine normally released each day by the thyroid gland. The body quickly decreases its production of thyroxine to balance the T3 dose taken and avoid hyperthyroidism. The end result is that the ratio of T3 to thyroxine is increased while total thyroid hormone activity remains unchanged. This affects the brain because it can use thyroxine but not T3. It is enigmatic why making the brain slightly hypothyroid causes TCAs to work faster and in a greater percentage of cases, and also why this potentiation works reliably only in females.

Several drugs besides T3 raise the T3/T4 ratio. However, they have other hormonal or psychotropic effects that might interfere with tricyclic potentiation. Further, they have additional side effects and risks. These drugs include lithium, carbamazepine, phenytoin, and barbiturates. A study comparing lithium and tricyclic against tricyclic alone in treating or preventing depression would be incomplete unless it accounted for changes in T3/T4 ratios. This might be done by adding T3 to the nortriptyline alone group. Unfortunately, the comparison studies did not measure the T3/T4 ratio. Incidentally, the common thyroid test "T3 uptake" does not measure T3 levels; "T3 by RIA" does.

Studies show that T3 doses potentiate tricyclics in female patients with severe melancholic depression. This meshes with coauthor Conrad Swartz's long clinical experience in treating psychotic melancholic depression. Still, there are no published clinical trials of treating psychotic depression with T3 potentiation. Only the melancholic type of psychotic depression is appropriate for T3 potentiation. Swartz says: Although I saw T3 potentiation bring remission in 2 days in a 19-year-old female with extreme catatonic psychotic depression, it never succeeded in my catatonic female patients after that one.

The negative studies on T3 potentiation included male patients. Yet, including males dilutes the positive results with females and can explain the results. Further dilution occurs by including patients who are not melancholic. The negative studies signify the importance of selecting only female patients with melancholia.

Lithium

Lithium alone is rarely effective in treating unipolar melancholic depression, whether psychotic or not. Some psychiatrists have recommended lithium as worth trying in patients with psychotic depression that is steroid induced or part of a bipolar I illness; that makes sense to us. If ECT is simply not available to treat a patient with catatonia, it is reasonable to try lithium. Lithium by itself can treat tardive psychosis if antipsychotic drugs are entirely discontinued, as described in Chapter 8.

Adding lithium to TCAs can bring remission in melancholic psychotic depression (Pai et al., 1986) and seems well worth trying, especially with a personal or family history of bipolar disorder. Adding lithium to an antimelancholic-antipsychotic combination, as a third concurrent drug, has been reported effective in several case studies, as noted below.

Besides these focused acute treatment uses, lithium is generally effective in preventing recurrence of psychotic depression after achieving remission by giving ECT or AMMs. Lithium should be started a few days after the final ECT because giving lithium together with ECT sometimes causes disorientation. With AMMs lithium can be started at any time.

Lithium has several treatable minor nuisance side effects. Excessive thirst is important because it brings frequent urination and possible weight gain if calorie-containing fluids are increased. This thirst can be substantially mitigated or blunted by potassium supplements, 15 meq one to two times daily (Musa and Tripuraneni, 1993). This potassium dose is small compared to the ordinary dietary intake of about 100 meq/day, and should be easily tolerated by patients with normal kidney function. Other common side effects include resting tremor and early muscle fatigue, both of which are worse if the patient also takes antipsychotic drugs. The resting tremor can be decreased by the CNS-active generic beta-blocker betaxolol; it can usually be taken as 5 mg (one-half tablet) once daily at bedtime.

Antipsychotic drugs alone

The numbers do not look good for antipsychotic drugs alone in psychotic depression. In summing over seventeen studies, the response rate of psychotic depression to dopamine-blocking antipsychotic drugs was 51 percent (Spiker et al., 1985b). With perphenazine alone, over 5 weeks the response rate in psychotic depression was 19 percent (64 mg/day equal to 800 mg/day chlorpromazine) (Spiker et al., 1985b). Besides variable efficacy, there are several reasons that antipsychotic drugs alone are not a desirable treatment for psychotic depression.

When given alone in high doses, antipsychotic tranquilizers suppress some symptoms of psychotic depression in many patients. Of course, the effects of these powerful drugs are not specific to depression, or to any illness, and they alter the patient's persona. Because of the fundamental importance that psychiatry assigns to personality defects, it is peculiar that the psychological effects of antipsychotic drugs on normal people and on nonpsychotic patients are not mentioned in psychiatric textbooks. When this is mentioned to other doctors and nurses, they wonder whether the question might not be appropriate for ethical examination. In reality, the FDA mandates "phase I" studies of new psychotropic drugs in which they are given in substantial doses to normal volunteers. Many publications describe the body metabolism of antipsychotic drugs in normal volunteers. Thus, we can find published measurements of the half-life, time to peak blood level, and volume of distribution of these drugs in normal volunteers, but not their psychological effects.

Stigma exists in the eye of the beholder. Antipsychotic drugs cause more stigma than ECT. This is because they reinforce the suggestion of other-ness by causing visible peculiarities of movement and personality changes. By these visible peculiarities, stigmata become stigma. The easily seen often permanent physical deformities caused by antipsychotics such as tardive dyskinesia provide evidence of personal peculiarity to casual acquaintances and even passers-by. This is immeasurably larger than subjective stigma. Stigmata is what antipsychotic tranquilizers, benzodiazepines, and undertreated illness deliver. Ethically, psychiatrists should explain how ECT compares with such stigma. When properly given with modern technique, ECT side effects are usually negligible, and even when not negligible they are brief, generally 4–10 days (Swartz, 2005).

There are internal inconsistencies in the basic idea of using antipsychotic drugs to treat psychotic major depressive disorder (and other serious nonatypical major depression). This inconsistency involves both behavior and neurotransmitters in the same way.

Behaviorally, antipsychotic drugs typically cause losses of initiation, willpower (abulia), strength (asthenia), alertness (somnolence), self-discipline (orbital-frontal symptoms), and appreciation of complexity (dysexecutive symptoms). Serious depression causes precisely the same losses. The motivation and reward for these behaviors are missing. So, from the perspective of behavior there is a clear inconsistency in giving antipsychotic drugs.

Neurochemically, antipsychotic drugs block dopamine or other catecholamines. However, serious major depression appears to involve a deficiency of dopamine and other catecholamines (Meyer et al., 2001; Bremner et al., 2003).

Although they come from two different perspectives, the behavioral and neurochemical inconsistencies are fundamentally the same problem. The neurotransmitters involved with motivation and reward prominently involve dopamine and other catecholamines. In blocking these neurotransmitters, antipsychotic drugs resemble the pathology of depression itself.

In using antipsychotic drugs for depression, the highest you can aim is for quietude of depressive and psychotic symptoms and subtlety of the side effects of abulia, asthenia, and thought simplicity. The expectation is that the patient who responds to antipsychotic drugs will take care of his own personal needs and not demonstrate disturbed behavior or state distressed thoughts. This is not a true recovery.

When psychiatrists explain the oversimplistic kind of judgment shown by patients taking antipsychotic drugs, it is too easy to blame the illness, instead of the drugs. This shifting of the cause from the drug to the patient gives the drug the benefit of the doubt instead of the patient. There is little doubt that olanzapine and other antipsychotic tranquilizers have powerful effects on the personality. Anyone unsure of this can test it by videotaping himself before and after a week of taking olanzapine at just 10 mg/day, less than the average dose. Please see the following section for details about drug-induced personality changes, and also the section in Chapter 3 on "treatment vs. management."

The psychiatric literature contains abundant reports of how antipsychotic drugs improve certain kinds of psychological performance in patients with schizophrenia. It goes without saying that unmedicated psychotic patients do not perform well; yet medicated patients with schizophrenia remain with markedly impaired functioning compared to medicated nonpsychotic patients (Jager et al., 2005). Some publications tacitly suggest that because antipsychotic drugs improve psychological performance in severely disturbed psychotic patients, they improve psychological performance for all patients generally. They do not. What they do is greatly impair the psychological performance of normal people, bringing them approximately to the performance level of the medicated patients with schizophrenia. But this is not the level we want in depression: the standard of psychological performance in patients with depression is normality.

In a recent 18-month study, most patients given an antipsychotic drug discontinued it because of side effects or lack of effectiveness (Lieberman et al., 2005). The discontinuation rate varied between 64 percent and 82 percent, including the costly patented antipsychotics risperidone, ziprasidone, olanzapine, and quetiapine. These rates indicate patient dissatisfaction with these drugs.

Antipsychotic drugs can worsen stuporous (i.e., catatonic) psychotic depression into lethal catatonia, which resembles neuroleptic malignant syndrome (NMS) (Ries and Bokan, 1979; Fricchione et al., 1983; Lew and Tollefson, 1983; Casey, 1987; Bowers and Swigar, 1988). Lethal catatonia can include either extreme agitation or weakness with prostration, fever, autonomic instability with tachycardia or fluctuating heart rate, diaphoresis, obtundation, or severe muscle enzyme elevations.

With short-term use, antipsychotic drugs have a clear place in the acute tranquilization of dangerous or troublesome agitation in patients with psychotic depression. The "sedation plan" section describes the details.

Antipsychotic drugs are also useful as a last resort. At a veterans hospital in the mid-1980s, one of us (CS) met a 65-year-old man who had been there since the end of World War II because of resistant melancholic psychotic depression. He was referred for ECT because of inanition. His motor retardation was severe and he would not speak without crudely insulting the interviewer. After each course of standard bilateral ECT, he experienced a complete remission, showing an affable and pleasant persona. However, it would last for only 1–3 weeks, when his conversation would revert to a croaking "go away, leave me alone, drop dead." Before ECT, he failed to respond to full trials of tricyclics with and without lithium. After ECT, phenelzine 60 mg/day failed to help. Because continuing weight loss was problematic, I placed him on a combination of perphenazine and lorazepam. With this he gained weight and stopped all irritable behavior, although he remained sad and slowed. He continued this way for many years.

Clozapine alone strongly diminished symptoms of both psychosis and depression in three patients with drug-resistant psychotic depression (Ranjan and Meltzer, 1996). None relapsed over 4 or more years of followup. Clozapine on top of occasional courses of ECT was the only effective means of managing a 54-year-old female referred to me for ECT after spending 30 continuous years at a state hospital. The patient had spent the last few years in restraint or seclusion because of uncontrollable agitation, despite receiving every mood stabilizer and antipsychotic available except clozapine. Before ECT her speech and behavior were thoroughly disorganized, undirected, and incoherent. Although she recovered with ECT, she began cycling between psychotic mania and psychotic depression every 3–6 months. When she was well she was friendly, kind, and gentle. When she relapsed her screaming and severe agitation were nerve-wracking for everyone involved. Clozapine did not stop the cycling or the need for ECT, but it stopped the screaming and greatly diminished the agitation, so the patient could participate in her care and did not require intense supervision.

Antipsychotic-antimelancholic combination

APA guidelines for treating psychotic depression start with the combination of antipsychotic tranquilizer and antidepressant. In a meta-analysis of forty-four treatment studies, the antipsychotic-tricyclic combination tended to be more effective than antipsychotic alone and TCA alone, but this conclusion was tentative because statistical significance was not reached (Parker et al., 1992). In a summation of data from seventeen studies, the tricyclic-antipsychotic combination produced substantial clinical improvement in 77 percent of patients (Kroessler, 1985); still, the difference between substantial improvement and complete remission can lead to suicide.

Starting the antipsychotic drug first and adding the antidepressant 2–3 days later helps keep clear the relationship between each drug and its adverse effects. The beneficial effects of the two drugs are separately observable because the effects from a steady dose of an antipsychotic drug largely occur within a few days while TCAs act over several weeks. A small dose of lorazepam such as 0.5 mg three times daily restricted to the first week should help the patient (except perhaps for the elderly) feel more comfortable.

In this combination large doses of antipsychotic tranquilizers are required, equivalent to 600–1,000 mg/day of chlorpromazine per day (Dubovsky and Thomas, 1992). Such doses include perphenazine 48–64 mg/day, risperidone 6–10 mg/day, thiothixene 25–40 mg/day, and haloperidol 9–16 mg/day, but one-quarter to one-half of these doses in the elderly. This need for high doses is illustrated by comparing outcomes between high-dose and low-dose perphenazine studies.

In a high-dose study over 5 weeks with combination amitriptyline and perphenazine 64 mg/day, the response rate of psychotic depression was 78 percent (Spiker et al., 1985b). This large dose of perphenazine is equivalent to 800 mg/day chlorpromazine. In a similar study in patients over 50 years old, with a lower perphenazine dose (average 19 mg/day, maximum 24 mg/day) and controlled nortriptyline blood levels, response rates after 4 weeks were only 47 percent both for nortriptyline alone and nortriptyline with perphenazine (Mulsant et al., 2001). In other words, perphenazine doses of up to 24 mg/day were equivalent to placebo, when combined with a TCA. In a retrospective study, responders received higher doses of antipsychotic drug than nonresponders (Nelson et al., 1986).

Psychiatrists rarely employ such high doses. This is according to a survey of the medical records of patients with psychotic depression who were referred for ECT after failing to respond to drug treatment. Moreover, these patients were treated at university hospitals, where treatment is presumably more aggressive, that is, higher drug doses are more readily given. The typical antipsychotic doses used in psychotic depression were equivalent to 200 mg/day chlorpromazine or less (Mulsant et al., 1997). About half of the patients received either less than 3 weeks of antipsychotic dosage or none at all before referral for ECT. This clinical practice behavior suggests that the university psychiatrists prefer to give ECT instead of giving high doses of antipsychotics. Antipsychotic drug discontinuation after 2 weeks is associated with inadequate response and relapse (Perry et al., 1982).

Are recently introduced antipsychotic drugs such as risperidone better for psychotic depression than older antipsychotics such as perphenazine? Over 6 weeks of treatment, depression severity (Bech-Rafaelsen Melancholia Rating score) fell by 70 percent with the combination of amitriptyline 180 mg/day and haloperidol (average 9 mg/day). This was significantly more than the 50 percent fall with an average of 7 mg/day risperidone, slightly higher than the haloperidol-equivalent dose. The 61 patients studied had several conditions that included both psychotic and depressive symptoms, but mostly psychotic depression

(Muller-Siecheneder et al., 1998). Memorably, extrapyramidal symptoms were more severe with risperidone than the haloperidol-amitriptyline combination. This is presumably because of the anticholinergic effects of amitriptyline. The efficacy results suggest that risperidone is not substantially better than older antipsychotic drugs in treating psychotic depression, and not the equivalent of an antimelancholic-antipsychotic combination.

Special considerations apply for the elderly. Although antipsychotic doses for patients over age 70 should be about half the usual adult dose to obtain equal blood levels, elderly patients are more sensitive to equal blood antipsychotic drug levels. They more readily develop persistently severe rigidity, falling down, trouble swallowing, and tardive dyskinesia. In turn these provoke tendon and muscle contractures, strokes, bone fractures, and aspiration pneumonia, besides the physical disfigurements of tardive dyskinesia. Accordingly, frail patients and those over 70 years old should take even lower antipsychotic doses. About 5 percent of elderly patients placed on antipsychotic drugs per year of drug exposure will develop the physical deformity of tardive dyskinesia, whether from a costly patented antipsychotic drug or a generic drug (Lee et al., 2005). The yearly rate of tardive dyskinesia onset is higher, about 7 percent, in elderly patients who have depression rather than dementia (Yassa et al., 1992). Another study reported an appalling 43 percent incidence of tardive dyskinesia after just 6 months of treatment with low-dose perphenazine (average 10 mg/day) in patients treated for psychotic depression, with average age 72 years (Meyers et al., 2001). In elderly patients response rates to an antipsychotic-antidepressant combination have been reported as 25 percent overall, and that took a lengthy 7 weeks to develop, on average (Flint and Rifat, 1998a).

Amoxapine (Asendin), a single drug said to have antidepressant effects besides definite antipsychotic effects, appeared in the late 1980s. The recommended antidepressant dose included as much antipsychotic effect as 15 mg/day of haloperidol, a potent portion equivalent to 900 mg/day chlorpromazine. Conversely, amoxapine is a high-concentration metabolite of the antipsychotic drug loxapine (Burch and Goldschmidt, 1983). There are no apparent advantages of amoxapine over taking both a dopamine-blocker antipsychotic tranquilizer and an antidepressant drug. There is the disadvantage of an unalterably high level of antipsychotic activity. This means that after an initial (but insufficient) improvement an increase in amoxapine dose can cause excessive tranquilization, seen as apathy and hypoactivity. Indeed, the peculiarity of deterioration with dose increase after initial improvement occurs (Signer and Billings, 1984). Moreover, in using antipsychotic-antidepressant combinations, the antipsychotic is routinely tapered out after 4–6 months while the antidepressant dose is maintained – and amoxapine does not allow this. This inflexibility pushes all patients into the same mold, regardless of the need to fine-tune levels of antipsychotic drug effect. Because amoxapine is a potent dopamine-blocker, patients routinely develop all the corresponding side effects, including writhing tardive dyskinesia.

It is not clear whether amoxapine has more effect on depression than the equivalent dose of an antipsychotic drug alone; we found no direct study of this. A large randomized study found amitriptyline alone more effective in inducing full recovery from depression than amoxapine; amoxapine also trended to more relapse (Mason et al., 1990). However, this study was not restricted to psychotic depression. In the treatment of psychotic depression alone, the response to amoxapine was about the same as or slightly less than the combination of amitriptyline and perphenazine, about 70 percent overall (Anton and Burch, 1990). Several studies claimed faster symptom relief with amoxapine than a TCA alone, but this is attributable to tranquilization by amoxapine and this effect was not accounted for (e.g., Donlon et al., 1981).

Adding a third drug to antimelancholic-antipsychotic

After the combination of tricyclic and antipsychotic failed to improve psychotic depression in 6–8 patients, adding lithium led to marked improvement in half (Price et al. 1983; Flint and Rifat, 1998a). In a further study, the Yale group found that lithium augmentation succeeded in eight of nine bipolar depressives but only three of twelve unipolars, a significant difference (Nelson and Mazure, 1986). Although the antipsychotic drug was not then withdrawn, the circumstances suggest that adding lithium to a tricyclic might reduce symptoms of psychotic depression as much as adding an antipsychotic tranquilizer, especially in bipolar patients. Important advantages of lithium addition over antipsychotic addition include bona fide remission rather than tranquilization of symptoms, and no large changes to personality and performance abilities. Moreover, it is routine to add lithium to tricyclics for maintenance, even when a good remission is obtained from the tricyclic alone.

In contrast to the success of lithium addition, adding carbamazepine to the combination of antidepressant and antipsychotic was rarely tolerated (Cullen et al., 1991). Further, carbamazepine and valproate have no clear rationale for use in patients who have never experienced mania.

Monoamine Oxidase Inhibitors (MAOIs)

The drugs phenelzine, tranylcypromine, and isocarboxazid are irreversible inhibitors of the enzyme monoamine oxidase, which inactivates catecholamine and serotonin neurotransmitters. This inhibition of inactivation increases brain levels of catecholamines, which presumably treats melancholia, and increases serotonin, which probably soothes worrying. Reversible inhibitors of monoamine oxidase such as moclobemide are available in Europe but not in the United States; they appear to be weaker and not effective against psychotic depression.

Response to phenelzine was obtained in 68 percent of patients with nonpsychotic depression, 43 percent with probably psychotic depression, and 21 percent of definitely psychotic depression (Janicak et al, 1988). The average of probably and definitely psychotic is 32 percent, about the same as in studies of TCAs alone. Nevertheless, this responsive one-third might be a substantially different group of patients than that which responds to tricyclics. The associated phenelzine dose was incompletely specified as at least 30 mg/day in half the patients and at least 60 mg/day in half the patients but no more than 90 mg/day. The minimum phenelzine dose in melancholic or psychotic depression is 45 mg/day, except 30 mg/day in the elderly.

Accordingly, some psychiatrists have used the combination of amitriptyline and an MAOI. Because amitriptyline is a potent alpha-adrenergic blocker, this combination is less likely to produce the notorious but uncommon hypertensive "cheese reaction" (Pare et al., 1982). Patients studied with this combination had resistant rather than severe depressions. Of 94 inpatients receiving the MAOI tranylcypromine with a tricyclic, 68 percent responded, and side effects were no greater than from a tricyclic alone (Schmauss et al., 1988). Similar results occurred in a study of atypical depression (McGrath et al., 1994); this is attributable to diminished psychological anxiety from the MAOI with decreased tension and insomnia from the sympatholytic amitriptyline. In psychotic depression ECT was superior to the combination of phenelzine and amitriptyline (Davidson et al., 1978).

Lamotrigine

Complete remission of paranoid symptoms in three females who probably had psychotic depression suggests that high-dose lamotrigine might have a bona fide effect in psychotic depression (Erfurth et al., 1998). The effective lamotrigine dose was 400 mg/day. Using the expected method of gradual lamotrigine dose increases to decrease toxicity of adverse skin eruptions, it should take nearly 4 months to reach that dose level. Because the diagnosis used on those patients was schizoaffective, they were apparently not melancholic. Similarly, addition of lamotrigine to antipsychotic drugs led to marked reduction in severity of "confusion psychosis" in four patients (Dietrich et al., 2004). The lamotrigine doses used were 75–175 mg/day. This takes 2–6 weeks to achieve, respectively, because the starting dose is 25 mg/day and increases are by 25 mg/day once weekly. The patients in these case studies had either psychotic catatonic depression or epileptic psychotic depression. Antiepileptic effect by lamotrigine is no surprise. The intriguing implication we see in this is that lamotrigine has an anticatatonia effect, whether similar to lorazepam or additive.

Serotonin Reuptake Inhibitors (SRIs, SSRIs)

wDrug companies are licensed by the FDA to promote sales of SSRIs to treat major depression. Although major depression includes several different conditions, the FDA did not differentiate among types of major depression. Yet they should have because the drug-company clinical testing of SSRIs excluded patients with psychotic depression. Drug companies are run by sales decisions, and typically their sales representatives are paid according to sales volumes in their territories. This means that the drug reps – who personally visit physicians in their offices and speak with them at meetings – encourage use of SSRIs for all major depressions. So it is natural to expect that physicians widely prescribe SSRIs for psychotic depression. Because they are ineffective for this, antipsychotic tranquilizers must be given together with SSRIs to decrease symptoms. However, this combination is equal in benefits to the antipsychotic tranquilizer alone.

SSRIs such as sertraline do not reliably treat psychotic depression. Specifically, in an 8-week open trial of sertraline in doses rising to 200 mg/day (Simpson et al., 2003), the 16 percent remission rate in patients with psychotic depression matched the expectations for placebo described earlier in this chapter. The remission rate for patients with nonpsychotic depression was 64 percent, substantially higher. In elderly patients treated for 12 weeks, nortriptyline alone was significantly more effective than the SSRI citalopram alone, particularly in psychotic depression (Navarro et al., 2001). Nevertheless, a group of psychiatrists in

Milan, Italy, have reported exceptionally high response rates – exceeding 75 percent – to fluvoxamine and sertraline in psychotic depression (Gatti et al., 1996; Zanardi et al., 1996, 1997, 1998, 2000). These rates are much higher than for any antidepressants alone in any studies elsewhere. Moreover, the response rate of nonpsychotic depression to SSRIs is repeatedly reported as barely higher than placebo, for example, 35 percent versus 26 percent for placebo (e.g., Schneider et al., 2003), 56–60 percent versus 42–47 percent for placebo (Arroll et al., 2005). These figures indicate that only about 10 percent of patients with mild depression respond to the specific pharmacological effects of SSRI drugs. In one large multisite study the response rate was higher for placebo than for SSRI at six of the nine study sites (Roose et al., 2004).

Accordingly, Rothschild and Phillips (1999) suggested that the patients in the Milanese studies would not have been diagnosed with psychotic depression elsewhere. They speculated that these patients rather had anxiety disorders or dissociative disorders. This is a profound discrepancy in diagnosis. It results from *DSM* allowing diagnosis to be given without evidence, purely on a subjective basis. The rebuttal from Milan was that pindolol accelerates response to fluvoxamine, and that similar results were seen in Brescia, Italy (Zanardi et al., 1999). However, Brescia is only a few kilometers from Milan, while the sole psychotropic effect of pindolol is as a beta-blocker, decreasing body tension anxiety. Specifically, pindolol effects on serotonin are too weak for corresponding clinical activity (Rabiner et al., 2001). In other words, the psychotropic effects of pindolol decrease anxiety only, and if adding pindolol improves response this points to anxiety disorder as the primary diagnosis.

Just as SSRIs do not treat psychotic depression they do not induce manic episodes. We could not find any reports describing use of s-adenosyl methionine (SAMe) or St. John's wort in psychotic depression. Several case reports describe onset of mania in people taking St. John's wort (Stevinson and Ernst, 2004) but this primarily suggests that some patients with serious mood disorders try St. John's wort before seeing a psychiatrist, not causality.

Combination antipsychotic-fluoxetine and -paroxetine

Let us come immediately to the point: This combination is a bad idea. Because SSRIs do not treat psychotic depression, giving an SSRI together with an antipsychotic tranquilizer is therapeutically equivalent to the antipsychotic alone, but has additional side effects. SSRIs decrease worrying and dissatisfaction, so these symptoms might be somewhat less with the combination, but for psychotic depression this is not the same as treatment. Of forty patients with psychotic depression who took perphenazine with fluoxetine for 5 weeks, thirty showed response. Response does not mean remission. Perphenazine was tapered out after 4 months and twenty-two patients showed no relapse over an additional 11 months, an overall success rate of 55 percent (Rothschild and Duval, 2003). This suggests that 4 months of antipsychotic drugs is not long enough for reliability. Although this study allows us to understand the effects of antipsychotic drug usage alone, it does not extrapolate to the use of an antimelancholic antidepressant such as nortriptyline with an antipsychotic drug. In an earlier and similar study the same authors excessively praised the fluoxetine-perphenazine combination by equating a 73 percent rate of 50-percent-symptom reduction to ECT effect (Rothschild et al., 1993); however upward of 73 percent is the remission rate from ECT, not merely the symptom reduction rate.

Fluoxetine and paroxetine inhibit elimination of most antipsychotic drugs, causing them to accumulate in the body just as if the patient were taking a larger dose. The equivalence of this larger dose varies with the antipsychotic drug. With perphenazine and other drugs eliminated by the 2D6, 3A3, or 3A4 pathways of the cytochrome P450 system, the drug blood level should rise on average somewhere between 200 percent and 900 percent, equivalent to 3–10 times the prescribed dose. For perphenazine this predisposes to excessive if not toxic drug exposure.

With olanzapine or clozapine the dose increase equivalence caused by fluoxetine or paroxetine is 50 percent on average. This can make the difference between calmness and apathy. Accordingly, comparing the combination of antipsychotic with paroxetine or fluoxetine against the antipsychotic alone is not valid without examining and accounting for the higher blood antipsychotic levels when fluoxetine or paroxetine is administered. Because these dose effects are large and highly variable, it is far riskier to combine antipsychotic drugs with fluoxetine or paroxetine than with other SSRIs such as venlafaxine. Again, because fluoxetine and paroxetine do not treat psychotic depression in any of its forms, the combination is equivalent to the antipsychotic drug alone. In contrast, the combination of venlafaxine, bupropion, or a TCA with an antipsychotic drug should be more effective than the antipsychotic alone.

The peculiar circumstances of the pill marketed as Symbyax deserve special mention – and caution. Symbyax packages olanzapine and fluoxetine in a single tablet. The basis for Lilly's claim of greater efficacy for Symbyax than olanzapine alone is that the HAM-D scale was lower with Symbyax than with olanzapine. However, the fluoxetine in Symbyax inhibits olanzapine elimination and raises olanzapine levels about 50 percent (Nelson and Swartz, 2000; Swartz, 2002). This is equivalent to a 50 percent larger dose of olanzapine, and it can account for Lilly's reports of greater efficacy of Symbyax than olanzapine alone. Although fluoxetine can decrease feelings of worry and dissatisfaction, it does not treat psychotic depression. Symbyax should decrease the symptoms of anxiety disorders and atypical major depression (itself a mislabeled anxiety disorder), but it is inappropriately strong and impairing for anxiety disorders except as a last resort. One of us (CS) says that prescribing Symbyax prematurely is analogous to attacking a mosquito with a brick. This method was mine as a 11 year old in boy scout camp; although the mosquito was huge the legend that followed was humongous. More recently I dispatched nearly a hundred three-inch red wasps in my home with a cardboard record sleeve entitled "Bugaloo." This corresponds to appropriate precision in treatment.

Although olanzapine by itself commonly causes weakness (so-called asthenia) and tiredness (somnolence), these symptoms should routinely be worse when given with fluoxetine because of higher olanzapine blood levels. Response of psychotic depression to Symbyax is highly variable; one of a pair of studies published by Eli Lilly Company itself showed response no better than placebo (Rothschild et al., 2004).

An Internet search revealed several individuals (not physicians) lauding Symbyax without mentioning taking it. The sales advantages of combining an antipsychotic with an antidepressant in one tablet began 30 years ago with the marketing of Triavil, combining perphenazine with amitriptyline. "Does-it-all" Triavil was widely prescribed by primary care physicians because it promptly decreased most psychiatric complaints and it was promoted as an antidepressant. Triavil diminished symptoms on a gamut from insomnia to worry, panic, agitation, psychosis, and depression. In taking Triavil patients paid the price of experiencing muscle stiffness and weakness, thought simplification, impaired problem solving, and tardive dyskinesia. Symbyax adds apathy, weight gain, and childlike oversimplicity, but has little muscle or movement problems, except in the elderly.

Other SSRIs in combination with antipsychotics

Citalopram in doses of 20–40 mg/day given with haloperidol in doses of 5–9 mg/day reduced symptom severity over 50 percent in seven patients with psychotic depression (Bonomo and Fogliani, 2000). As previously discussed, symptom reduction is crucially different from remission, and this degree of symptom reduction can be explained by antipsychotic tranquilization alone. We were unable to find any reports of studies of patient groups that reported success in using sertraline or fluvoxamine in combination with antipsychotic drugs to treat psychotic depression. Several reports noted that fluvoxamine causes doubling of olanzapine blood levels by inhibiting the cytochrome P450–1A2 metabolic pathway, equivalent to doubling the antipsychotic dose (Bergemann et al., 2004). When sertraline was given to four patients already taking antipsychotic medication, psychosis appeared (Popli et al., 1997).

Anticorticoids

Antagonists of cortisol receptors have recently been tried in treatments of psychotic depression. The background is that psychotic depression is accompanied by higher than normal production of corticotropin releasing hormone (CRH) and cortisol. The presumption is that these high levels of CRH and cortisol mediate all the symptoms of depression, and correcting them will treat the depression. An alternative hypothesis is that high levels of CRH and cortisol are only some symptoms of depression, and that correcting them might decrease some symptoms without treating the illness, analogous to aspirin for pneumonia. About half of patients with psychotic depression show a slight (average 10%) but definite excess of body cortisol production. In depressed patients with this cortisol excess, the anticortisol medication ketoconazole decreased the severity of depressive symptoms, while it had no effect in patients without cortisol excess (Wolkowitz et al., 1999).

After taking the anticorticosteroid mifepristone for 7 days, two-thirds of nineteen patients showed a mild decrease in depressive symptoms, and 42 percent showed response (but not remission) compared to 27 percent of the nominal dose placebo equivalent group (Belanoff et al. 2002). This high placebo response is peculiar for a one-week trial in psychotic depression. Moreover, a 1-week trial is peculiarly short; it was apparently necessitated by the health risks from continuing a body deficiency in cortisol for longer. Mifepristone (Corlux) showed effects no different from placebo in its first randomized, double-blind study for diminishing the severity of psychotic symptoms in psychotic depression. As with the 1-week open trial this 8-week study showed a remarkably high rate of improvement on placebo, specifically that 80 percent of patients receiving placebo showed 50 percent improvement (Corcept Therapeutics, Inc., 2006; DeBattista et al., 2006). The high placebo response reflected by the Hamilton Depression rating suggests that results were influenced by anxiety disorders or atypical depression, which were not excluded, and that the diagnosis of "psychotic depression" is not sufficient. Results for mifepristone in psychotic depression to date are distant from being clinically useful, and well behind those for TCAs and bupropion. Mifepristone was said to show promise in treating the psychosis of psychotic depression, but psychosis is just a symptom, so this is analogous to aspirin showing promise in treating the fever of pneumonia. Mifepristone is well known for its effects in preventing pregnancy; it is part of RU-486, the "morning after" birth control pill.

Mirtazapine, Nefazodone, Topiramate

Evidence suggests that mirtazapine, a drug marketed as an antidepressant, is not useful in psychotic depression. In a study of ninety-seven severely depressed inpatients, some of whom were psychotic, response occurred in 50 percent of those given imipramine alone but in only 22 percent of those who received mirtazapine (Brujin et al., 1996). An opinion article mentioned that mirtazapine is not effective in psychotic depression but provided no data (Birkenhager and Moleman, 1999).

The lone report on nefazodone in psychotic depression provides insight into investigator dissatisfaction with clinical results despite reductions in depression rating scores. This report described a retrospective study of ten patients on nefazodone and ten on amitriptyline-haloperidol, as well as a prospective study of the same. In the retrospective study, nefazodone brought one remission (10%) while amitriptyline-haloperidol brought none. Similar symptom reduction occurred with both treatments. In the prospective study, the HAM-D rating indicated remission (i.e., at least 60% fall and final score 8 or less) in five patients (50%) receiving nefazodone and three patients (30%) on amitriptyline-haloperidol. However, some of the prospective nefazodone patients showed continuing psychotic symptoms despite low depression ratings and the authors stated that their results do not support monotherapy with nefazodone in psychotic depression (Grunze et al., 2002). They also do not reflect well on the combination of amitriptyline and haloperidol.

Topiramate decreases somatic tension anxiety. There is no good evidence that it is an antidepressant. In patients with bipolar depression who were already taking a mood stabilizer, topiramate decreased the HAM-D score (McIntyre et al., 2002), but it could do this by decreasing somatic tension anxiety symptoms.

Repetitive Transcranial Magnetic Brain Stimulation (TMS)

In transcranial magnetic brain stimulation (TMS, rTMS), a rapidly changing intense magnetic field is applied to a small area of the head. In treating major depression this area is the left or right temple. Inside the brain this changing magnetic field induces an electric current through brain neurons. It is this electric current, not magnetism, that causes brain neurons to depolarize. A brain seizure is avoided rather than induced. Accordingly, TMS is similar to giving unilateral ECT at an electrical dose that is too low to induce a seizure. Such a "subthreshold" ECT procedure is not effective in treating depression. Even a unilateral ECT that includes a full tonic-clonic grand mal seizure but whose electrical dose is minimized has low effectiveness, working in only about one-third of patients who would respond to higher electrical dose (Sackeim et al., 1993). The similarity of TMS to subthreshold ECT suggests that for psychotic depression TMS is at best weak and unreliable. Perhaps TMS can treat some conditions that are not appropriate for ECT, such as vertigo, anxiety disorders, or the auditory hallucinations of some chronic psychoses.

Studies have not found TMS useful in psychotic depression. Meta-analysis of all fourteen data-based trials of transcranial magnetic brain stimulation discerned no clear evidence of clinically significant benefit in treating major depression of any kind (Martin et al., 2002). The few studies with positive results are outnumbered by the many reports of marginal or no substantial benefit. The overall weak effect speaks against TMS usefulness in the severe illnesses represented by psychotic depression. One study specifically studied rTMS for psychotic depression, comparing it against ECT. ECT superiority was "striking" and statistically significant, with ECT response in ten of ten and rTMS response in two of nine patients (Grunhaus et al., 2000). Conversely, a patient with depression and no history of psychotic symptoms developed "recurrent severe delusions" during a course of TMS (Zwanzger et al., 2002); fortunately, this is rare.

Surgery, deep brain stimulation, vagal nerve stimulation

Surely the group of treatments last to be chosen involves surgery. Even among these, there are two general groups, reversible and permanent. The possibilities include implantation of a vagal nerve electrical stimulator, implantation of deep brain electrodes, and destruction of brain tissue by surgery or gamma radiation.

The idea of vagal nerve stimulation for treating depression sprouted from its use in patients with severe epilepsy resistant to anticonvulsant medication. Some of these patients said that their mood was better with vagal nerve stimulation. This is partially attributable to higher morale from experiencing fewer epileptic seizures, with less frustration, and partially attributable to the deleterious mood effects of complex partial seizures. Even if vagal nerve stimulation improved mood directly, the connection with psychotic depression is speculative. Company-sponsored studies of vagal stimulation in patients with major depression have shown that the average clinical benefit is clinically insignificant (Rush et al., 2005). Although the results were also statistically insignificant, the vagal nerve stimulator was approved for marketing because there is no FDA standard for effectiveness of medical devices comparable to standards for new drugs. Perhaps predictors of good and reliable response to vagal nerve stimulation will eventually be discovered, but they are not yet known.

Deep brain stimulation for psychotic depression is an experimental procedure that involves implanting electrodes underneath the brain cortex (Slater, 2005). Uncontrolled OCD accounts for most of the hundred psychiatric patients who underwent this procedure. The electrical wires that connect to the electrode are brought through the skull and scalp and are attached to an electrical stimulator programmed by the psychiatrist. This procedure began in the management of intractable epilepsy and Parkinson's disease. Generally, the electrodes are located in the same brain regions where psychosurgery has been done, in the prefrontal cingulate gyrus or in the internal capsule just below the caudate nucleus. The electrical currents interrupt brain activity near the electrodes, mimicking surgical ablation.

At first glance, the deep brain stimulation method seems reversible, but long-term use should cause persistent if not permanent changes in the structure and function of the neurons exposed to persistent electrical currents. There is supposed to be negligible brain injury, except for about 1 percent of implantations complicated by hemorrhage or infection, but brain tissue can be damaged (Gimsa et al., 2006). This procedure should be reserved for patients whose condition could not be controlled by trials of medications and ECT. Still, it seems preferable to ablative psychosurgery and gamma radiation.

In a small series of undifferentiated cases of treatment-resistant depression, antidepressant effects were associated with a marked reduction in blood flow in white matter tracts adjacent to the cingulate gyrus (Mayberg et al., 2005). That is, deep brain stimulation blocked brain function near the electrodes, as ablative brain surgery does. Cingulate gyrus abnormalities are associated with OCD, so there is no clear relationship to treating psychotic depression. Conversely, deep brain stimulation for Parkinson's disease has caused depression and aggressive behavior (Piasecki and Jefferson, 2004). Surely the effects of deep brain stimulation are highly dependent on location; a location effective in treating psychotic depression has not been reported.

Along with treating chronic pain disorders and resistant OCD, psychosurgery is reported to alleviate chronic depression. However, we were unable to find any reports in the modern literature of psychosurgery for psychotic depression. An odium has clung, perhaps unfairly, to the procedure from the days of indiscriminate prefrontal lobotomy and even less clear diagnosis (Valenstein, 1987). Modern psychosurgery lesions are far smaller than the 1950s prefrontal lobotomy. They are generally confined to the cingulum, the basal ganglia, or the internal capsule. These lesions share side effects with antipsychotic tranquilizers, specifically simplification of the personality and loss of abilities in handling social complexity, solving problems, and multitasking. Of course these same abilities are impaired by illness. Psychosurgery is particularly risky for patients over age 70; their death rate within 1 year is 25 percent (Hodgkiss et al, 1995). Psychosurgery or gamma-ray neuronal ablation might conceivably provide important therapeutic benefits to patients with psychotic depression who remain unrelieved from other treatment methods. It is just that there is no published precedent for them.

8

Treatment by Type of Psychotic Depression

BECAUSE THERE ARE DIFFERENT TYPES OF PSYCHOTIC DEPRESSION, each must be treated appropriately. The reader will find here a practical guide born of years of experience – by author CS – plus an attentive reading of the literature. Few claims made in pharmaceutical advertising will be reflected in these pages.

Melancholic psychotic depression

Because this condition is usually long standing with multiple episodes of illness that come and go, treatment has two phases: acute and preventive. We will review these in order.

There are three kinds of acute treatments for this. We will summarize them first and then explain. They are antidepressant medication alone, combination antidepressant and antipsychotic medication, and ECT. Antidepressant medication brings remission in only about a third of

Table 8.1 Strategy for melancholic psychotic depression

If urgent start ECT. If ECT not available, start sedation plan, add antidepressant
If you can do 5-day trial, start both brief trial plan below and ECT workup. If no large improvement in 5 days, switch to ECT. If ECT not available, add quetiapine unless patient recently took substantial doses of another antipsychotic drug
With well-supervised elderly patients where the only urgency is frustration, there are several choices

patients, so a trial to see if it might suffice should be limited to a few days. Antipsychotic medication causes impairment and serious adverse effects so it is desirable only if limited to a few months or as a last resort. ECT requires more physician expertise and hospital resources, but expertise and hospital resources are modern medicine. ECT nearly always works promptly. With maintenance medication or continuation ECT, relapse is not more common after ECT than after medications alone.

The typical treatment strategy (Table 8.1) begins with deciding how urgently improvement is needed. If response is particularly important within 5 days start with ECT. If ECT is not available start the "sedation plan" (Table 8.2), then add antidepressant medication in a day or two. If you have 5 days or more for a medication trial, begin the short medication trial plan given below, while starting the medical evaluation procedures in preparation for ECT. This is to avoid delays in starting ECT if the medication is not effective.

Except as a last resort, the sedation plan is temporary and an adjunct to treatment. The problem in starting tranquilizers is in stopping them because it risks agitation. Accordingly, whenever starting tranquilizers, write the tentative plan for discontinuation.

As an unbendable rule benzodiazepines should be used for no longer than 2 weeks, not counting up to two more weeks of gradually lowering doses for discontinuation. Longer use promotes impairment. Avoid

Table 8.2 Sedation plan

For adults who are not elderly

1 Mild: lorazepam 0.25–0.5 mg orally 3–4 times/day. Avoid alprazolam. This is for 2 weeks or less.

2 Moderate: lorazepam 0.5–1 mg + quetiapine 50–100 mg 2–3 times/day.

3 Moderately intense: lorazepam 0.5–0.75 mg + quetiapine 100–200 mg 4 times/day

4 Intense: lorazepam 0.5–0.75 mg + molindone 10–20 mg 4 times/day. Molindone persists less than others after discontinuation.

5 Emergency: lorazepam 1.5 mg + droperidol IV or IM 5–10 mg.

In the above lorazepam should be discontinued or tapered within 2 weeks.

For elderly adults

1 Mild: hydroxyzine (Atarax) 10 mg every 4–6 hours. Quetiapine 12.5–25 mg 2–4 times daily.

2 Moderate: quetiapine 50–100 mg 2–4 times daily.

3 Intense: quetiapine 100–150 mg 4 times daily + olanzapine 2.5–5 mg 2–3 times daily oral or parenteral.

4 Emergency: droperidol 5 mg possibly with olanzapine instant disintegration (zydis) 10 mg.

In emergency droperidol efficacy outweighs cardiac QTc risks and alternatives. Strictly avoid haloperidol.

alprazolam because it is far too difficult to decrease. For nonelderly adults, using low-dose benzodiazepines for up to 2 weeks is reliable and has few side effects. For elderly adults, benzodiazepines too easily provoke delirium and falling.

The quality of sedation with antipsychotic tranquilizers varies enormously by drug, and so do risky side effects. Whenever possible, try to use oral quetiapine or a mixture of lorazepam and quetiapine. This corresponds to having at least an hour for the medication to work. If quietude is needed sooner, parenteral droperidol is reliable; if needed immediately, droperidol is labeled for intravenous use. Droperidol is sedating and has milder side effects than haloperidol, which is not sedating. Moreover, droperidol effects rarely persist more than 24 hours and Parkinsonian side effects are much milder than haloperidol.

Hydroxyzine is strong enough to take the edge off but not for much else. This can provide enough comfort for mildly tense patients, but will not reliably decrease problematic agitation.

The usual initial treatment for this type is a short medication trial. If improvement is urgently needed or the patient is elderly, ECT is generally the desirable first treatment. Elderly patients usually have difficulty tolerating TCAs because of a tendency to fall, delirium, or cardiac arrhythmia.

For females who are not frail and elderly and have no history of mania, start triiodothyronine 25 μg (not mg) in the morning together with nortriptyline 75–125 mg/day, aiming for serum levels of 60–150 ng/ml. At the same time obtain an ECG and draw tests to screen out hyperthyroidism (e.g., T4 and T3 uptake). This is a 3–4-day trial; if there is clearly no improvement by then with a serum nortriptyline level in range, switch to ECT; likewise if clinical response does not match an urgent need. If the patient was taking only a TCA and has not responded, adding the latter can bring substantial improvement. If there is continuing but incomplete improvement without urgency, adjust nortriptyline dose if needed and continue until either remission success or inadequate improvement plateau nonsuccess. If serum nortriptyline level is out of range after 3–4 days without clear clinical improvement or urgency, adjust dose for 3–4 more days of trial. If these medications can bring remission, it will happen within a week. If in a previous episode a female patient failed to respond to a TCA with triiodothyronine, treat in the same way as described for male under 40 years old or below or start with ECT. For bipolar females, treat in the same wasy as described for males under 40 years old.

Frail and elderly generally means either frail and of age 65–80 or over 80 years of age regardless. Below age 80, frail generally means weak, physically ill, or easily injured. If there is any urgency at all, the first choice treatment for frail and elderly females is ECT. If there is no urgency, start venlafaxine sustained release and gradually increase the dose to 150–225 mg/day. If the patient is agitated or does not respond to venlafaxine, add quetiapine 12.5–25 mg twice daily.

If the patient was already taking thyroxine tablets but not triiodothyronine to correct hypothyroidism (e.g., Synthroid), adjust the doses of both equally. In collaboration with the treating internist, decrease the daily thyroxine dose by 25 μg/day while adding the equal triiodothyronine dose.

For males 40 or older with no history of seizure or traumatic brain injury, start bupropion 200 mg/day (100 mg/day for most men over 70 years). If the patient had a previous episode of mania or mixed manic-depressive state, start lithium as well, as described in the paragraph for males under 40. This is a 5-day trial. If no improvement occurs within 5 days, switch to ECT. Higher bupropion dosage is unlikely to make a difference and is not worth trying if there is any urgency for response. If bupropion is undesirable for a patient, and the patient is not frail and elderly, treat as males under age 40. If the patient is frail and elderly, start venlafaxine sustained release and gradually increase the dose to 150–225 mg/day. If that fails, switch to ECT.

For males under 40 or who have a history of seizure or traumatic brain injury, start regular doses of nortriptyline (75–125 mg/day) and lithium. This also applies for females with a previous episode of mania or mixed manic-depressive state who are not frail and elderly. Start nortriptyline first, then add lithium the next day. Start a lithium dose you expect to be the eventual steady-state dose. Check serum lithium after 48 hours; the eventual steady-state lithium level should be about 1.33 times that particular spot lithium level. A prompt lithium adjustment at this time should prevent excessive lithium levels from developing later. Check serum nortriptyline level after 4 days (96 hours) together with a second lithium level. The eventual steady-state nortriptyline and lithium levels should be about 1.14 times these fourth-day levels. If the patient experiences increased thirst or urination on lithium, start potassium chloride supplements 15 meq 1–2 times daily (Musa and Tripuraneni, 1993). Adjust lithium and nortriptyline doses according to the expected steady-state level. This should be a 5–7-day trial. If substantial clinical improvement occurs, continue the trial. If no substantial response occurs or if drug response later plateaus at an inadequate level, switch to ECT.

CSwartz says: When I was a resident psychiatrist on the ward at the University of Iowa Hospitals we received many patients with melancholic depression. None of these patients was well enough to manage outside the hospital. Except for a few relatively moderately or briefly ill females who responded to the combination of triiodothyronine (Cytomel) and a TCA, all failed to respond to tricyclics and went on to have ECT. ECT worked. This path was followed whether or not psychosis was present. Sometimes it seemed that tricyclics never worked and most patients on the ward were taking ECT. Eventually it was obvious that using TCAs alone was an exercise in futility that simply prolonged patient stay. My routine for treating females was to immediately draw screening thyroid blood tests (total T4, T3 uptake) and an ECG, start nortriptyline and triiodothyronine, and proceed with the routine ECT workup. If the patient showed no improvement at all in about 4 days, I would start ECT. The beauty of using nortriptyline and triiodothyronine is that it is a fast trial; when it works, clear improvement is usually seen in 1–3 days. Unlike most TCAs, the nortriptyline dose is usually limited according to its serum blood level (150 ng/ml) and not by side effects such as dizziness.

A range for serum nortriptyline levels is not established for psychotic depression. If the patient does not respond within the usual range of 50–150 ng/ml , there is no data precedent against increasing the dose to reach a serum level within 200–275 ng/ml.

Despite about twenty trials I have never seen a male hospitalized for melancholia respond to a tricyclic with triiodothyronine. My routine for treating males eventually became starting bupropion and proceeding to ECT if no improvement at all developed within 5 days. This avoids the need to check thyroid tests. However, bupropion can provoke seizures in some patients, so an EEG is needed in patients who become confused or develop what seems to be catatonia on it (because it might be delirium).

Patients whose melancholia is not severe enough to require hospitalization typically respond to tricyclics or bupropion. However, psychotic melancholics nearly always need hospitalization because of impaired judgment, self-care abilities, or suicidality.

Although side effects from nortriptyline should be less than with amitriptyline or imipramine, some elderly patients still cannot tolerate it. This is usually because of orthostatic hypotension, cardiac arrhythmia, or delirium. The approach is to use nortriptyline, not to avoid it, but to routinely screen for these particular side effects.

If the treatments above do not succeed, four ordinary alternatives remain. These are using MAOIs, the combination of an antimelancholic antidepressant and quetiapine, the combination of an antimelancholic antidepressant with another antipsychotic drug, and clozapine.

Of these, the one most likely to produce a true remission is the MAOI. The advantage of a true remission is that the thought disorder and suicidality generated by the psychotic depression disappear. In the seeming remission achieved with the other agents, these problems can remain.

MAOIs can treat psychotic depression (Swartz, 1979), although doses are higher than needed for atypical depression and anxiety disorders. Appropriate doses of phenelzine start at 15 mg three times daily and can progress to twice that. The dose is usually limited by orthostatic hypotension. All patients who take MAOIs must maintain a special tyramine-free diet 48 hours before the first dose, for example, excluding aged cheeses, red wine, and several uncommon particular foods. They must scrupulously avoid a variety of over-the-counter and prescribed medications, including SSRIs, buspirone, bupropion, stimulants, and decongestants. These precautions aim to prevent a dangerous rapid rise in blood pressure. After stopping fluoxetine, at least 5 weeks must pass before starting an MAOI. In my experience, response to MAOI is abrupt, in contrast to the gradual day-by-day improvement seen with other medications. Patients show no clear change, then suddenly overnight 2–3 weeks later they are back to normal. MAOIs can induce mania in a dose-related manner, for example, the patient is manic at 60 mg/day but not at 45 mg/day (or an elderly patient is manic at 45 but not at 30).

If the patient does not show remission on MAOI, it is risky to combine with an antipsychotic drug or other tranquilizer. This is because MAOIs are extremely deadly in overdose, and reducing symptoms with a tranquilizer does not reliably remove suicidality symptoms. Prudence indicates ensuring that before hospital discharge either the patient on MAOI is no longer suicidal or the MAOI is stopped.

Of the four remaining alternatives noted above, the easiest to prescribe is the combination of quetiapine and an antimelancholic antidepressant. This is because these medications are familiar and relatively safe from extrapyramidal symptoms, tardive dyskinesia, and tardive psychosis. Although overdose can be deadly with this combination, it should be least dangerous with venlafaxine and worst with a TCA. Accordingly, if the patient has any risk of self-injury, a desirable combination is quetiapine with venlafaxine in the range of 200–300 mg/day, or 150–200 mg in the elderly. The daily dose of quetiapine would be 600–800 mg/day, or a quarter to half that in the elderly. Achieving these doses requires a gradual build-up from low starting doses, 37.5 mg/day of venlafaxine, and 12.5–50 mg twice daily of quetiapine. If the patient has no risk of self-injury, it is reasonable to simply add quetiapine to the antimelancholic antidepressant the patient was taking.

If the combination of quetiapine and an antidepressant fails to succeed, it is reasonable to replace quetiapine with loxapine starting at 10 mg twice daily. Loxapine would be increased as needed up to 40 mg twice daily, half that in the elderly. The use of a dopamine-blocking antipsychotic drug for no more than 4 months should sharply decrease the possibility of Parkinsonian symptoms and tardive phenomena. Still, patients over age 65 at least occasionally show extreme sensitivity to low doses of dopamine blockers, with symptoms that persist for several months, after taking and stopping just a few doses. Octogenarians can develop fatal neuroleptic malignant syndrome after just a few haloperidol 2 mg doses.

Clozapine is generally reserved as the ordinary last choice, for the most resistant and serious cases, to be used for at least several years. It is the last choice because of its risks and its potent psychological side effects. Patients who take clozapine are not unhappy, but they do not realize how it has changed their personalities and capabilities. The dose is usually started at 25 mg twice daily. Maintenance doses should be 200–800 mg/day, a quarter to half that in the elderly. With clozapine the white blood cell count is monitored weekly, and eventually every 2 weeks, to prevent agranulocytosis.

Preventing recurrence of the melancholic type

In most patients with psychotic depression, recurring episodes of depression or mania are major personal intrusions and problems. They disrupt all aspects of life including career, marriage, and family, and they risk death and injury from suicide and from pulmonary and cardiac illnesses. Here we identify three different philosophies to prevent recurrence of depression. Two or all can be used together.

The continuation philosophy is that the treatment that was effective will prevent recurrence. This generally means that nortriptyline is continued to prevent depression. Despite its simplicity, TCA continuation does not work reliably. However, after a course of ECT imipramine strongly prevented relapse in patients who failed to respond to imipramine before ECT (van den Broek, et al., 2006). The continuation philosophy for a patient who relapses on TCAs after ECT sometimes means outpatient ECT every 2–4 weeks for months to years; this works reliably but is time consuming when counting transportation.

The bipolar philosophy is that addition of lithium will prevent further depression as well as the development of mania. Although lithium by itself does not reliably treat psychotic depression, it prevents relapse. Some studies indicate the combination of TCA and lithium is not more effective than lithium alone in preventing bipolar depression (Ghaemi et al., 2001); psychotic depression should be the same. Likewise, a worse outcome resulted from discontinuing lithium but not from discontinuing the tricyclic imipramine (Prien et al., 1984). The routine plan for a patient who responded to a TCA would be to continue the tricyclic and add lithium, then taper out the tricyclic after 3–6 months.

Separate from the above is the stress-related philosophy, that episodes of psychotic depression are triggered in susceptible people by activation of the sympathetic nervous system. This is the fight-or-flight panic-related emergency excitement system. Its persistent activation without a real threat is a core problem in anxiety disorders and can be called body tension anxiety.

This philosophy suggests that patients with both psychotic depression and an anxiety disorder (such as PTSD or GAD) will have more depression than patients who have no anxiety disorder. The most effective and specific body tension anxiety reducers are long-acting beta-blockers that reach the brain (betaxolol given twice daily or bisoprolol thrice daily) and certain anticonvulsants (topiramate, lamotrigine).

Patients who have recently recovered from psychotic depression and do not have a problem with body tension anxiety can probably prevent it from starting by taking an antiobsessive drug alone. People who already have an anxiety disorder need both an antiobsessive drug and a body tension reducer. Antiobsessives include buspirone and SRIs such as venlafaxine or SSRIs such as fluvoxamine. The stress-related philosophy might explain how lamotrigine prevents recurrence of depression. Preventing or treating anxiety symptoms seems a logical step for patients with a concurrent anxiety disorder or a particularly difficult life course of psychotic depression. What we mean by a difficult course is disappointing response to basic prevention, frequent recurrence, or repeatedly inadequate response to antidepressant medication.

The sympathetic nervous system is connected to the body's circadian rhythm system, that is, the biological day clock. Disturbing the circadian rhythm should cause body tension anxiety and – in susceptible people – serious depression. Indeed, jet lag can provoke serious depression. Total sleep deprivation has temporary antidepressant effects, despite its annoying qualities. Maintaining a regular daily schedule for sleeping and meals should valuably prevent stress on the circadian rhythm system and decrease body tension anxiety. We would not spoil the fun of staying out late, but an episode of psychotic depression would.

Patients with earlier onset of illness, greater severity of thought disorder (Wilcox et al., 2000), or frequent past relapses stand greater risk of relapse. Those with serious suicidality or dangerous agitation bear greater risk if relapse occurs. These patients with excessive risk of relapse, or risk from relapse, should be considered for maintenance with concurrent lithium and antimelancholic antidepressant or maintenance ECT.

Psychosis-dominant depression

The two subtypes, bipolar mixed state and deteriorative, are discussed separately.

Bipolar mixed state subtype

If the patient seems to have a mixed manic-depressive episode, had a previous manic or mixed manic-depressive episode, or had a psychosis or severe depression within 2 months of childbirth or abortion, treat the patient as bipolar. If response is urgently needed, the promptness and reliability of ECT make it appropriate. If ECT is needed but not available, start the "sedation plan" described earlier, then add acute treatment medications. If five or more days are available for a medication trial, start lithium carbonate or valproic acid. The presence of psychosis or irritability does not detract from selecting lithium or point toward valproic acid.

Start a lithium dose you expect to be the eventual steady-state dose. With normal kidney function, for males between 40 and 65, this is typically 1,200 mg/day and for females 900 mg/day. Check serum lithium after 48 hours; the eventual steady-state lithium level should be about 1.33 times this. A lithium dose adjustment at this time should prevent high lithium levels later. After another 24 hours check a second lithium level; the steady-state lithium level should be about 1.14 times this level. If the patient experiences increased thirst or urination, start potassium chloride 15 meq 1–2 times daily. Aim to exceed a serum lithium level of 0.7 within 4 days of starting lithium, but avoid exceeding 1.0 meq/l. Draw blood frequently enough to assure this, even if daily. The patient should reach maximal improvement within 3 days of entering this range. This should be a 5–7-day trial. If no substantial response occurs or if clinical improvement plateaus at an inadequate level, add valproic acid, unless the patient prefers the higher reliability of ECT.

To use valproic acid, start a dose that is 30 mg/kg per day, rounded down to the nearest 250 mg. For frail or elderly patients, start 20 mg/kg instead. For generic valproic acid, divide the daily dose so that each individual dose is 750 mg or less. The more costly Depakote ER can be taken once daily. Draw the first serum valproic acid level within 2 days. If drawn 16 hours after the first dose, the eventual steady-state serum level should be about twice that spot level. If drawn 32 hours after the first dose, and the first day's dose was repeated on the second day, the steady-state level should be about 1.33 times that level. Aim to bring the serum valproic acid level into the range of 70–100. Draw blood frequently enough to assure this, even if daily. The patient should achieve maximal improvement within 2 days of entering this range. This should be a 4–7-day trial. If no substantial response occurs or if clinical improvement plateaus at an inadequate level, add lithium, unless the patient prefers ECT. If the combination was already tried, ECT should be desirable.

Deteriorative subtype

If the patient has cerebrovascular disease or strong risks for it, and if an anxiety disorder is not present, ECT is the treatment of choice. If somatic tension anxiety is present but the delusions or hallucinations are bizarre, ECT is still desirable. This is not only because ECT should succeed, but because the likely ineffectiveness of medication makes it truly second best. If ECT is not available, start the "sedation plan" and treat with lithium or valproate as described above.

Method of antipsychotic management

If none of the methods above is successful, it seems that only management by antipsychotic tranquilization remains, such as described here. If the patient did not recently take antipsychotic drugs for more than 3 months, start quetiapine at 25 mg to 100 mg twice daily. Elderly patients should receive half that dose. Increase the dose every 3–7 days until stabilized, with a maximum of 800 mg/day. Perhaps more than 800 mg/day might be appropriate for a few patients, but we cannot advise for or against that. If the patient has taken antipsychotic drugs for the past 2 years or longer, consider the possibility of tardive psychosis, and please see that section. If quetiapine is not effective under these circumstances, switch to another antipsychotic drug, such as loxapine 10–30 mg twice daily, or perphenazine 8–32 mg/day. If the antipsychotic drug you choose is not effective, switch to olanzapine in doses of 10–25 mg/day, half that with elderly patients. After olanzapine, clozapine is appropriate, prescribed as in the treatment of schizophrenia.

Treating severe anxiety disorder

Occasionally, psychosis-dominant depression represents the severe expression of an anxiety disorder. When this happens, it should be treated as an anxiety disorder. This should be suspected if the patient has an anxiety disorder with strong somatic tension anxiety: if the patient's affect is contagiously tense or concerned but otherwise normal and not blunted; if the delusions or hallucinations are paranoid and not bizarre; if the patient is worried and unhappy about the delusions or hallucinations (they are "ego-dystonic"); if the patient's speech is normal excepting signs of tension; and if the content of the delusions or hallucinations is circumscribed rather than pervasive. In such cases, and when there is no risk of dangerous behavior, consider a trial of the antianxiety treatment plan. If there is dangerous behavior or a risk for it, add the "sedation plan" described earlier to the antianxiety treatment plan.

This section describes the treatment plan for severe anxiety disorder. At the minimum, both an antitension drug and an antiobsessive drug are needed. First, start an antitension drug, if the patient does not have asthma, congestive heart failure, bradyarrhythmia, peripheral vascular insufficiency or Raynaud's disease and does not already take a beta-blocker. If the patient has congestive heart failure, consult with an internist; a beta-blocker might be desirable for that as well. The best psychotropic beta-blocker is betaxolol 2.5–5 mg twice daily. It is the best because it enters the brain at moderate speed, has a long half-life (about 19 hours), is beta-1 selective, does not disturb sleep architecture, and does not cause depression. Everyone who takes care of patients with anxiety disorder should be familiar with what betaxolol can do in reducing somatic tension anxiety. Check blood pressure at baseline and after at least 3 days. Caution the patient to avoid falling. If you have little experience working with betaxolol, the single best dose is 2.5 mg in the morning and 5 mg at bedtime. This requires a pill splitter because the tablet is 10 mg. In treating tension the minimum is 5 mg/day and the maximum is 10 mg/day. If the patient has not had an ECG recently, one should be obtained.

If the patient is already taking metoprolol (or Toprol) because of cardiovascular disease, collaborate with the internist to change the dose to metoprolol sustained release given twice daily or bisoprolol 2.5–5 mg three times daily. For psychotropic purposes, these drugs should not be taken less frequently over the day because this will not give a smooth enough blood level for good antitension effect. Bisoprolol relieves tension better than metoprolol sustained release does. These drugs have proven cardiac benefits that led internists to prescribe them for many patients.

Nadolol and atenolol are ineffective as psychotropic agents because they do not enter the brain. Propranolol works quickly but often causes rebound effects. Pindolol avoids rebound effects but has a short half-life, so must be taken four times daily (occasionally three times daily in the elderly).

If the patient cannot take a beta-blocker, or if tension remains problematic despite the beta-blocker, add topiramate 25 mg twice daily. Good topiramate dosage varies enormously among patients, from 25 mg once daily to 100 mg three times daily. Topiramate dose increases are typically every 3 or 4 days. In CS's clinical work, clear improvement on topiramate consistently occurs within 1 day of reaching an effective dose. The observable improvement plateaus in about a day. Patients typically report feeling this improvement, and some experience further subjective improvements over several weeks. Avoid topiramate in patients with kidney stones. If topiramate is not tolerated or ineffective, consider replacing it with lamotrigine, which also has an anxiolytic profile (Mirza et al., 2005); start 25 mg/day, increase by 25 mg/day no faster than once per week.

When the dose of topiramate or beta-blocker is too large, the patient feels tired, weak, or uncoordinated; blurry vision is possible. A patient who experiences this will usually demand to stop the medication. This is an important reason why excessive doses should be avoided. If you cannot convince the patient to take a lower dose, switch to a similar medication, such as bisoprolol instead of betaxolol, or lamotrigine instead of topiramate.

After the antitension drug is started, add an antiobsessional drug. When an antitension drug is given first, buspirone can make a large and easily appreciated improvement. Merely 7.5–15 mg twice daily of buspirone is sufficient.

With severe anxiety disorders, a second and different antiobsessional drug is usually desirable. Using two medications that operate in different ways on the same target is typically much more effective, analogous to combining sulfamethoxazole and trimethoprim to stop bacterial growth in treating urinary tract infections. More simply, it is analogous to picking up a large box with two hands in different positions on the box, rather than one hand underneath the other. Because of safety reasons, we recommend the nonprescription over-the-counter drug SAMe, S-adenosyl methionine, as the first or second choice antiobsessional drug, that is before or after buspirone, but before an SSRI. SAMe has been shown useful as an "antidepressant" (Papakostas et al., 2003). Whether it is an antiobsessional drug (as SSRIs are) or an antimelancholic (as tricyclics) or both is not established. In Swartz's clinical experience it has antiobsessional activity. In Europe SAMe is a prescription antidepressant. Typically start 400 mg once daily, increase to 600 mg/day after several weeks, and consider increasing to 800 mg/day. The maximum dose is 800 mg twice daily. When the SAMe dose is increased too rapidly it can provoke insomnia. Unfortunately, few hospital pharmacies will supply SAMe, and medical insurance will not pay for it. It should cost less than SSRIs.

If SAMe is not available, together with buspirone and one or more antitension drugs add an SSRI. The SSRI that Swartz prefers is generic fluvoxamine 50 mg/day because it is not known to cause cancer, as some SSRIs can (Swartz, 2004b), and medication interactions are rare and at most mild. An alternative is venlafaxine sustained release 75–150 mg/day; it has no known medication interactions.

Preventing recurrence of psychosis-dominant type

The preventive plan has two to three aspects. The first part is to continue the primary treatment. If it was ECT, lithium is a good selection, aiming for serum lithium level in the range 0.6–0.9 meq/l. The second part is to treat anxiety disorder, if present. The third part is to diminish cerebrovascular risks. This means stop smoking, lose weight if there is any tendency toward diabetes (as with high fasting glucose level), lower systolic blood pressure to 100–120 mmHg, decrease blood cholesterol, decrease homocysteine levels (e.g., with methylcobalamin tablets), and treat hypogonadism if present. Unfortunately, there is uncertainty about how best to treat female hypogonadism so as to decrease vascular risks; hopefully, this will be determined. Likewise, the treatment of male hypogonadism requires specific knowledge and experience with the risks and benefits.

Catatonic psychotic depression

The only treatment shown effective for catatonia is ECT, followed by maintenance with either more ECT, lithium, or TCA, or several of these. Based on case experience, clozapine probably also prevents recurrence after ECT, but other antipsychotic drugs do not.

Routinely for patients with catatonia, give a test dose of lorazepam, typically 1.5 mg by mouth or intramuscular injection. Then interview the patient yourself 60 minutes later. This will demonstrate the most that lorazepam can do to decrease symptoms. If you delegate the observation to someone else and they do not see an improvement, you cannot be sure of a lack of effect. Lorazepam will often, but not always, allow the patient to hold a conversation. The improvement will last for a period between 2 and 24 hours, on average about 6 hours. This temporary improvement represents a valuable opportunity to explain the patient's condition to him and obtain written informed consent for ECT. Give additional doses of lorazepam with the first two to three ECTs, to help the patient pay attention and assist in his treatment. At bedtime before ECT, give the patient a tablet or injection of lorazepam, typically 1 mg, and likewise about 2 hours before the ECT session. It is important to discontinue lorazepam early in the ECT course, such as after two or three sessions because it diminishes the ECT treatment, which weakens itself naturally along the course.

ECT is so effective in treating catatonic depression that if the patient does not improve it is reasonably likely that the patient has a coarse neurological disease causing the catatonic symptoms. Further evaluation might involve EEG, serum VDRL, sed rate, neurology consultation, thyroid panel, additional family history, genetics consultation, brain MRI, or spinal tap if not done before ECT.

Although some benzodiazepines (lorazepam, clonazepam, triazolam) temporarily decrease symptoms, no tests of the value of continued benzodiazepine use in catatonia have been reported. This means that no one knows what happens to patients with catatonia on benzodiazepines after hospital discharge or with long-term use. This is a serious shortcoming because patients who take benzodiazepines for anxiety typically become tolerant to drug benefits within weeks to months; that is, the drug stops working. Then, effects opposite to the benefits begin and get worse; that is, drug tolerance and rebound make anxiety worse. The same problem might well happen when a benzodiazepine is given for catatonia. The few catatonic psychotic patients that Swartz treated who declined to take ECT and were discharged on lorazepam 2 mg/day or more did not stay well; all were soon rehospitalized with prominent depression, psychosis, or catatonia. Nevertheless, there are a few exceptions. Perhaps 1 percent of patients with catatonia achieve good function on small doses of lorazepam, 0.5–1 mg/day; they deserve a trial of lorazepam maintenance without ECT.

If ECT cannot be given there are no established good alternatives, only a tiny number of case reports. Accordingly, these non-ECT alternatives are mentioned only as last and desperate resorts; even among these there are priorities. The first to try is lorazepam up to 1 mg/day. You should know what lorazepam can do from giving test doses. If this is not sufficient, change the dose to 2 mg/day and add lithium. If you see improvement within 48 hours of the serum lithium rising over 0.7 meq/l, attribute it to lithium and taper the lorazepam. If lithium levels are in the therapeutic range without bringing improvement, stop lithium and start lamotrigine 25 mg/day, then raise the dose every 7 days by 25 mg/day until remission is achieved or 200 mg/day is reached.

Recently a few case reports describe partial but meaningful improvement in patients with psychotic catatonia by administration of memantine (e.g., Carroll et al., 2005). Most of these reports are complicated by concurrent dopaminergic or antidopaminergic medication, serious medical conditions, and possibilities of delirium. These could interact with memantine, a medication whose FDA indication is cognitive impairment from Alzheimer's disease. Nevertheless, a trial of memantine is rapid and low risk and if the previously mentioned therapies do not bring improvement it should be considered.

Some psychiatrists prescribe antipsychotic tranquilizers for patients with catatonia, whether or not it is catatonic depression. In the hospital, CS has seen some patients improve rapidly with this regimen and others become much worse, developing excited catatonia or lethal catatonia. Lethal catatonia has many symptoms in common with neuroleptic malignant syndrome. As with benzodiazepines, no tests of the value of continued outpatient antipsychotic drug use in catatonic depression have been reported. Concurrent use of lorazepam or clonazepam with the antipsychotic drug might mitigate worsening if it occurs. The least risky antipsychotic tranquilizer to use in catatonia is probably quetiapine, followed by clozapine.

The preventive plan for catatonic psychotic depression after recovery with ECT is the same as for melancholic psychotic depression. The emphasis is on lithium, or maintenance ECT if lithium was not effective.

Psychotic-equivalent depression

This condition occurs primarily in elderly patients. Accordingly, delirium and deteriorative dementia must be considered at the same time. Often this includes examining for delirium tremens, scrutinizing the list of drugs taken for anticholinergic effects and benzodiazepines, and checking EEG, brain CT scan, blood oxygen saturation, urine cultures, erythrocyte sedimentation rate, and serum electrolytes and thyroid hormone levels. Evaluation for delirium and dementia are complex topics outside the purview of this book. Once these have been ruled out or found attributable only to depression, the only reliable treatment is ECT. If ECT cannot be given, a distant second plan is to treat with medications as for melancholic depression.

The preventive plan includes the same steps as for melancholic depression, along with measures to slow cerebrovascular deterioration.

This is because psychotic-equivalent depression predicts the development of Alzheimer's disease or cerebrovascular dementia, even when the cognitive difficulties disappear with treatment. Several actions might prevent or delay the dementia; these are the same steps that decrease heart attacks and strokes. They are stopping smoking, losing weight if there is any tendency to diabetes, lowering blood pressure, decreasing blood cholesterol and homocysteine levels, and referring for treatment of hypogonadism if present.

Tardive psychotic depression

This is an area without established treatment; that is, all treatment plans are speculative. Nevertheless, consideration of principles, literature reports, and case experiences suggest four different treatment plans. These are better than dismissing this diagnosis and overlooking this common and debilitating chronic condition. They are presented below in ranked order.

The lithium method for tardive psychosis

This method probably has the best combination of efficacy and safety. Start lithium carbonate, as described under psychosis-dominant depression. Once therapeutic serum lithium level has been reached, stop antipsychotic drugs entirely and at once. If agitation occurs, use the "sedation plan" described earlier. If you find that you cannot discontinue the sedation, even gradually, add carvedilol as below. If this does not succeed, switch to the clozapine method described below.

Strictly avoid all antipsychotic drugs, excepting quetiapine and clozapine. This method has worked well in each of the highly selected but severely disturbed cases that CS has used it with, without any need for sedatives (Swartz, 1995). Still, all his experience is with inpatients, and it seems risky for outpatients.

The carvedilol method for tardive psychosis

Carvedilol is a drug with several active pharmacological effects, none of which separately explains its benefits. It is a beta-adrenergic blocker, an alpha-adrenergic blocker, a calcium channel blocker, and a powerful antioxidant. It rapidly decreases several tardive phenomena including dyskinesia, vomiting, hiccupping, obsessions, and depression (Stueber and Swartz, 2006). Carvedilol should not be used if the patient has asthma, bradyarrhythmia, peripheral vascular insufficiency or Raynaud's disease. If the patient already takes a beta-blocker, you should collaborate with the prescriber to switch to carvedilol. If the patient has cardiac problems, collaboration with an internist is prudent. A good starting dose is 6.25 mg four times daily, for an elderly patient half that. Check the blood pressure and pulse before and after starting carvedilol. Start the carvedilol while the patient is still taking the antipsychotic drug. After a day, discontinue the antipsychotic drug entirely and abruptly. If agitation occurs, use the "sedation plan" described above, then double the carvedilol dose if tolerated and try to taper out sedation.

The clozapine method for tardive psychosis

Start clozapine while the patient is still taking the antipsychotic drug, at 25 mg twice daily. If the patient is taking a benzodiazepine, respiratory failure can occur, so try to minimize the dose and consider using pulse-oximetry monitoring. Then start tapering the antipsychotic drug while increasing the clozapine dose, every 2–3 days. At 300 mg/day clozapine, stop any other antipsychotic drugs. You can continue gradually increasing the clozapine dose to as high as 800 mg/day. Monitoring serum clozapine levels to guide the dose is helpful. A white cell count must be drawn weekly for at least several months, then at least every 2 weeks, to prevent deadly agranulocytosis (nonproduction of white blood cells). If the white blood cell count falls below 2,000, promptly consult a hematologist about administering granulocyte-stimulating factor, which is commercially available.

The antipsychotic method for tardive psychosis

This method is for short-term symptom management. It is not good treatment because it makes tardive psychosis worse. It consists of giving the patient more of the same type of medication that caused the tardive psychosis, the dopamine-blocking antipsychotic drug. The method is simple: just raise the dose until the symptoms respond. A strong response to slightly higher doses of dopamine-blocking medication is said to be the clinical archetype characteristic of tardive psychosis (Chouinard and Steinberg, 1984). With time the dose should need further increase. Of course, the psychological impairments of taking dopamine-blocking antipsychotic tranquilizers continue.

Drug-induced and hormone-induced psychotic depression

The general treatment approach starts with stopping or reducing as much as possible the offending medication or hormone. Although this may prove inadequate, it can bring remission if what appears to be depression is actually delirium. Psychotic depression induced by hormones or hormone deficiency typically persists despite hormone level correction. It can be caused by excesses, deficiencies, or rapid drops in corticosteroids, thyroid hormones, and androgenic or estrogenic steroids.

If the psychotic depression was induced by hypothyroidism, it is often risky to administer the combination of triiodothyronine and nortriptyline until at least several weeks have passed. This is because these patients typically have cardiac problems from the hypothyroidism and administration of triiodothyronine increases thyroid hormone activity too rapidly, provoking arrhythmias. Although this seems to suggest using

ECT, hypothyroidism unfortunately predisposes to weaker ECT seizures. Nevertheless, this is only a tendency and not a rule, and ECT remains desirable if prompt response is urgent. Swartz says: After responding quickly to ECT I gave 2 years prior, a 70-year-old man experienced recurrence of depression with new onset of severe hypothyroidism. He was in uncompensated congestive heart failure. I was unable to obtain good quality ECT seizures similar to the previous course apparently because of hypothyroidism and the patient showed no improvement. Further ECT was postponed after three unsuccessful sessions, but the patient died 6 weeks later.

Corticosteroid-induced psychotic mood disorders can respond to lithium. If the patient is stable enough to permit a 5-day medication trial, you might try the lithium method as described under psychosis-dominant type, with the sedation plan if necessary. If this is not successful, your next recommended treatment plan might depend on the goal for the patient. If the patient is chronically impaired with medical conditions, using an antipsychotic tranquilizer might possibly not decrease the quality of life or add to impairment. If the patient does not have such chronic impairment, ECT might be much more desirable than an antipsychotic drug.

If the patient with drug- or hormone-induced psychotic depression appears to be in a catatonic state, an EEG should help to distinguish between catatonia and delirium. As one example, disulfiram (Antabuse) toxicity can include a delirium with prominent posturing, grimacing, staring, muteness, and waxy flexibility. This delirium should disappear spontaneously in half a week. If the patient has catatonia rather than delirium, treat as per the catatonia section given above.

Psychotic depression in epilepsy and epileptic psychotic depression – other coarse brain disease

There is no established treatment of the psychosis of epilepsy outside the treatment of epilepsy itself. Patients vary enormously in their response to anticonvulsants. On average, in groups of patients one anticonvulsant drug is as good as another; however, individual patients will respond differently to specific anticonvulsant drugs. New patented anticonvulsants have fewer side effects than phenytoin, primidone, and phenobarbital, but the psychiatric response is sometimes better to the old drugs.

Anticonvulsant drugs have three separate uses: anticonvulsant, antimanic, and antitension anxiety. Antimanic and antitension actions are often blended into "mood stabilization." However, these two actions are different and some strong antitension agents are not antimanic (e.g., topiramate, lamotrigine), while other strong antimanic agents decrease tension little or none (e.g., lithium, valproate). In treating epileptic depression, the antimanic and antitension actions are not primary considerations.

If the patient is not on an anticonvulsant, you will need to start one. If the patient remains symptomatic on an anticonvulsant, you will need to either add a second anticonvulsant or change the anticonvulsant.

The once-famous concept of "forced normalization" is misleading and an oversimplification. Its idea is that giving an anticonvulsant to a patient with seizure disorder induces psychosis or exacerbates one already present (Flor-Henry, 1983). The incorrect implied suggestion is to give only antipsychotic drugs and avoid anticonvulsants. A more complete explanation is that half-treating a seizure disorder can produce more psychotic behavior than the disorder itself created. Starting an anticonvulsant can change seizure activity from generalized grand mal seizures into complex partial seizures. This decreases the amount of seizure activity but can increase the amount of disordered behavior and psychosis. Grand mal seizures tend to be antipsychotic, although they can cause delirium. In contrast, complex partial seizures can be psychotogenic and can also cause delirium. What the patient needs is treatment that is more effective and not incomplete. If epileptic psychosis becomes worse during treatment with an anticonvulsant drug, consider increasing the dose, adding a second anticonvulsant, or changing the anticonvulsant.

Olanzapine can so powerfully diminish disordered behavior that it sometimes may suppress psychosis, depression, and all disturbed behavior caused by ongoing complex partial seizures (Swartz, 2001a). This is a clear example of how antipsychotics can decrease symptoms without treating the illness causing the symptoms. It illustrates how symptom reduction from antipsychotic drugs implies nothing about the nature of the patient's illness. Of course, it is inappropriate to withhold anticonvulsant treatment from patients with active seizure disorders.

Conversely, olanzapine and other antipsychotic drugs can induce seizures with delirious symptoms resembling depression and psychosis (Swartz, 2001b). In such cases it is not appropriate to continue antipsychotic drugs to try to reduce these symptoms because they are manifestations of delirium, not of major depression or a functional psychotic disorder such as psychotic depression or schizophrenia.

Treatment of psychotic depression in Alzheimer's and Parkinson's diseases is similar to its treatment without these diseases, except the goal is usually palliative and there is no clear meaning in the concept of returning to baseline function. We discussed basic management in the diagnosis section. Some patients will simply not respond to medication, despite intensive doses. ECT can ameliorate the symptoms of Parkinson's disease along with the depression, although Parkinsonian symptoms typically return within a few weeks of the last ECT. Although literature reports about ECT in Alzheimer's disease are sparse, Swartz has seen some psychiatrists frequently and successfully use ECT to treat resistant agitated depression in psychotic demented patients. The goal of decreasing agitated behavior to obtain patient safety, and manageability was reached.

Pseudopsychosis

Consider treating patients with pseudopsychosis for anxiety disorder, excepting those patients who have antisocial personality disorder.

Patients with anxiety disorders often have trouble identifying and explaining their distress as anxiety. They often claim to have major depression, bipolar-II disorder, adult attention-deficit hyperactivity disorder, or a medical condition to explain their symptoms. This claim can extend to psychotic depression. They are often dismissed as having borderline personality disorder, factitious disorder, or some other personality disorder. These patients should be evaluated for anxiety disorder. Treatment is outlined in the section above on psychosis-dominant type.

Untyped, Unknown, Unclear

Generally, these cases seem to call for more evaluation. Because your medical notes are likely to reflect uncertainty, you might want to get a second opinion from a respected colleague if the mystery drags on for several days. Swartz says: Speaking for myself, several circumstances seem to produce unclear cases. One is where the patient withholds essential history or it is not obtainable. Some of these patients I treated were abusing alcohol but hid this because, as one said, "I didn't want to be treated as just another alcoholic." When the patient cannot communicate accurately and collateral information is not available for several days, the "sedation plan" can be useful to buy time. Delirium can easily continue as an unclear diagnostic puzzle for hours to days. Mysterious cases with both psychosis and depressive symptoms are sometimes neurological, for example, Huntington's Disease. The absence of any information about biological relatives is peculiar enough to suggest such an illness.

When acute catatonia is seen only through staring behavior and partial mutism (such as sparse irrelevant speech), the diagnosis is easily missed, especially when a psychosis is also present. Catatonia is still more likely missed when the patient has a concurrent medical condition that can cause delirium or if the patient has experienced traumatic brain injury. Distinguishing between delirium and catatonia due to a medical condition often requires an EEG and a brain MRI. Twice recently CS diagnosed catatonia on patients hospitalized on a medical ward while a neurologist diagnosed delirium. The normal EEG was on the side of catatonia, and so was the fact that the symptoms persisted stably for several weeks. Sometimes the psychiatrist might be hesitant to diagnose catatonic depression because ECT is indicated yet difficult to arrange.

Patients who experienced traumatic brain injury can exhibit symptoms of any psychiatric illness acutely or chronically, and the symptom picture can change over time to seemingly visit different conditions. If seizure activity is occurring, the symptoms can be of delirium. I have seen enough cases of seizures occurring despite normal EEGs and a dismissive neurology consultation to know that every psychiatrist will see them too. Nevertheless, traumatic brain injury can produce psychotic depression, with or without catatonia; this is not delirium and does not respond to anticonvulsant medication. These nondelirium cases are generally treated according to their psychopathology as described above.

If the patient continues with a mysterious diagnosis, there is sense in conducting sequential trials of various treatments until something succeeds. However, diminishing the symptoms with antipsychotic tranquilizers suggests nothing about diagnosis because these drugs can suppress symptoms of depression, mania, delirium, most psychoses, anxiety, and epilepsy. The general principles remain that antipsychotic drugs are the last resort and sometimes a culprit, ECT is not a last choice but sometimes comes first; concurrent neurological illness, delirium, or anxiety disorder often contribute symptoms that appear to be depression or psychosis.

Residual depressive symptoms and PTSD

Serious illness – including psychotic depression – causes anxiety disorders such as PTSD. PTSD is a long-lasting condition of troubling memories, unhappy feelings, tension, and demoralization. PTSD becomes more likely with increasing numbers of stressful episodes. The psychiatric literature typically overlooks the development of anxiety disorders from psychotic depression and other serious depressions. Instead, psychiatrists attribute the symptoms of the anxiety disorder to the depression itself. Recently used terms for this are "chronic subsyndromal depression," "residual depression," or "nonresponsive depression." This is a basic problem because anxiety disorders such as PTSD are treated differently than psychotic depression.

As usual, before treatment comes diagnosis. Anxiety disorders are usually shown by both dissatisfaction and tension. Dissatisfaction is not observable, only reported by the patient. The patient believes he deserves better. Tension is usually observable as need to ventilate, irritability, hyperreactivity or impatience, fidgeting, restlessness, restless insomnia, or grating voice. Of course, dissatisfaction and tension can arise from frustrations, losses, or threats; it is when they continue and persist that they deserve treatment. Most "residual symptoms" of depression are aspects of tension.

The treatment of anxiety disorders is not easy and methods for effective treatment are not widely understood. This is part of the reason that anxiety disorders are typically not looked for once a depression is observed. Of course, anxiety disorders need to be diagnosed before they can be properly treated.

Both the dissatisfaction and the tension require treatment. Treating one does not treat the other. Removing dissatisfaction does not remove tension, except for mild cases. The treatment outline is described above under the psychosis-dominant type. The many details of these treatments are outside the scope of this book. However, it is worth repeating that SSRIs and buspirone do not calm the sympathetic nervous system and so do not decrease tension. The tension must be treated.

Appendix 1

Summary Guide to Psychiatric Concepts

For medication issues see Appendix 2: Summary Guide to Psychotropic Medication and Treatment.

History of illness and mental status examination

Much as in life, in medicine including psychiatry the understanding of the patient's complaint begins with listening to the history of the illness. Understanding the history often leads to the diagnosis.

The history of the present illness starts with understanding the dissatisfactions and complaints of the patient and family. Distinguishing between dissatisfaction and depression is important. The history identifies the very first onset of disturbances in behavior and speech and the time course of symptom disappearances and recurrences, hospitalizations, and medications.

The mental status examination is a description of the patient, perhaps similar to an observant character description in a book. It includes general appearance such as hygiene and amount of distress, attitude to the interviewer (helpful, passive, sarcastic), alertness, reliability, stated mood, observed emotional expression (affect), amount and peculiarities of muscle activity, rate and peculiarities of speech, basic intellectual function, peculiarities of expressed thoughts, and amount of insight. The study of these characteristics is called psychopathology.

Alertness is excessive in patients who are hypervigilant and hyperreactive. Progressively less alertness leads to somnolence (drowsiness), obtundation (decreased response), stupor (only slightly responsive), and coma. Diminished alertness is associated with catatonia or delirium.

The patient's mood is what he says it is. In contrast, affect is the nonverbal bodily expression of emotions, including rapport. A flat affect is mechanical. A labile affect changes rapidly. Several affects are joy, anger, concern, sadness, puzzlement, fatigue, tension, and surprise.

Observed muscle activity and speech patterns are important in assessing melancholia and catatonia. Initiation, response, and repetition are three different perspectives on expression of thoughts and movements. In depression there is typically little or no initiation of new thoughts or movements and only brief responses. These are referred to as poverty of thought and bradykinesia, respectively. A few patients will show agitation for no reason, that is, without a stimulus. Bradykinesia often includes a mask-like face and a bulging muscle just above the nose, called the "omega sign" because it looks like the upper or lowercase Greek letter omega, Ω or a rounded w.

Body tension anxiety is generally seen in the muscles. It points to an activated sympathetic nervous system, a switched-on emergency panic system when there is no emergency. Tension includes fidgeting, trembling, jumpiness, irritability, agitation, anger, loud or harsh voice, talkativeness, repetitiveness, muscle tightness, or restless insomnia. Tension anxiety can exist by itself or be caused by another condition such as psychotic depression. Observable tension is uncomfortable, like pain. Patients with tension of this nature need relief and might act unpredictably or dangerously to obtain relief. Most suicidal people are tense.

Basic intellectual function is called cognitive function. It includes orientation, which means accurate statement of name, place, date, and present circumstances. The "mini-mental state" exam (MMSE) concerns only intellectual function, and includes knowledge of current news events, basic arithmetic, simple recall, naming items, and following simple directions. A good MMSE score is 28–30, an adequate score for a person of little education is 23–27, and under 23 is abnormal.

Delusions and hallucinations are peculiarities of expressed thoughts. Delusions are unshakeable unrealistic statements the patient appears to genuinely believe. They are sometimes called fixed false beliefs, not related to real politics or an existing religion. Delusions cannot be changed by discussion. Hallucinations are false sensations when nothing was present, usually of hearing voices or noises, and sometimes of seeing or feeling something that is not there. Some hallucinations are not psychotic: such as when half-asleep, hearing one's name called, and seeing things after two nights without any sleep. Distortion of a face or image is not a hallucination. A firm meaning given to a hallucination is considered a delusion. If a patient obeys an auditory hallucination's demand he has a "command hallucination"; it typically indicates a dangerously low quality of judgment.

Psychiatrists distinguish between bizarre and nonbizarre delusions. A bizarre delusion is unrelated to ordinary life, for example, green men will come through the walls to take me. The delusion that the police or IRS are looking for the patient is not bizarre. Such nonbizarre delusions are common in psychotic depression.

Other thought problems of psychotically depressed patients might include obsessions (persistently repetitive thoughts), compulsions (persistently repetitive actions), paranoia (which can be delusional or just anxious), derailment of speech, and overinclusive speech (circumstantiality).

Insight refers to the patient's awareness of his illness and his need for treatment. As with the other parts of the examination there are many levels of insight. A psychotic patient who admits he is ill but maintains he would be fine if he could just get some good sleep is denying that his condition is an illness.

Psychiatric diagnosis

Physicians treat diseases, not symptoms, although diseases cause symptoms. When a disease goes into remission the symptoms should disappear. If a disease responds to treatment but does not go into remission the symptoms remain at a lower level. The book published by the APA that attempts to describe each diagnosis in a standard manner is the *DSM*; the current version is the fourth edition referred to as the *DSM*-IV. To qualify for a diagnosis a series of criteria must be met. Most criteria can be met in several different ways. *DSM* diagnoses were constructed by committees, are not based on evidence, and do not require hard findings except for catatonia or neurological conditions such as dementia.

Many diagnoses in psychiatry have historic robustness, antedating modern science. Many are coins with two sides, psychological and physical. For example, catatonia can be described in these two ways. Physically it includes such features as an affect of puzzlement, bewilderment, emotional vacancy or somnolence; slap-back muscle rigidity; nearly continual staring; grimacing or moldable posturing; and word echoing or partial muteness. Psychologically what do these have in common? They apparently represent extreme impairment of attentiveness, as in delirium. Most catatonia occurs with depression, but it can occur from a medical illness (such as traumatic brain injury) or with schizophrenia.

Melancholia is a sickly depression with marked slowness of thought production and bodily movements. The patients seem exhausted, stiff, and beyond caring. Melancholic patients usually do not respond happily to good news.

Schizophrenia is a diagnosis from a hundred years ago. It means a psychosis that lasts for at least 1 month (but sometimes at least 6 months) that cannot be attributed to a particular cause or to a mood disorder such as depression. Schizophrenia means nothing more than the patient is psychotic and we do not know why. Correspondingly, schizophrenia has no treatment, only palliation with antipsychotic tranquilizers. Schizophrenia should not be stated if the patient could have psychotic depression instead.

Schizophreniform disorder is a diagnosis that resembles schizophrenia in its features but it has not been present for as long. It is virtually impossible to reliably distinguish between a psychotic mood disorder (such as psychotic depression) and schizophreniform illness or schizophrenia. A basic reason for this unreliability is that the distinction is made on the basis of the patient's self-report of symptoms. Yet the patient's ability to report symptoms completely and accurately is impaired by illness, medications, and perhaps incomplete self-awareness. Under these circumstances it may harm the patient to apply a diagnosis of schizophreniform or schizophrenia rather than psychotic mood disorder.

Schizoaffective disorder is a diagnosis that has no reliability. Its meaning keeps changing with each edition of the *DSM*. A proper diagnosis of this condition requires observation of the patient without the effects of psychotropic medication, but this is virtually never feasible. This diagnosis should not be stated if the patient could have psychotic depression. A patient said to have schizoaffective disorder should be treated as if he has psychotic depression unless evidence is presented that this is not the case.

Laboratory tests in psychiatry

Both MRI and CT are methods of producing an anatomical image of the brain. The MRI resembles a black- and-white photo of the brain in cross-section. The CT looks like an X-ray picture, which it actually is. These images can reveal brain abnormalities that can cause confusion or depression, such as accumulation of blood or other fluid inside the brain, a stroke, a swelling, shrinkage or a growth. In psychotic depression and other forms of serious psychiatric illness, the MRI typically shows no abnormalities but some peculiarities. These peculiarities are highly intense white spots in the white matter around the cerebral ventricles. Sometimes the CT shows these spots. These spots have been known since the mid-1980s and are thought to represent changes in the walls of the small arteries (arterioles) that bring blood to the brain. Although some people show these MRI bright spots and do not develop psychiatric illness, the spots are associated with psychiatric illness, analogous to how smoking is associated with heart disease. Microscopic examination of the brain has not found visible changes that correspond to these MRI bright spots; their anatomical nature remains mysterious but their presence is verifiable.

EEG is a way of studying the electrical activity of the brain. The EEG is nearly always abnormal in epilepsy or delirium. It is usually normal in psychiatric illness, including in melancholic or catatonic depression. If a patient with psychotic depression has an abnormal EEG, the physical cause needs to be identified and treated.

Several blood tests are important in identifying medical illnesses that cause psychiatric problems. Hypothyroidism can cause psychotic depression; when the hypothyroidism is corrected the depression might leave or it might continue unchanged. Syphilis, AIDS, lupus, hyponatremia (low sodium), hypernatremia (high sodium), and diabetes are medical conditions that blood tests can reveal that can cause confusion (delirium) or depression.

Dexamethasone suppression test (DST) results are abnormal in about half of patients with psychotic depression. This abnormality reflects a distinct although small excessive amount (typically 10%) of cortisol in the body.

Appendix 2

Summary Guide to Psychotropic Medication and Treatment

THIS IS A SKETCH OF PSYCHOTROPIC DRUGS used in treating or managing psychotic depression. We list the generic name of the drug first. Using only the generic name directs focus to the patient and away from drug advertising. It prevents the costly suggestion associated with mentioning the brand name. Some drugs identified below as costly should soon cost less, as generics become available.

Antipsychotic tranquilizers

The drug type "antipsychotic" is a misnomer. All antipsychotics powerfully affect thought processes in everyone who takes them. They do not make thoughts normal and they are not specifically antipsychotic. Rather, they generally decrease the complexity and amount of thinking. Most patients discontinue their antipsychotic drug, probably because it decreases feelings of pleasure in life experience and reward in accomplishment overall, including for taking medication properly. Other side effects vary; for example, some antipsychotics cause grogginess but others do not. Drugs that are still on patent typically cost several times as much as generics.

The original antipsychotics were called neuroleptics (the commonest class of which were phenothiazines). These drugs block the effects of the neurotransmitter dopamine, causing dopamine deficiency. Dopamine blockade decreases outflow of nerve cell activity from the prefrontal lobes of the brain, analogous to a faucet decreasing water flow. The prefrontal lobes house the complex thinking of the human brain. Dopamine deficiency is part of Parkinson's disease. Ordinary side effects of neuroleptics resemble Parkinson's disease: deficiency of movements, thoughts, and emotional expressions; muscular rigidity, tremor, and involuntary movement; difficulties balancing, walking, and swallowing; and eventually anxiety, depression, and loss of motivation. The first neuroleptic, chlorpromazine, was launched in 1954. It is no less effective than later drugs (except clozapine) but is undesirable because of unusual toxic effects.

Antipsychotic drugs introduced since 1990 have been called "atypical type" or "second generation" but these terms have no specific or consistent medical meaning. They do refer to drugs highly promoted by drug companies, in style, still patented, and costly. Some recent antipsychotics block dopamine strongly, some moderately, and others negligibly. The antipsychotics that do not block dopamine directly inhibit the functioning of parts of the prefrontal lobe. Some antipsychotics moderately block dopamine and moderately inhibit prefrontal lobe functioning. With some antipsychotics we have no physiological evidence to explain their effects, so we can only presume their mechanisms. We group drugs by mechanism because side effects correspond to it.

Dopamine-blocker drugs

These drugs block the neurotransmitter dopamine from working, mostly in a deep and central part of the brain called the basal ganglia. This part of the brain acts like faucet valves and switches to control nerve conduction from the prefrontal lobes to the muscles and to the reasoning and consciousness parts of the brain. When dopamine-blocker drugs are given in doses large enough to diminish symptoms of psychotic depression, both obvious and subtle side effects usually occur. Side effects are more severe and longer-lasting in older patients. The common obvious side effects are (a) muscle rigidity and loss of spontaneous movements (called akinesia), together referred to as Parkinsonism, (b) restlessness (called akathisia), and eventually (c) involuntary writhing movements (called tardive dyskinesia), and (d) psychosis and depression (tardive psychosis and tardive depression). Some doctors are unaware of tardive psychosis and tardive depression, and instead unknowingly attribute these effects to the psychiatric condition instead of to the antipsychotic drug. Definite but hopefully rare side effects include (e) neuroleptic malignant syndrome with fever, weakness, and stupor (often mistaken for pneumonia), and (f) cancer, particularly breast cancer. Some dopamine blockers make people groggy because they also inhibit the sympathetic nervous system; specifically they block alpha-1 or histamine-1 receptors. Other dopamine blockers do not make people drowsy. These drugs also decrease nausea, and some are used mostly for that effect.

Dopamine blockers that rarely cause drowsiness

Aripiprazole (Abilify). The sales promotion of this on-patent drug as a dopamine balancer rather than dopamine blocker overstates benefits and underestimates side effects, as does the brand name. This drug causes severe side effects in elderly patients. Extremely costly and rarely worth it. No generic in the near future.

Fluphenazine (Prolixin) and haloperidol (Haldol). Used as tablets, liquid, injection, or long-acting once-monthly injection. Generally more potent and longer-acting than needed for psychotic depression. Generic.

Molindone (Moban). Each tablet lasts for not much more than a day, and has little interaction with other drugs. This facilitates rapid adjustments in dose including quick discontinuation. It is unlikely to cause weight gain and is suitable for managing psychotic depression. Generic.

Perphenazine (Trilafon). A well-tolerated dopamine blocker of medium potency, suitable for psychotic depression. Generic.

Pimozide (Orap). Particularly long acting and potent, this drug continues to accumulate for weeks, longer than any other antipsychotic. So, dose adjustment is slowest and most difficult. Excessive accumulation can slow the heart.

Risperidone (Risperdal). Potent but tolerable. It has antidepressant activity and makes some patients with mania worse. Suitable for psychotic depression but extremely costly and rarely worth it.

Thiothixene (Navane). Used as tablets, liquid, or injection. About as potent as haloperidol but with fewer side effects. Suitable for psychotic depression. Generic.

Thiethylperazine (Torecan). Widely used for nausea but a potent antipsychotic. Generic.

Dopamine blockers that often cause drowsiness

These usually decrease tension anxiety, which helps achieve calmness and decreases impulsive behavior. Excepting chlorpromazine and prochlorperazine, side effects (a) through (e) above are less than from other dopamine blockers, but still occur. These drugs cause weight gain. They can slow heart conduction, sometimes seriously, so ECGs are needed to check the "QTc interval." All are available as generics. These are particularly deadly in overdose.

Amoxapine (Asendin). This was marketed as an antidepressant, not as an antipsychotic. The typical 200 mg/day dose is equivalent to 13 mg/day of haloperidol, a potent antipsychotic dose.

Chlorpromazine (Thorazine). Its side effects are out of proportion to its other effects. It can cause extreme constipation.

Metoclopramide (Reglan). Prescribed for gastrointestinal problems, when patients over 50 take it for longer than a couple of months, psychosis, involuntary movements, or depression can develop either while the drug is taken or within a day or two of stopping it.

Prochlorperazine (Compazine). Prescribed for nausea.

Thioridazine (Mellaril). Dose limit for a few weeks 800 mg/day, for a few months 300 mg/day. In higher doses it can permanently impair vision. Highly calming. Lowers testosterone in males, which decreases sex drive and function. Its possible slowing of the electrical conduction system of the heart requires an ECG to measure what is called the QTc interval.

Prefrontal inhibitors

These drugs do not cause the first four side effects listed under dopamine blockers, and the other two side effects are probably negligible. This kind of drug decreases prefrontal lobe functioning. Side effects include apathy, weakness, weak willpower ("abulia"), drowsiness, weight gain, diminished problem solving, disorganization, and childlike oversimplicity. These drugs are safer than dopamine blockers to use with patients who are elderly or with Parkinson's disease.

Quetiapine (Seroquel). This is the safest antipsychotic drug, with fewest adverse effects. It does not decrease white blood cells as clozapine does. Quetiapine works well for patients who were not taking a different antipsychotic drug before it was started. This is because, at least in ordinary doses, quetiapine does not reliably treat the lingering problems caused by dopamine-blocking antipsychotic drugs, such as tardive psychosis. Weight gain is often 15 pounds, average 5 pounds. Typical dose is 200–800 mg/day. Very costly.

Clozapine (Clozaril). Like olanzapine but probably also has lithium-like action as a true antimanic and antidepressant. Studies suggest this as the most effective antipsychotic drug and the only antipsychotic drug to work on some patients who do not improve with other antipsychotics. This is partially explained by its lithium-like action. Clozapine alleviates tardive psychosis. It is not widely used because it decreases bacteria-fighting white blood cells to a life-threatening degree in 1–2 percent of patients. To try to prevent death from this, blood is tested every 1–2 weeks for as long as the drug is taken. Clozapine causes marked or extreme apathy or sedation, which adds to such effects from other drugs. Weight gain is often 30 pounds, average 10 pounds. Typical dosage is 100–800 mg/day. Very costly, even for generic drug.

Mixed dopamine blockers – prefrontal inhibitors

Olanzapine (Zyprexa). Particularly effective at quieting thinking. This comes at the expense of causing notable apathy, physical weakness (asthenia), willpower weakness (abulia), somnolence (anergia), and the other prefrontal inhibitor side effects. In the elderly or at high doses it also causes the side effects of the dopamine blockers. It often brings a 30-pound weight gain but 10 pounds is average, sometimes inducing diabetes, a severe side effect. Typical dose for psychotic depression is 15–20 mg/day. Very costly.

Loxapine (Loxitane). Available as a generic and much less costly than all others in this group. Works well at low doses (10–20 mg/day) in elderly without causing muscle rigidity. Typical dose up to 40 mg/day. If the patient is not particularly dangerous or agitated, loxapine is a good economical choice. Generic.

Ziprasidone (Geodon). Mild, gradual, and nonsedating, ziprasidone also has antiobsessional activity similar to buspirone. It causes little to no weight gain. If urgent action is needed, this is not a good choice.

If quetiapine is not appropriate this might be the next choice, especially in elderly or patients with Parkinson's disease. Very costly.

Antimelancholic antidepressants

This group includes the first-choice medications for psychotic depression when medication is appropriate. In overdose all antimelancholics are deadly; tricyclics readily cause apnea (stopping breathing) and MAOIs cause either hypotension and bradycardia or the opposite. Of course there is no overdose risk from ECT. All are available as generics.

Amitriptyline (Elavil). Amitriptyline is highly effective but has strong side effects. It is extremely anticholinergic, which causes marked confusion in elderly patients. This clears when the drug is stopped. Patients on amitriptyline often gain 20–30 pounds, so it is hard to recommend over nortriptyline. Orthostatic hypotension and drowsiness are common. A typical antidepressant dose is 150–300 mg/day. Amitriptyline is widely used to treat insomnia, given 25–50 mg at bedtime.

Bupropion (Wellbutrin). Antimelancholic, mild stimulant. Provokes seizures in people with history of epilepsy or current stimulant use, including theophylline. It is a first choice antimelancholic drug for males over age 40 who have no seizure risk. Higher doses do not produce greater effects. Typical dose is 100 mg/day in elderly, 150 mg/day in others. Elderly patients generally tolerate bupropion better than other antimelancholics. Bupropion raises blood pressure and pulse, more so with higher doses; blood pressure should be checked regularly.

Clomipramine (Anafranil). Similar to amitriptyline but more extreme in every way. It might be the strongest antimelancholic but its hypotension and sedation are the most difficult to tolerate. Dosage 100–250 mg/day. Antiobsessional as well as antidepressant, also somewhat decreases tension.

Desipramine, protriptyline. These drugs make patients restless rather than sedated and patients do not gain weight on them. Still, there are no apparent advantages over nortriptyline in treating psychotic depression. 150–300 mg/day.

Doxepin (Sinequan). Similar to amitriptyline.

Imipramine (Tofranil). Imipramine sedates some people, activates others, has anticholinergic activity, and causes hypotension. Still, it works well. It is our second choice among tricyclics and that is why we do not use it. Dosage 150–300 mg/day.

Isocarboxazid (Marplan) is similar to phenelzine.

Nortriptyline (Aventyl, Pamelor). This is highly effective and generally well tolerated. It is a first choice antimelancholic in females, especially when given with triiodothyronine. Its dose is usually limited by its blood concentration rather than side effects. Serum nortriptyline should be in the range of 50–150 ng/ml after a week. One must bear in mind that nortriptyline has anticholinergic activity and causes some orthostatic hypotension, sedation, and weight gain. Typical dosage is 50–125 mg/day.

Phenelzine (Nardil). This is an MAOI. It requires maintaining a special diet and avoiding stimulants, decongestants, and SSRI drugs. It can be taken together with amitriptyline, nortriptyline, or a beta-blocker. It is moderately less effective than other antimelancholics but probably works with different patients. Because of higher medical risks and remission in only about 25 percent of patients, it is rarely used. Still, it is also antiobsessional. It does not sedate, and people do not gain weight on it. Typical dosage is 45–60 mg/day.

Venlafaxine (Effexor). In doses 150–200 of mg/day for elderly patients and 200–300 mg/day for adults it is probably antimelancholic as bupropion is, and similarly raises blood pressure and pulse. Generic, but if not given in a sustained- or slow-release formulation nausea can be a problem. Nausea might be prevented by 7.5–15 mg of generic mirtazapine. Venlafaxine is also antiobsessional.

ECT: A special note

ECT is widely used because it has no equal, and there is no reasonable substitute. Selecting ECT means that you expect the highest quality result, you want the most reliable treatment, and you aim to minimize the chance of anxiety disorder developing or self-injury. ECT is a first-line treatment for psychotic depression, nonpsychotic melancholia, and catatonia, and sometimes for mania. These virtues are documented supra.

Antiobsessionals

These drugs decrease worry, obsessions, and dissatisfaction. One of the early SSRI drugs, fluvoxamine (Luvox) was originally introduced to treat obsessive-compulsive disorder (OCD), but sales were low because OCD is rare. However, dissatisfaction and worrying are extremely common, and SSRIs sold well when dissatisfaction was relabeled depression and later SSRIs were promoted as antidepressants. Although their use for dissatisfaction and worry as part of anxiety disorders is appropriate, they do not treat psychotic depression. By diminishing anxiety they might possibly prevent the recurrence of psychotic depression after remission is achieved, but this is only hypothetical. Side effects of SSRIs (but not buspirone) include low sodium (hyponatremia) with possible delirium, excessive bleeding tendency (especially during surgery), and nausea. Some can cause cancer. All are dangerous in overdose.

Buspirone (Buspar). Generic. Not an SSRI.

Citalopram (Celexa). SSRI. Occasionally causes restlessness. Generic.

Duloxetine (Cymbalta). Very costly. Claimed second action as SNRI besides SSRI, it is unclear whether SNRI per se has useful clinical effect.

Escitalopram (Lexapro). A very costly version of citalopram.

Fluoxetine (Prozac). An SSRI. Obsolete because it interferes with the body's removal of some other drugs. Often causes restlessness. Generic.

Fluvoxamine (Luvox). A generally safe SSRI. Generic. Avoid taking with clozapine, theophylline, or high doses of NSAIDS (such as ibuprofen, naproxen).

Paroxetine (Paxil). An SSRI. Obsolete because it interferes with the body's removal of some other drugs. Clear withdrawal effect. Appears to cause cancer.

Sertraline (Zoloft). SSRI. Costly.

Venlafaxine (Effexor). SSRI. Safe. Generic. In higher doses it raises blood pressure and pulse.

Miscellaneous psychotropics

Lithium (Eskalith, Lithobid). Also treats tardive psychosis and mania. Occasionally treats catatonia. Its primary use in depression is to make TCAs more effective and to prevent recurrence of depression after ECT. There is no benefit known for using lithium and triiodothyronine together, rather the lore is they prevent each other from working. Typically makes patients urinate more and feel more thirst, which can lead to weight gain if one is not careful; this effect is stopped by potassium supplements 15 meq 1–2 times daily, and potassium might decrease other side effects such as body tremors, loss of muscle endurance, and scars in the kidney.

Triiodothyronine (Cytomel). This is a type of thyroid hormone. Its only use in psychiatry is to make TCAs more effective in treating melancholic or psychotic depression. The standard dose is 25 μg/day (please note: not mg/day)

Carvedilol (Coreg). Treats tardive dyskinesia, tardive vomiting, and tardive hiccups. Probably treats tardive psychosis.

Trazodone (Desyrel). No efficacy known or expected for psychotic depression. Widely given to treat insomnia, but not studied for that. Avoid taking more than 200 mg/day in any case or more than 50 mg/day with fluoxetine or paroxetine because it can cause blood clotting in the genitals.

Mirtazapine (Remeron). No efficacy known or expected for psychotic depression.

Nefazodone (Serzone). No efficacy known or expected for psychotic depression.

Methylphenidate (Ritalin) is a stimulant and sometimes an antidepressant. It treats poststroke depression and posttraumatic brain injury depression, and it can make other antidepressants work better in elderly patients. Like such stimulants as caffeine and nicotine, it helps concentration but can worsen tension anxiety such as restlessness or agitation.

Anti-Parkinson agents

These drugs decrease the side effects of dopamine-blocker antipsychotic drugs. This list is not complete.

L-DOPA (Sinemet) increases dopamine in the brain, to treat the symptoms of Parkinson's disease, such as muscle rigidity. It acts opposite to most antipsychotic drugs. It can cause anxiety and possibly psychotic symptoms.

Amantadine (Symmetrel) increases dopamine in the brain. It can cause visual hallucinations but is not known to cause auditory hallucinations.

Benztropin (Cogentin) is an anticholinergic drug that decreases rigidity. As with any anticholinergic drug, marked confusion in elderly patients is likely.

Biperiden (Akineton) is an anticholinergic drug that decreases rigidity.

Diphenhydramine (Benadryl) is an anticholinergic that decreases rigidity.

Trihexyphenidyl (Artane) is an anticholinergic that decreases rigidity.

Tension reducers

The safest and smoothest-acting drugs that reduce somatic tension anxiety (body anxiety such as agitation, restlessness, edginess, being too easily upset by small things) are long-acting beta-blockers that enter the brain or certain anticonvulsant drugs. Beta-blockers should generally be avoided by patients with currently active asthma, bradyarrhythmias, hypotension, symptomatic congestive heart failure, or peripheral artery disease.

Betaxolol (Kerlone) is a long-acting beta-blocker that enters the brain, of average half-life 20 hours. It can be taken once daily at bedtime but works best twice daily. Range: 5–15 mg/day, average 10 mg/day.

Bisoprolol (Zebeta) is a medium-acting beta-blocker that enters the brain, of average half-life 10 hours. It can be taken twice daily but works best three times daily. Range: 2.5–5 mg 2–3 times daily.

Topiramate (Topamax) is an anticonvulsant. Dose is 25 mg once to twice daily in elderly patients, up to 100 mg three times daily in adults. It is generally safer than other anticonvulsants; its side effects are nuisances rather than threats.

Lamotrigine (Lamictal) is an anticonvulsant that is promoted for the treatment of bipolar depression. It does not treat mania and is probably not an antimelancholic. Causes problematic allergic rashes in 5–10 percent of patients, which are occasionally life threatening. To minimize risks from rashes, the dose must be started very low and increased very gradually.

Metoprolol (Toprol, Toprol-XL) is a short-acting beta-blocker that enters the brain. This drug is commonly given to people who have had a heart attack, to diminish the chance of another. Its antitension effects are usually strongest during the first month, then they become inconsistent unless the extended release (XL) form of metoprolol is taken every 12 hours. Its benefits are not as consistent or persistent as those from betaxolol or bisoprolol.

Propranolol (Inderal, Inderal LA) is a very short-acting beta-blocker that rapidly enters the brain. Its short half-life and rapid brain penetration make its effects inconsistent after about a month unless the long acting (LA) form is taken every 12 hours. Not recommended for longer than a week.

Antimanics

These can be useful in mixed manic-depressive episode. All have inexpensive generic versions and costly brand name versions.

Valproate, valproic acid, divalproex. (Depakote, Depakene). The brand name version is heavily promoted as more tolerable, yet most patients tolerate the inexpensive generic. Common side effects are weight gain and tremor. Possible side effects include fatigue, liver irritation, pancreatitis, hair loss. Hair loss can be reversed by taking zinc 25 mg/day and selenium 100 μg/day over-the-counter supplements. The drug is an anticonvulsant. Pregnant women should avoid this.

Lithium (Eskalith, Lithobid). See miscellaneous psychotropics section.

Carbamazepine (Tegretol). An anticonvulsant. Oxcarbamazepine (Trileptal) is similar. They can cause dangerous hyponatremia or decrease in bacteria-fighting white blood cells.

Benzodiazepine tranquilizers

These drugs decrease brain function including learning, memory, attention, and coordination. Higher doses decrease brain function further and bring unconsciousness. They often cause delirium and falls in the elderly. People who take these should not drive within 24 hours. If injected intravenously or if taken in any way with alcohol they can cause apnea (respiratory arrest).

Alprazolam (Xanax). This drug is the most addictive benzodiazepine. It is a trap: once started it is nearly impossible to stop because it causes drug withdrawal in between doses.

Clonazepam (Klonopin). Can temporarily decrease catatonia.

Diazepam (Valium). Can temporarily decrease catatonia. Highly addictive. When injected intramuscularly, it is not reliably absorbed, and it causes excessive pain and some muscle injury.

Lorazepam (Ativan). Can temporarily decrease catatonia. Lorazepam is the only psychotropic benzodiazepine available that is reliably absorbed when injected intramuscularly.

Oxazepam (Serax). Short acting and without metabolites, so safer than other benzodiazepines.

Temazepam (Restoril). Used mostly for insomnia.

Triazolam (Halcion). Used mostly for insomnia. Temporarily decreases catatonia. Powerfully interferes with learning, including remembering events after taking it.

References

Aarsland, D., Larsen, J. P., Cummings, J. L., and Laake, K. 1999. Prevalence and clinical correlates of psychotic symptoms in Parkinson Disease. A community-based study. *Arch Neurol* 56: 595–601.

Abrams, R. 2002. *Electroconvulsive therapy*, 4th edn. New York: Oxford University Press.

Abrams, R. and Taylor, M. A. 1983. The importance of mood-incongruent psychotic symptoms in melancholia. *J Affect Disord* 5: 179–81.

Alexopoulos, G. S., Meyers, B. S., Young, R. C., et al. 1993. The course of geriatric depression with "reversible dementia": A controlled study. *Am J Psychiatry* 150: 1693–9.

American Psychiatric Association (APA) 1994. *Diagnostic and statistical manual of mental disorders*, 4th edn. Washington, DC: APA, pp. 348, 384–6.

Amsterdam, J. D. and Shults, J. 2005. Fluoxetine monotherapy of bipolar type II and bipolar NOS major depression: A double-blind, placebo-substitution, continuation study. *Int Clin Psychopharmacol* 20: 257–64.

Andreassen, O. A., Ferrante, R. J., Aamo, T. O., et al. 2003. Oral dyskinesias and histopathological alterations in substantia nigra after long-term haloperidol treatment of old rats. *Neuroscience* 122: 717–25.

Angst, F., Stassen, H. H., Clayton, P.J., and Angst, J. 2002. Mortality of patients with mood disorders: Follow-up over 34–38 years. *J Affect Disord* 68: 167–81.

Anton, R. F., Jr. and Burch, E. A., Jr. 1990. Amoxapine versus amitriptyline combined with perphenazine in the treatment of psychotic depression. *Am J Psychiatry* 147: 1203–8.

Anton, R. F., Jr. and Burch, E. A., Jr. 1993. Response of psychotic depression subtypes to pharmacotherapy. *J Affect Disord* 28: 125–31.

Aronson, T. A., Shukla, S., and Hoff, A. 1987. Continuation therapy after ECT for delusional depression: A naturalistic study of prophylactic treatments and relapse. *Convuls Ther* 3: 251–9.

Aronson, T. A., Shukla, S., Hoff, A., and Cook, B. 1988. Proposed delusional depression subtypes: Preliminary evidence from a retrospective study of phenomenology and treatment course. *J Affect Disord* 14: 69–74

Arroll, B., Macgillivray, S., Ogston, S., et al. 2005. Efficacy and tolerability of tricyclic antidepressants and SSRIs compared with placebo for treatment of depression in primary care: A meta-analysis. *Ann Family Med* 3: 449–56.

Associated Press. 2006. Woman not guilty in retrial in the deaths of her 5 children. *New York Times*, July 27, p. A18.

Avery, D. and Lubrano, A. 1979. Depression treated with imipramine and ECT: The DeCarolis study reconsidered. *Am J Psychiatry* 136: 559–62.

Avery, D. and Winokur, G. 1976. Mortality in depressed patients treated with electroconvulsive therapy and antidepressants. *Arch Gen Psychiatry* 33: 1029–37.

Bakish, D. 2001. New standard of depression treatment: Remission and full recovery. *J Clin Psychiatry* 62(Suppl 26): 5–9.

Banken, R. 2002. *The use of electroconvulsive therapy in Quebec. Agence d'valuation des technologies et des modes d'intervention en sant (AETMIS).* Montreal: AETMIS.

Bassett, S. S. 2005. Cognitive impairment in Parkinson's Disease. *Prim Psychiatry* 12: 50–55.

Bayley, J. 1881. Case of recurrent melancholia. *Lancet* 2: 1041–2.

Beck, A. T. 1967. *Depression: Clinical, experimental, and theoretical aspects.* New York: Harper & Row.

Belanoff, J. K., Rothschild, A. J., Cassidy, F., et al. 2002. An open label trial of C-1073 (mifepristone) for psychotic major depression. *Biol Psychiatry* 52: 386–92.

Bellini, L., Gatti, F., Gasperini, M., and Smeraldi, E. 1992. A comparison between delusional and non-delusional depressives. *J Affect Disord* 25: 129–38.

Benziger, B. F. 1969. *The prison of my mind*. New York: Walker.

Bergemann, N., Frick, A., Parzer, P., and Kopitz, J. 2004. Olanzapine plasma concentration, average daily dose, and interaction with co-medication in schizophrenic patients. *Pharmacopsychiatry* 37: 63–8.

Birkenhager, T. K. and Moleman, P. 1999. Two new antidepressants: Mirtazapine and venlafaxine. *Ned Tijdscr Geneeskd* 143: 934–7.

Birkenhager, T. K., Pluijms, E. M., and Lucius, S. A. 2003. ECT response in delusional versus non-delusional depressed inpatients. *J Affect Disord* 74: 191–5.

Black, D. W. and Winokur, G. 1989. Psychotic and nonpsychotic depression: Comparison of response to ECT. *J Clin Psychiatry* 50: 186.

Bonomo, V. and Fogliani, A. M. 2000. Citalopram and haloperidol for psychotic depression. *Am J Psychiatry* 157: 1706–7.

Bowers, M. B. and Swigar, M. E. 1988. Psychotic patients who become worse on neuroleptics. *J Clin Psychopharmacol* 8: 417–21.

Bremner, J. D., Vythinlingam, M., Ng, C. K., et al. 2003. Regional brain metabolic correlates of alpha-methylparatyrosine-induced depressive symptoms: Implications for the neural circuitry of depression. *JAMA* 289: 3125–34.

Breslau, N. and Meltzer, H. Y. 1988. Validity of subtyping psychotic depression: Examination of phenomenology and demographic characteristics. *Am J Psychiatry* 145: 35–40.

Brockington, I. F., Roper, A., Copas, J., et al. 1991. Schizophrenia, bipolar disorder and depression. A discriminant analysis, using "lifetime" psychopathology ratings. *Br J Psychiatry* 159: 485–94.

Brown, G. W., Ni Bhrolchain, M., and Harris, T. O. 1979. Psychotic and neurotic depression. Part 3. Aetiological and background factors. *J Affect Disord* 1: 195–211.

Brown, R. P., Frances, A., Kocsis, J. H., and Mann, J. J. 1982. Psychotic vs. nonpsychotic depression: Comparison of treatment response. *J Nerv Ment Dis* 170: 635–7

Brown, T. A., Campbell, L. A., Lehman, C. L., et al. 2001. Current and lifetime comorbidity of the DSM-IV anxiety and mood disorders in a large clinical sample. *J Abnorm Psychol* 110: 585–99.

Brujin, J. A., Moleman, P., Mulder, P. G., et al. 1996. A double-blind, fixed blood-level study comparing mirtazapine with imipramine in depressed in-patients. *Psychopharmacol (Berlin)* 237: 231–7.

Burch, E. A. and Goldschmidt, T. J. 1983. Loxapine in the treatment of psychotic-depressive disorders: Measurement of antidepressant metabolites. *South Med J* 76: 991–5.

Cade, J. F. J. 1949. Lithium salts in the treatment of psychotic excitement. *Med J Aust* 2: 349–52.

Calabrese, J. R., Keck, P. B., MacFadden, W., et al. 2005. A randomized double-blind placebo-controlled trial of quetiapine in the treatment of bipolar I or II depression. *Am J Psychiatry* 162: 1351–60.

Carpenter, W. T. and Buchanan, R. W. 1994. Schizophrenia. *N Engl J Med* 330: 681–90.

Carroll, B. J. 1981. Review of Harold I. Kaplan, et al. (eds) *Comprehensive textbook of psychiatry*, 3rd edn. *Am J Psychiatry* 138: 705–7.

Carroll, B. J. 1982. The dexamethasone suppression test for melancholia. *Br J Psychiatry* 140: 292–304.

Carroll, B. J. 1983. Neurobiologic dimensions of depression and mania. In Jules Angst (ed.) *The origins of depression: Current concepts and approaches*. Berlin: Springer.

Carroll, B. J., Curtis, G. C., and Mendels, J. 1976. Cerebrospinal fluid and plasma free cortisol concentrations in depression. *Psychol Med* 6: 235–44.

Carroll, B. T., Thomas, C., Jayanti, K., et al. 2005. Treating persistent catatonia when benzodiazepines fail. *Curr Psychiatry* 4: 56–64.

Casey, D. A. 1987. Electroconvulsive therapy in the neuroleptic malignant syndrome. *Convuls Ther* 3: 278–83.

Cerletti, U. 1940. L'Elettroshock. *Rivista Sperimentale di Freniatria* 64: 209–310.

Chan, C. H., Janicak, P. G., Davis, J. M., et al. 1987. Response of psychotic and nonpsychotic depressed patients to tricyclic antidepressants. *J Clin Psychiatry* 48: 197–200.

Chelminski, I., Zimmerman, M., and Mattia, J. I. 2000. Diagnosing melancholia. *J Clin Psychiatry* 61: 874–5.

Chouinard, G. and Steinberg, S. 1984. New clinical concepts on neuroleptic-induced supersensitivity disorders: Tardive dyskinesia and supersensitivity psychosis. In H. C. Stancer, P. E. Garfinkel, and V. M. Rakoff (eds) *Guidelines for the use of psychotropic drugs*. New York: Spectrum, pp. 205–27.

Corcept Therapeutics, Inc. 2006. Corcept Therapeutics announces negative results from the first of three phase 3 studies evaluating CORLUX(R) for treating the psychotic features of psychotic major depression. *PR Newswire*, August 25, accessed September 13, 2006 at http://biz.yahoo.com/prnews/060825/laf018.html?.v=61

Cotard, J. 1880. Du délire des négations. *Archives de neurologie* 4: 152–70.

Coryell, W. and Tsuang, M. T. 1982. Primary unipolar depression and the prognostic importance of delusions. *Arch Gen Psychiatry* 39: 1181–4.

Coryell, W., Pfohl, B., and Zimmerman, M. 1984. The clinical and neuroendocrine features of pscyhotic depression. *J Nerv Ment Dis* 172: 521–8.

Coryell, W., Zimmerman, M., and Pfohl, B. 1986. Outcome at discharge and six months in major depression. The significance of psychotic features. *J Nerv Ment Dis* 174: 92–6

Cullen, M., Mitchell, P., Brodaty, H., et al. 1991. Carbamazepine for treatment-resistant melancholia. *J Clin Psychiatry* 52: 472–6.

Davidson, J., McLeod, M., Law-Yone, B., and Linnoila, M. 1978. A comparison of electroconvulsive therapy and combined phenelzine-amitriptyline in refractory depression. *Arch Gen Psychiatry* 35: 639–42.

DeBattista, C., Belanoff, J., Glass, S., et al. 2006. Mifeprisone versus placebo in the treatment of psychosis in patients with psychotic major depression. *Biol Psychiatry* 60: 1343–9.

De Montigny, C., Grunberg, F., Mayer, A., et al. 1981. Lithium induces rapid relief of depression in tricyclic antidepressant drug non-responders. *Br J Psychiatry* 138: 252–6.

DelBello, M. P., Carlson, G. A., Tohen, M., et al. 2003. Rates and predictors of developing a manic or hypomanic episode 1 to 2 years following a first hospitalization for major depression with psychotic features. *J Child Adolesc Psychopharmacol* 13: 173–85.

Denber, H. C. B. 1957. Treatment of chlorpromazine-diethazine in depression. *Dis Nerv Syst* 17: 76–9.

Denno, D. W. 2003. Who is Andrea Yates? A short story about insanity. *Duke J Gend Law Policy* 10: 1–139.

Dietrich, D. E., Godecke-Koch, T., Richter-Witte, C., and Emrich, H. M. 2004. Lamotrigine in the treatment of confusion psychosis, a case report. *Pharmacopsychiatry* 37: 88–90.

Donlon, P. T., Biertuemphel, H., and Willenbring, M. 1981. Amoxapine and amitriptyline in the outpatient treatment of endogenous depression. *J Clin Psychiatry* 42: 11–15.

Downs, J. M., Akiskal, H. G., and Rosenthal, T. L. 1993. Neuroleptic-induced pseudoschizoaffective disorder (abstract 146). *Proc Am Psychiatric Assoc Annual Meet*, p. 153 (full program on audiotape).

Dubovsky, S. L. and Thomas, M. 1992. Psychotic depression: Advances in conceptualization and treatment. *Hosp Comm Psychiatry* 43: 1189–98.

Eagles, J. M. 1983. Delusional depressive in-patients, 1892–1982. *Br J Psychiatry* 143: 558–63.

Erfurth, A., Walden, J., and Grunze, H. 1998. Lamotrigine in the treatment of schizoaffective disorder. *Neuropsychobiology* 38: 204–5.

Ernst K. 1983. Geisteskrankheit ohne institution: eine feldstudie im Kanton Fribourg aus dem jahr 1875. *Schweizer Archiv für Neurologie, Neurochirurgie und Psychiatrie* 133: 239–62.

Evans, D. L. and Nemeroff, C.B. 1987. The clinical use of the Dexamethasone Suppression Test in DSM-III affective disorders: Correlation with the severe depressive subtypes of melancholia and psychosis. *J Psychiatr Res* 21: 185–94.

Feighner, J. P., Robins, E., Guze, S. B., et al. 1972. Diagnostic criteria for use in psychiatric research. *Arch Gen Psychiatry* 26: 57–63.

Fenichel, O. 1945. *The psychoanalytic theory of neurosis.* New York: Norton.

Fink, M. 1979. A theory of convulsive therapy (chapter 14). In M. Fink (ed.) *Convulsive therapy: Theory and practice.* New York: Raven Press, p. 173.

Fink, M. and Taylor, M. A. 2003. *Catatonia: A clinician's guide to diagnosis and treatment.* New York: Cambridge University Press.

Fink, M., Klein, D. F., and Kramer, J. C. 1965. Clinical efficacy of chlorpromazine-procyclidine combination, imipramine and placebo in depressive disorders. *Psychopharmacologia* 7: 27–36.

Finlay-Jones, R. and Parker, G. 1993. A consensus conference on psychotic depression. *Aust NZ J Psychiatry* 27: 581–9.

Fish, F. 1964. Concluding observations. In E. Beresford Davies (ed.) *Depression: Proceedings of the symposium held at Cambridge 22 to 26 September 1959.* Cambridge, UK: Cambridge University Press, pp. 349–52.

Flint, A. J. and Rifat, S. L. 1998a. The treatment of psychotic depression in later life: A comparison of pharmacotherapy and ECT. *Int J Geriatr Psychiatry* 13: 23–8.

Flint, A. J. and Rifat, S. L. 1998b. Two-year outcome of psychotic depression in late life. *Am J Psychiatry* 155: 178–83.

Flor-Henry, P. 1983. Determinants of psychosis in epilepsy, laterality and forced normalization. *Biol Psychiatry* 18: 1045–57.

Freud, S. 1946. Trauer und melancholie (1916). In Freud (ed.) *Gesammelte Werke,* vol. 10. Frankfurt: M. Fischer, pp. 428–46.

Freyhan, F. A. 1959. Clinical effectiveness of tofranil in the treatment of depressive psychoses. *Can Psychiatr Assoc J* 4(Suppl): S86–S97.

Freyhan, F. A. 1961. The influence of specific and non-specific factors on the clinical effects of psychotropic drugs. *Neuropsychopharmacology* 2: 189–203.

Fricchione, G. L., Cassem, N. H., and Hooberman, D. 1983. Intravenous lorazepam in neuroleptic-induced catatonia. *J Clin Psychopharmacol* 3: 338–42.

Fritsch, J. 1882. Diagnostik und therapie der melancholischen krankheitsformen. *Zeitschrift für Diagnostik und Therapie* 1: 101–3.

Frueh, B. C., Knapp, R. G., Cusack, K. J., et al. 2005. Patients' reports of traumatic or harmful experience within the psychiatric setting. *Psychiatric Serv* 56: 1123–33.

Gatti, F., Bellini, L., Gasperini, M., et al. 1996. Fluvoxamine alone in the treatment of delusional depression. *Am J Psychiatry* 153: 414–6.

Gaupp, R. 1926. Krankheitseinheit und mischpsychosen. *Zeitschrift fur die gesamte Neurologie und Psychiatrie* 101: 1–15.

Ghaemi, S. N., Lenox, M. S., and Baldessarini, R. J. 2001. Effectiveness and safety of long-term antidepressant treatment in bipolar disorder. *J Clin Psychiatry* 62: 565–9.

Gillespie, R. D. 1926. Discussion comment. *BMJ* 2: 878.

Gimsa, U., Schreiber, U., Habel, B., et al. 2006. Matching geometry and stimulation parameters of electrodes for deep brain stimulation experiments – numerical considerations. *J Neurosci Meth* 150: 212–27.

Glassman, A. H. and Roose, S. P. 1981. Delusional depression: A distinct clinical entity? *Arch Gen Psychiatry* 38: 424–7.

Glassman, A. H., Kantor, S. J., and Shostak, M. 1975. Depression, delusions, and drug response. *Am J Psychiatry* 132: 716–19.

Glick, I. D., Murray, S. R., Vasudevan, P., et al. 2001. Treatment with atypical antipsychotics: New indications and new populations. *J Psychiatr Res* 35: 187–91.

Goldman, D. 1955. *The effect of chlorpromazine on severe mental and emotional disturbances. In Chlorpromazine and mental health: Proceedings of the symposium held under the auspices of Smith, Kline & French Laboratories, June 6, 1955.* Philadelphia: Lea & Febiger, pp. 19–40.

Goodwin, F. K., Prange, A. J., Post, R. M., Muscettola, G., and Lipton, M. A. 1982. Potentiation of antidepressant effects by L-triiodothyronine in tricyclic nonresponders. *Am J Psychiatry* 139: 34–8.

Goren, J. L. and Levin, G. M. 2000. Mania with bupropion: A dose-related phenomenon? *Ann Pharmacother* 34: 619–21.

Gournellis, R., Lykouras, L., Fortos, A., et al. 2001. Psychotic (delusional) major depression in late life: A clinical study. *Int J Geriatr Psychiatry* 16: 1085–91.

Grunhaus, L., Dannon, P. N., Schreiber, S., et al. 2000. Repetitive transcranial magnetic stimulation is as effective as electroconvulsive therapy in the treatment of nondelusional major depressive disorder: An open study. *Biol Psychiatry* 47: 314–24.

Grunze, H., Marcuse, A., Scharer, L. O., et al. 2002. Nefazodone in psychotic unipolar and bipolar depression: A retrospective chart analysis and open prospective study on its efficacy and safety versus combined treatment with amitriptyline and haloperidol. *Neuropsychobiology* 46(Suppl 1): 31–5.

Guze, S. B., Woodruff, R. A., Jr, and Clayton, P. J. 1975. The significance of psychotic affective disorders. *Arch Gen Psychiatry* 32: 1147–50.

Hamilton, M. 1989. Frequency of symptoms in melancholia (depressive illness). *Br J Psychiatry* 154: 201–6.

Hermann, R. C., Dorwart, R. A., Hoover, C. W., and Brody, J. 1995. Variation in ECT use in the United States. *Am J Psychiatry* 152: 869–75.

Hill, S. K., Keshavan, M. S., Thase, M. E., and Sweeney, J. A. 2004. Neuropsychological dysfunction in antipsychotic-naïve first-episode unipolar psychotic depression. *Am J Psychiatry* 161: 996–1003.

Hippius, H. and Jantz, H. 1959. Die heutige behandlung der depressionen. *Nervenarzt* 30: 466–73.

Hoch, A. and MacCurdy, J. T. 1922 The prognosis of involution melancholia. *Arch Neurol Psychiatry* 7: 1–37.

Hodgkiss, A. D., Malizia, A. L., Bartlett, J. R., and Bridges, P. K. 1995. Outcome after the psychosurgical operation of stereotactic subcaudate tractotomy, 1979–1991. *J Neuropsychiatry Clin Neurosci* 7: 230–4.

Hoff, H. 1959. Indications for electro-shock, tofranil and psychotherapy in the treatment of depressions. *Can Psychiatr Assoc J* 4(Suppl): S55–S68.

Hollister, L. E. and Overall, J. E. 1965. Reflections on the specificity of action of anti-depressants. *Psychosomatics* 6: 361–5.

Honoré, P., Moller, S. E., and Jorgensen, A. 1982. Lithium + l-tryptophan compared with amitriptyline in endogenous depression. *J Affect Disord* 4: 79–82.

Hordern, A., Holt, N. F., Burt, C. G., and Gordon, W. F. 1963. Amitriptyline in depressive states: Phenomenology and prognostic considerations. *Br J Psychiatry* 10: 815–25.

Jager, M., Bottlender, R., Strauss, A., and Moller, H. J. 2005. Fifteen-year follow-up of Diagnostic and Statistical Manual of Mental Disorders, Fourth Edition depressive disorders: The prognostic significance of psychotic features. *Compr Psychiatry* 46: 322–7.

Jain, V. and Swartz, C. M. 2002. Charcoal enhancement of treatment for tricyclic-induced mania. *Pharmacopsychiatry* 35: 197–9.

Janicak, P. G., Pandey, G. N., Davis, J. M., et al. 1988. Response of psychotic and nonpsychotic depression to phenelzine. *Am J Psychiatry* 145: 93–5.

Jaspers, K. 1913. *Allgemeine psychopathologie.* Berlin: Springer.

Jeste, D. V., Heaton, S. C., Paulsen, J. S., et al. 1996. Clinical and neuropsychological comparison of psychotic depression with nonpsychotic depression and schizophrenia. *Am J Psychiatry* 153: 490–6.

Joffe, R. T., MacQueen, G. M., Marriott, M., et al. 2002. Induction of mania and cycle acceleration in bipolar disorder: Effect of different classes of antidepressant. *Acta Psychiatr Scand* 105: 427–30.

Johnson, J., Horwath, E., and Weissman, M. M. 1991. The validity of major depression with psychotic features based on a community study. *Arch Gen Psychiatry* 48: 1075–81.

Joseph, K. S., Blais, L., Ernst, P., and Suissa, S. 1996. Increased morbidity and mortality related to asthma among asthmatic patients who use major tranquillisers. *BMJ* 312(7023): 79–82.

Judd, L. L., Akiskal, H. S., Schettler, P. J., et al. 2002. The long-term natural history of the weekly symptomatic status of bipolar I disorder. *Arch Gen Psychiatry* 59: 530–7.

Judd, L. L., Paulus, M. J., Schettler, P. J., et al. 2000. Does incomplete recovery from first lifetime major depressive episode herald a chronic course of illness? *Am J Psychiatry* 157: 1501–4.

Kahlbaum, K. 1863. *Die Gruppirung der Psychischen Krankheiten und die Eintheilung der Seelenstörungen.* Danzig: Kafemann.

Kalinowsky, L. B. 1941. The various forms of shock therapy in mental disorders and their practical importance. *NY State J Med* 41: 2210–15.

Kantor, S. J. and Glassman, A. H. 1977. Delusional depressions: Natural history and response to treatment. *Br J Psychiatry* 131: 351–60.

Kellner, C. H., Fink, M., Knapp, R., et al. 2005. Relief of expressed suicidal intent by ECT: A consortium for research in ECT study. *Am J Psychiatry* 162: 977–82.

Kendell, R. E., Chalmers, J. C., and Platz, C. 1987. Epidemiology of puerperal psychoses. *Br J Psychiatry* 150: 662–73.

Kielholz, P. 1954. Über die largactilwirkung bei depressiven zuständen und manien sowie bei der entziehung von morphin- und barbitursüchtigen. *Schweizer Archiv für Neurologie und Psychiatrie* 73: 291–309.

Kiloh, L. G. and Garside, R. F. 1963. The independence of neurotic depression and endogenous depression. *Br J Psychiatry* 109: 451–63.

Kiloh, L. G. and Garside, R. F. 1977. Depression: A multivariate study of Sir Aubrey Lewis's data on melancholia. *Aust NZ J Psychiatry* 11: 149–56.

Kinross-Wright, V. 1955. Chlorpromazine treatment of mental disorders. *Am J Psychiatry* 111: 907–12.

Kirk, S. A. and Kutchins, H. 1992. *The selling of DSM: The rhetoric of science in psychiatry.* New York: Aldine.

Kiser, S. 2004. An existential case study of madness: Encounters with divine affliction. *J Human Psychol* 44: 431–54.

Kivela, S. L. and Pahkala, K. 1989. Delusional depression in the elderly: A community study. *Zeitschrift fur Gerontologie* 22: 236–41.

Klein, D. and Fink, M. 1962. Behavioral reaction patterns with phenothiazines. *Arch Gen Psychiatry* 7: 449–59.

Klein, D. F. 1976. Differential diagnosis and treatment of the dysphorias. In Donald M. Gallant (ed.) *Depression: Behavioral, biochemical, diagnostic and treatment concepts*. New York: Spectrum, pp. 127–54.

Klerman G. L. 1974. Unipolar and bipolar depressions. In Jules Angst (ed.) *Classification and prediction of outcome of depression*. Stuttgart: F. K. Schattauer, pp. 49–74.

Klerman, G. L. and Cole, J. O. 1965. Clinical pharmacology of imipramine and related antidepressant compounds. *Pharmacol Rev* 17: 101–41.

Kocsis, J. H., Croughan, J. L., Katz, M. M., et al. 1990. Response to treatment with antidepressants of patients with severe or moderate nonpsychotic depression and of patients with psychotic depression. *Am J Psychiatry* 147: 621–4.

Kostiukova, E. G. 1989. Comparative features of the preventive action of carbamazepine and lithium carbonate in affective and schizoaffective psychoses. *Zhurnal Nevropatologii I Psikhiatrii Imeni S-S-Korsakova* 89: 64–71.

Kraepelin, E. 1913. *Psychiatrie: Ein lehrbuch fur studierende und aerzte*, 8th edn, vol. 3(2). Leipzig: Barth; 6th edn, 1899.

Kramer, B. A. 1999. Use of ECT in California, revised: 1984–1994. *J ECT* 15: 245– 51.

Kranz, H. 1955. Das thema des wahns im wandel der zeit. *Fortschritte der Neurologie und Psychiatrie* 23: 58–72.

Kreye, A. 2005. *Hausfrauenreport aus Hollywood*. Sueddeutsche Zeitung, April 9, p. 22.

Kroessler, D. 1985. Relative efficacy rates for therapies of delusional depression. *Convuls Ther* 1: 173–82.

Kuhs, H. 1991. Depressive delusion. *Psychopathology* 24: 106– 14.

La Rue, A., Spar, J., and Hill, C. D. 1986. Cognitive impairment in late-life depression: Clinical correlates and treatment implications. *J Affect Disord* 11: 179–84

Lambert, M. V. and Robertson, M. M. 1999. Depression in epilepsy: Etiology, phenomenology, and treatment. *Epilepsia* 40(Suppl 10): S21–S47.

Lancet, 1940. Editorial: Primum non nocere. *Lancet* 1: 275.

Lee, P. E., Sykora, K., Gill, S. S., et al. 2005. Antipsychotic medications and drug-induced movement disorders other than parkinsonism: A population-based cohort study in older adults. *J Am Geriatr Soc* 53: 1374–9.

Lenz, H. 1967. Themenwandel in der psychopathologie. *Wiener Zeitschrift für Nervenheilkunde* 25: 286–96.

Leonhard, K. 1957. *Aufteilung der endogenen Psychosen*. Berlin: Akademie-Verlag, pp. 185–217.

Lesser, I. M., Miller, B. L., Boone, K. B., et al. 1991. Brain injury and cognitive function in late-onset psychotic depression. *J Neuropsychiatry Clin Neurosci* 3: 33–40.

Lesser, I. M., Rubin, R. T., Rifkin, A., et al. 1989. Secondary depression in panic disorder and agoraphobia. II. Dimensions of depressive symptomatology and their response to treatment. *J Affect Disord* 16: 49–58.

Lew, T. Y. and Tollefson, G. 1983. Chlorpromazine-induced neuroleptic malignant syndrome and its response to diazepam. *Biol Psychiatry* 18: 1441–6.

Lewis, A. 1971. "Endogenous" and "exogenous": A useful dichotomy? *Psychol Med* 1: 191–6.

Lewis, A. J. 1934. Melancholia: A clinical survey of depressive states. *J Ment Sci* 80: 277–378.

Lewis, D. A. and Smith, R. E. 1983. Steroid-induced psychiatric syndromes. A report of 14 cases and a review of the literature. *J Affect Disord* 5: 319–32.

Lieberman, J. A., Stroup, T. S., McEvoy, J. P., et al. 2005. Effectiveness of antipsychotic drugs in patients with chronic schizophrenia. *N Engl J Med* 242: 1209–23.

Liu, Z. X. and Wang, D. C. 1992. A clinical and follow-up study in 33 cases of rapid cyclic affective psychosis. *Zhonghua Shen Jing Jing Shen Ke Za Zhi* 25: 341–3.

Lu, M. L., Pan, J. J., Teng, H. W., et al. 2002. Metoclopramide-induced supersensitivity psychosis. *Ann Pharmacother* 36: 1387–90.

Lykouras, E., Malliaras, D., Christodoulou, G. N., et al. 1986a. Delusional depression: Phenomenology and response to treatment. *Psychopathology* 19: 157–64.

Lykouras, E., Malliaras, D., Christodoulou, G. N., et al. 1986b. Delusional depression: Phenomenology and response to treatment. A prospective study. *Acta Psychiatr Scand* 73: 324–9.

Maj, M., Pirozzi, R., and Di Caprio, E. L. 1990. Major depression with mood-congruent psychotic features: A distinct diagnostic entity or a more severe subtype of depression? *Acta Psychiatr Scand* 82: 439–44.

Malla, A. K., Norman, R. M., Manchanda, R., et al. 2002. One year outcome in first episode psychosis: Influence of DUP and other predictors. *Schizophr Res* 54: 231–42.

Margolese, H. C., Chouinard, G., Beauclair, L., and Belanger, M. C. 2002. Therapeutic tolerance and rebound psychosis during quetiapine maintenance monotherapy in patients with schizophrenia and schizoaffective disorder. *J Clin Psychopharmacol* 22: 347–52.

Markowitz, J., Brown, R., Sweeney, J., and Mann, J. J. 1987. Reduced length and cost of hospital stay for major depression in patients treated with ECT. *Am J Psychiatry* 144: 1025–9.

Marsh, L., Williams, J. R., Rocco, M., et al. 2004. Psychiatric comorbidities associated with psychosis in patients with Parkinson's disease. *Neurology* 63: 293–300.

Marshall, M., Lewis, S., Lockwood, A., et al. 2005. Association between duration of untreated psychosis and outcome in cohorts of first-episode patients. *Arch Gen Psychiatry* 62: 975–83.

Martin, J. L., Barbanoj, M. J., Schlaepfer, T. E., et al. 2002. Transcranial magnetic stimulation for treating depression. *Cochrane Database Syst Rev* 2: CD003493.

Mason, B. J., Kocsis, J. H., Frances, A. J., and Mann, J. J. 1990. Amoxapine versus amitriptyline for continuation therapy of depression. *J Clin Psychopharmacol* 10: 338–43.

Masters, K. M. and Wandless, D. 2005. Use of pulse oximetry during restraint episodes. *Psychiatr Serv* 56: 1313–14.

Maudsley, H. 1867. *The physiology and pathology of mind.* New York: Appleton.

Mayberg, H. S., Lozano, A. M., Voon, V., et al. 2005. Deep brain stimulation for treatment-resistant depression. *Neuron* 45: 651–60.

McDonald, C., Bullmore, E., Sham, P., et al. 2005. Regional volume deviations of brain structure in schizophrenia and psychotic bipolar disorder. *Br J Psychiatry* 18: 369–77.

McGrath, P. I., Stewart, J.W., Nunes, E.N., and Quitkin, F.M. 1994. Treatment response of depressed outpatients unresponsive to both a tricyclic and a monoamine oxidase inhibitor antidepressant. *J Clin Psychiatry* 55: 336–9.

McIntyre, R., Mancini, D. A., McCann, S., et al. 2002. Topiramate versus bupropion SR when added to mood stabilizer therapy for the depressive phase of bipolar disorder: A preliminary single-blind study. *Bipolar Disord* 4: 207–13.

Meyer, J. H., Kruger, S., Wilson, A. A., et al. 2001. Lower dopamine transporter binding potential in striatum during depression. *Neuroreport* 12: 4121–5.

Meyers, B. S., Klimstra, S. A., Gabriele, M., et al. 2001. Continuation treatment of delusional depression in older adults. *Am J Geriatr Psychiatry* 9: 415–22.

Mingazzini, G. 1926. Die modifikationen der klinischen symptome, die einige psychosen in den letzten jahrzehnten erfahren haben. *Psychiatrisch-Neurologische Wochenschrift* 28: 68–72.

Mirza, N. R., Bright, J. L., Stanhope, K. J., et al. 2005. Lamotrigine has an anxiolytic-like profile in the rat conditioned emotional response test of anxiety: A potential role for sodium channels? *Psychopharmacol (Berlin)* 180: 159–68.

Mueser, K. T., Goodman, L. B., Trumbetta, S. L., et al. 1998. Trauma and posttraumatic stress disorder in severe mental illness. *J Consult Clin Psychol* 66: 493–9.

Muller-Siecheneder, F., Muller, M. J., Hillert, A., et al. 1998. Risperidone versus haloperidol and amitriptyline in the treatment of patients with a combined psychotic and depressive syndrome. *J Clin Psychopharmacol* 18: 111–20.

Mulsant, B. H., Haskett, R. F., Prudic, J., et al. 1997. Low use of neuroleptic drugs in the treatment of psychotic major depression. *Am J Psychiatry* 154: 559–61.

Mulsant, B. H., Sweet, R. A., Rosen, J., et al. 2001. A double-blind randomized comparison of nortriptyline plus perphenazine versus nortriptyline plus placebo in the treatment of psychotic depression in late life. *J Clin Psychiatry* 62: 597–604.

Munro, T. A. 1949. On depression. *Edinburgh Med J* 56: 530–43.

Musa, M. N. and Tripuraneni, B. R. 1993. Lithium-induced polyuria ameliorated by potassium supplementation. *Lithium* 4: 199–203.

Myers, B. S. and Greenberg, R. 1986. Late-life delusional depression. *J Affect Disord* 11: 133–7.

Naidu, P. S. and Kulkarni, S. K. 2001. Excitatory mechanisms in neuroleptic-induced vacuous chewing movements (VCMs): Possible involvement of calcium and nitric oxide. *Behav Pharmacol* 12: 209–16.

Naimark, D., Jackson, E., Rockwell, E., and Jeste, D. V. 1996. Psychotic symptoms in Parkinson's disease patients with dementia. *J Am Geriatr Soc* 44: 296–9.

Navarro, V., Gasto, C., Torres, X., et al. 2001. Citalopram versus nortriptyline in late-life depression: A 12-week randomized single-blind study. *Acta Psychiatr Scand* 103: 435–40.

Nelson, J. C. and Bowers, M. B., Jr. 1978. Delusional unipolar depression: Description and drug response. *Arch Gen Psychiatry* 35: 1321–8.

Nelson, J. C. and Charney, D. S. 1981. The symptoms of major depressive illness. *Am J Psychiatry* 138: 1–13.

Nelson, J. C. and Mazure, C. M. 1986. Lithium augmentation in psychotic depression refractory to combined drug treatment. *Am J Psychiatry* 143: 363–6.

Nelson, J. C., Charney, D. S., and Quinlan, D. M. 1981. Evaluation of the DSM-III criteria for melancholia. *Arch Gen Psychiatry* 38: 555–9.

Nelson, J. C., Price, L. H., Jatlow, P. I. 1986. Neuroleptic dose and desipramine concentrations during combined treatment of unipolar delusional depression. *Am J Psychiatry* 143: 1151–4.

Nelson, L. A. and Swartz, C. M. 2000. Melancholic symptoms from concurrent olanzapine and fluoxetine. *Ann Clin Psychiatry* 12: 167–70.

Niskanen, P. and Achte, K. A. 1972. Disease pictures of depressives psychoses in the decades 1880–89, 1900–09, 1930–39, and 1960–69. *Psychiatria Fennica* 95–100.

Olfson, M., Marcus, S., Sackeim, H. A., Thompson, J., and Pincus, H. A. 1998. Use of ECT for the inpatient treatment of recurrent major depression. *Am J Psychiatry* 155: 2–29.

Overall, J. E., Hollister, L. E., Johnson, M., and Pennington, V. 1966. Nosology of depression and differential response to drugs. *JAMA* 195: 946–8.

Overall, J. E., Hollister, L. E., Pokorny, A. D., et al. 1962. Drug therapy in depressions: Controlled evaluation of imipramine, isocarboxazide, dextroamphetamine-amobarbital, and placebo. *Clin Pharmacol Ther* 3: 16–22.

Pai, M., White, A. C., and Deane, A. G. 1986. Lithium augmentation in the treatment of delusional depression. *Br J Psychiatry* 148: 736–8.

Papakostas, G. I., Alpert, J. E., and Fava, M. 2003. S-adenosyl-methionine in depression: A comprehensive review of the literature. *Curr Psychiatry Rep* 5: 460–6.

Pare, C. M., Kline, N., Hallstrom, C., and Cooper, T. B. 1982. Will amitriptyline prevent the "cheese" reaction of monoamine oxidase inhibitors? *Lancet* 2(8291): 183–6.

Parker, G. 2000. Classifying depression: Should paradigms lost be regained? *Am J Psychiatry* 157: 1195–203.

Parker, G. 2004. Evaluating treatments for the mood disorders: Time for the evidence to get real. *Aust NZ J Psychiatry* 38: 408–14.

Parker, G., Hadzi-Pavlovic, D., Brodaty, H., et al. 1995. Sub-typing depression, II. Clinical distinction of psychotic depression and non-psychotic melancholia. *Psychol Med* 25: 825–32.

Parker, G., Hadzi-Pavlovic, D., Hickie, I., et al. 1991a. Distinguishing psychotic and non-psychotic melancholia. *J Affect Disord* 22: 135–48.

Parker, G., Hadzi-Pavlovic, D., Hickie, I., et al. 1991b. Psychotic depression: A review and clinical experience. *Aust NZ J Psychiatry* 25: 169–80.

Parker, G., Roussos, J., Mitchell, P., et al. 1997. Distinguishing psychotic depression from melancholia. *J Affect Disord* 42: 155–67.

Parker, G., Roy, K., Hadzi-Pavlovic, D., and Pedic, F. 1992. Psychotic (delusional) depression: A meta-analysis of physical treatments. *J Affect Disord* 24: 17–24.

Parvin, M. M., Swartz, C. M., and LaMontagne, B. 2004. Patient education by ECT experienced volunteer. *J ECT* 20: 127–9.

Perry, P. J., Morgan, D. E., Smith, R. E., and Tsuang, M. T. 1982. Treatment of unipolar depression accompanied by delusions. ECT versus tricyclic antidepressant – antipsychotic combinations. *J Affect Disord* 4: 195–200.

Petrides, G., Fink, M., Husain, M. M., et al. 2001. ECT remission rates in psychotic versus nonpsychotic depressed patients: A report from CORE. *J ECT* 17: 244–53.

Piasecki, S. D. and Jefferson, J. W. 2004. Psychiatric complications of deep brain stimulation for Parkinson's disease. *J Clin Psychiatry* 65: 845–9.

Placidi, G. F., Lenzi, A., Lzzerini, F., et al. 1986. The comparative efficacy and safety of carbamazepine versus lithium: A randomized, double-blind 3-year trial in 83 patients. *J Clin Psychiatry* 47: 490–4.

Plath, S. 1996. *The bell jar* (1971), 25th anniversary edn. New York: HarperCollins.

Pollak, P., Tison, F., Rascol, O., et al. 2004. Clozapine in drug induced psychosis in Parkinson's disease: A randomised, placebo controlled study with open follow up. *J Neurol Neurosurg Psychiatry* 75: 689–95.

Pope, H. G. and Katz, D. L. 1994. Psychiatric and medical effects of anabolic-androgenic steroid use. A controlled study of 160 athletes. *Arch Gen Psychiatry* 51: 375–82.

Popli, A. P., Fuller, M. A., and Jaskiw, G. E. 1997. Sertraline and psychotic symptoms: A case series. *Ann Clin Psychiatry* 9: 15–17.

Price, J. P. 1978. Chronic depressive illness. *BMJ* 1: 1200–1.

Price, L. H., Conwell, Y., and Nelson, J. C. 1983. Lithium augmentation of combined neuroleptic-tricyclic treatment in delusional depression. *Am J Psychiatry* 140: 318–22.

Prien, R. F., Kupfer, D. J., Mansky, P. A., et al. 1984. Drug therapy in the prevention of recurrences in unipolar and bipolar affective disorders. Report of the NIMH Collaborative Study Group comparing lithium carbonate, imipramine, and a lithium carbonate-imipramine combination. *Arch Gen Psychiatry* 41: 1096–104.

Quitkin, F., Klein, D. F., and Rifkin, A. 1978. Imipramine response in deluded depressive patients. *Am J Psychiatry* 7: 806–11

Rabheru, K. and Persad, E. 1997. A review of continuation and maintenance electroconvulsive therapy. *Can J Psychiatry* 42: 476–84.

Rabiner, E. A., Bhagwagar, Z., Gunn, R. N., et al. 2001. Pindolol augmentation of selective serotonin reuptake inhibitors: PET evidence that the dose used in clinical trials is too low. *Am J Psychiatry* 158: 2080–2.

Raja, M. and Azzoni, A. 2003. Oxcarbazepine vs. valproate in the treatment of mood and schizoaffective disorders. *Int J Neuropsychopharmacol* 6: 409–14.

Ranjan, R. and Meltzer, H. Y. 1996. Acute and long-term effectiveness of clozapine in treatment-resistant psychotic depression. *Biol Psychiatry* 40: 253–8.

Rapaport, M. H., Judd, L. L., Schettler, P. J., et al. 2002. A descriptive analysis of minor depression. *Am J Psychiatry* 159: 637–43.

Ries, R. and Bokan, J. 1979. Electroconvulsive therapy following pituitary surgery. *J Nerv Ment Dis* 167: 767–8.

Robinson, A. D. T. 1988. A century of delusions in south west Scotland. *Br J Psychiatry* 153: 163–7.

Roose, S. P., Glassman, A. H., Walsh, B. T., et al. 1983. Depression, delusions, and suicide. *Am J Psychiatry* 140: 1159–62.

Roose, S. P., Sackeim, H. A., Krisnan, K. R. R., et al. 2004. Antidepressant pharmacotherapy in the treatment of depression in the very old: A randomized, placebo-controlled trial. *Am J Psychiatry* 161: 2050–9.

Ropacki, S. A. and Jeste, D. V. 2005. Epidemiology of and risk factors for psychosis of Alzheimer's disease: A review of 55 studies published from 1990 to 2003. *Am J Psychiatry* 162: 2022–30.

Rothschild, A. J. and Duval, S. E. 2003. How long should patients with psychotic depression stay on the antipsychotic medication? *J Clin Psychiatry* 64: 390–6.

Rothschild, A. J. and Phillips, K. A. 1999. Selective serotonin inhibitors and delusional depression. *Am J Psychiatry* 156: 977–8.

Rothschild, A. J., Samson, J. A., Bessette, M. P., et al. 1993. Efficacy of the combination of fluoxetine and perphenazine in the treatment of psychotic depression. *J Clin Psychiatry* 54: 338–42.

Rothschild, A. J., Williamson, D. J., Tohen, M. F., et al. 2004. A double-blind, randomized study of olanzapine and olanzapine/fluoxetine combination for major depression with psychotic features. *J Clin Psychopharmacol* 24: 365–73.

Rush, A. J., Marangell, L. B., Sackeim, H. A., et al. 2005. Vagus nerve stimulation for treatment-resistant depression: A randomized, controlled acute phase trial. *Biol Psychiatry* 58: 347–54.

Ruskin, D. B. and Goldner, R. 1959. Treatment of depressions in private practice with imipramine. *Dis Nerv Syst* 20: 391–9.

Sackeim, H. A., Prudic, J., Devanand, D. P., et al. 1993. Effects of stimulus intensity and electrode placement on the efficacy and cognitive effects of electroconvulsive therapy. *N Engl J Med* 328: 839–46.

Sanchez-Ramos, J. R., Ortoll, R., and Paulson, G. W. 1996. Visual hallucinations associated with Parkinson disease. *Arch Neurol* 53: 1265–8.

Sands, J. R. and Harrow, M. 1995. Vulnerability to psychosis in unipolar major depression: Is premorbid functioning involved? *Am J Psychiatry* 152: 1009–15.

Santora, M. and Carey, B. 2005. Depressed? New York screens for people at risk. *New York Times*, April 13, p. 1, 16.

Sareen, J., Cox, B. J., Afifi, T. O., et al. 2005. Anxiety disorders and risk for suicidal ideation and suicide attempts. *Arch Gen Psychiatry* 62: 1249–57.

Schatzberg, A. F. and Rothschild, A. J. 1992. Psychotic (delusional) major depression: Should it be included as a distinct syndrome in DSM-IV? *Am J Psychiatry* 149: 733–45.

Schatzberg, A. F., Posener, J. A., DeBattista, C., et al. 2000. Neuropsychological deficits in psychotic versus nonpsychotic major depression and no mental illness. *Am J Psychiatry* 157: 1095–100.

Schildkraut, J. J. 1965. The catecholamine hypothesis of affective disorders: A review of supporting evidence. *Am J Psychiatry* 122: 509–22.

Schmauss, M., Kapfhammer, H. P., Meyr, P., and Hoff, P. 1988. Combined MAO-inhibitor and tri- (tetra) cyclic antidepressant treatment in therapy resistant depression. *Prog Neuropsychopharmacol Biol Psychiatry* 12: 523–32.

Schneider, K. 1920. Die schichtung des emotionalen lebens und der aufbau der depressionszustände. *Zeitschrift für die gesamte Neurologie und Psychiatrie* 59: 281–6.

Schneider, L. S., Dagerman, K. S., and Insel, P. 2005. Risk of death with atypical antipsychotic drug treatment for dementia. *JAMA* 294: 1934–43.

Schneider, L. S., Nelson, J. C., Clary, C. M., et al. 2003. An 8-week multicenter, parallel-group, double-blind, placebo-controlled study of sertraline in elderly outpatients with major depression. *Am J Psychiatry* 160: 1277–85.

Schneider, P. B. and Villa, J. L. 1961. Essai d'un nouveau médicament antidépressif: Le G 33040 [Opipramol]. *Praxis* 50: 1378–81.

Schulz, S. C. 1986. The use of low-dose neuroleptics in the treatment of "schizo-obsessive patients." *Am J Psychiatry* 143: 1318–19.

Schwartz, A. C., Bradley, R. L., Sexton, M., et al. 2005. Posttraumatic stress disorder among African Americans in an inner city mental health clinic. *Psychiatr Serv* 56: 212–15.

Seach, J. 2005. How dangerous are volcanoes? http: //www.volcanolive.com/eruption3.html, accessed November 4, 2005.

Shepherd, M. 1959. Evaluation of drugs in the treatment of depression. *Can Psychiatr Assoc J* 4: 120–8.

Shiraishi, H., Koizumi, J., Hori, M., et al. 1992. A computerized tomographic study in patients with delusional and non-delusional depression. *Jap J Psychiatry Neurol* 46: 99–105.

Shorter, E. 1990. Private clinics in central Europe 1850–1933. *Soc Hist Med* 3: 159–95.

Shorter, E. 1997. *A history of psychiatry from the era of the asylum to the age of Prozac*. New York: John Wiley.

Shorter, E. 2005. *A historical dictionary of psychiatry*. New York: Oxford University Press.

Signer, S. F. and Billings, R. F. 1984. Amoxapine failure – a neuroleptic property? *Can J Psychiatry* 29: 510–2.

Sigwald, J. and Bouttier, D. 1953. L'utilisation des propriétés neuroplégiques du chlorhydrate chloro-3-(diméthylamino-3'-propyl)-10-phénothiazine en thérapeutique neuro-psychiatrique. *Presse Médicale* 61: 607–9.

Sigwald, J., Bouttier, D., and Nicolas-Charles, P. 1956. Ambulatory treatment with chlorpromazine. *J Clin Exp Psychopathol* 17: 57–69.

Simeon, D., Stanley, B., Frances, A., et al. 1992. Self-mutilation in personality disorders: Psychological and biological correlates. *Am J Psychiatry* 149: 221–6.

Simpson, G. M., El Sheshai, A., Rady, A., et al. 2003. Sertraline as monotherapy in the treatment of psychotic and nonpsychotic depression. *J Clin Psychiatry* 64: 959–65.

Simpson, S., Baldwin, R. C., Jackson, A., and Burns, A. 1999. The differentiation of DSM-III-R psychotic depression in later life from nonpsychotic depression: Comparisons of brain changes measured by multispectral analysis of magnetic resonance brain images, neuropsychological findings, and clinical features. *Biol Psychiatry* 45: 193–204.

Sims, J. 1799. Pathological remarks upon various kinds of alienation of mind. *Memoirs Med Soc Lond* 5: 372–406.

Slater, L. 2005. Who holds the clicker? *Mother Jones* (magazine), November, 30(6), pp. 62–7, 90, 92.

Solan, W. J., Khan, A., Avery, D. H., and Cohen, S. 1988. Psychotic and nonpsychotic depression: Comparison of response to ECT. *J Clin Psychiatry* 49: 97–9

Spiker, D. G., Dealy, R. S., Hanin, I., et al. 1986. Treating delusional depressives with amitriptyline. *J Clin Psychiatry* 47: 243–6.

Spiker, D. G., Stein, J., and Rich, C. L. 1985a. Delusional depression and electroconvulsive therapy: One year later. *Convuls Ther* 1: 167–72.

Spiker, D. G., Weiss, J. C., Dealy, R. S., et al. 1985b. The pharmacological treatment of delusional depression. *Am J Psychiatry* 142: 430–6.

Spitzer, R. L., Endicott, J., and Robins, E. 1978. Research diagnostic criteria: Rationale and reliability. *Arch Gen Psychiatry* 35: 773–82.

Spitzer, R. L., Endicott, J., Robins, E., et al. 1975. Preliminary report of the reliability of research diagnostic criteria applied to psychiatric case records. In Abraham Dusilovsky et al. (eds) *Predictability in psychopharmacology: Preclinical and clinical correlations*. New York: Raven, pp. 1–47.

Starkstein, S. E., Jorge, R., Mizrahi, R., and Robinson, R. G. 2005. The construct of minor and major depression in Alzheimer's Disease. *Am J Psychiatry* 162: 2086–93.

Stephens, J. H. and McHugh, P. R. 1991. Characteristics and long-term follow-up of patients hospitalized for mood disorders in the Phipps Clinic, 1913–1940. *J Nerv Ment Dis* 179: 64–73.

Stevinson, C. and Ernst, E. 2004. Can St. John's wort trigger psychosis? *Int J Clin Pharmacol Ther* 42: 473–80.

Stoll, A. L., Mayer, P. V., Kolbrener, M., et al. 1994. Antidepressant-associated mania: A controlled comparison with spontaneous mania. *Am J Psychiatry* 151: 1642–5.

Strakowski, S. M., Flaum, M., Amador, X., et al. 1996. Racial differences in the diagnosis of psychosis. *Schizophrenia Res* 21: 117–24.

Stueber, D. and Swartz, C. M. 2006. Carvedilol suppresses intractable hiccups. *J Am Board Fam Med* 19: 418–21.

Swartz, C. M. 1979. Depression with nonauditory hallucinations: Success with phenelzine. *Psychosomatics* 20: 286–7.

Swartz, C. M. 1982. Dependency of antidepressant efficacy on thyroid hormone potentiation: Case studies. *J Nerv Ment Dis* 170: 50–2.

Swartz, C. M. 1984. The justification for ECT. *Behav Brain Sci* 7: 37.

Swartz, C. M. 1989. Safety and ECT stimulus electrodes: I. Heat liberation at the electrode-to-skin interface. *Convuls Ther* 5: 171–5.

Swartz, C. M. 1995. Tardive psychopathology. *Neuropsychobiology* 32: 115–19.

Swartz, C. M. 2000. Physiological response to ECT stimulus dose. *Psychiatry Res* 97: 229–35.

Swartz, C. M. 2001a. Misdiagnosis of schizophrenia for a patient with epilepsy. *Psychiatr Serv* 52: 109.

Swartz, C. M. 2001b Olanzapine-lithium encephalopathy. *Psychosomatics* 42: 370.

Swartz, C. M. 2002. Olanzapine-induced depression. *J Pharm Technol* 18: 321–3.

Swartz, C. M. 2003a. Antipsychotics as thought simplifiers. *Psychiatric Times*, January, 20(1), pp. 12–14.

Swartz, C. M. 2003b. Simplicity as a complication: Antipsychotics. *Psychiatric Times*, February, 20(2): 44–6.

Swartz, C. M. 2003c. Pseudomania. *Psychiatric Times*, June, 20, pp. 23–5.

Swartz, C. M. 2004a. Antipsychotic psychosis. *Psychiatric Times*, October, 21 (11), pp. 17–20.

Swartz, C. M. 2004b. Iatrogenic cancer. *Psychiatric Times*, September, 21(10), pp. 21–4.

Swartz, C. M. 2005. Aspiration and postictal agitation after electroconvulsive therapy with propofol but no succinylcholine or atropinic agent. *J ECT* 21: 50–1.

Swartz, C. M. and Galang, R. L. 2001. Adverse outcome with delay in catatonia identification in elderly patients. *Am J Geriatric Psychiatry* 9: 78–80.

Swartz, C. M. and Guadagno, G. 1998. Melancholia with onset during treatment with SSRIs. *Ann Clin Psychiatry* 10: 177–9.

Swartz, C. M. and Manly, D. T. 2000. Efficiency of the stimulus characteristics of ECT. *Am J Psychiatry* 157: 1504–6.

Swartz, C. M. and Nelson, A. I. 2005. Rational electroconvulsive therapy electrode placement. *Psychiatry* 2: 37–43.

Swartz, C. M., Morrow, V., Surles, L., and James, J. F. 2001. Long-term outcome after ECT for catatonic depression. *J ECT* 17: 180–3.

Sweeney, D., Nelson, C., Bowers, M., et al. 1978. Delusional versus non-delusional depression: Neurochemical differences. *Lancet* 2: 100–1.

Taylor, M. A., Berenbaum, S. A., Jampala, V. C., and Cloninger, C. R. 1993. Are schizophrenia and affective disorder related? Preliminary data from a family study. *Am J Psychiatry* 150: 278–85.

Taylor, M. A. and Fink, M. 2006. *Melancholia: The diagnosis, pathophysiology, and treatment of depressive illness.* Cambridge, UK: Cambridge University Press.

Tsuang, D. and Coryell, W. 1993. An 8-year follow-up of patients with DSM-III-R psychotic depression, schizoaffective disorder, and schizophrenia. *Am J Psychiatry* 150: 1182–8.

Tsuang, M. T., Dempsey, M., and Rauscher, F. 1976. A study of atypical schizophrenia. *Arch Gen Psychiatry* 33: 1157–60.

Tsuang, M. T., Woolson, R. F., and Fleming, J. A. 1979. Long-term outcome of major psychoses. *Arch Gen Psychiatry* 36: 1295–304.

Tsuang, T., Woolson, R. F., and Fleming, J. A. 1979. Long-term outcome of major psychoses. *Arch Gen Psychiatry* 36: 1295–304.

Valenstein, E. S. 1987. *Great and desperate cures: The rise and decline of psychosurgery and other radical treatments for mental illness.* New York: Basic Books.

van den Broek, N.W., Birkenhager, T.K., Mulder, P.G., et al. 2006. Imipramine is effective in preventing relapse in electro convulsive therapy-responsive depressed inpatients with prior pharmacotheraphy treatment failure: a randomized, placebo-controlled trial. *J Clin Psychiatry* 67: 263–8.

Viguera, A. C., Baldessarini, R. J., Hegarty, J. D., et al. 1997. Clinical risk following abrupt and gradual withdrawal of maintenance neuroleptic treatment. *Arch Gen Psychiatry* 54: 49–55.

Von Orelli, A. 1954. Der Wandel des Inhaltes der depressiven Ideen bei der reinen Melancholie, unter besonderer Berücksichtigung des Inhaltes der Versündigungsideen. *Schweizer Archiv für Neurologie und Psychiatrie* 73: 217–87.

Vythilingam, M., Chen, J., Bremner, J. D., et al. 2003. Psychotic depression and mortality. *Am J Psychiatry* 160: 574–6.

Wada, H., Nakajoh, K., Satoh-Nakagawa, T., et al. 2001. Risk factors of aspiration pneumonia in Alzheimer's disease patients. *Gerontology* 47: 271–6.

Walen, S. 2002. It's a funny thing about suicide: A personal experience. *Br J Guid Couns* 30: 415–30.

Weiss, E., Hummer, M., Koller, D., et al. 2000. Off-label use of antipsychotic drugs. *J Clin Psychopharmacol* 20: 695–8.

Weissman, M. M., Prusoff, B. A., and Merikangas, K. R. 1984. Is delusional depression related to bipolar disorder? *Am J Psychiatry* 141: 892–3.

Wernicke, C. 1900. *Grundriss der Psychiatrie*. Leipzig: Thieme.

Wheatley, D. 1972. Potentiation of amitriptyline by thyroid hormone. *Arch Gen Psychiatry* 26: 229–33.

Whitty, P., Clarke, M., McTigue, O., et al. 2005. Diagnostic stability four years after a first episode of psychosis. *Psychiatr Serv* 56: 1084–8.

Wilcox, J. A., Ramirez, A. L., and Baida-Fragoso, N. 2000. The prognostic value of thought disorder in psychotic depression. *Ann Clin Psychiatry* 12: 1–4.

Wolkowitz, O. M., Reus, V. I., Chan, T., et al. 1999. Antiglucocorticoid treatment of depression: Double-blind ketoconazole. *Biol Psychiatry* 45: 1070–4.

World Health Organization (WHO) 1967. *Research in psychopharmacology: Report of a WHO Scientific Group*. WHO Technical Report Series No. 371. Geneva: WHO.

Yassa, R., Nastase, C., Dupont, D., and Thibeau, M. 1992. Tardive dyskinesia in elderly psychiatric patients: A 5-year study. *Am J Psychiatry* 149: 1206–11.

Zanardi, R., Franchini, L., Gasperini, M., et al. 1996. Double-blind controlled trial of sertraline versus paroxetine in the treatment of delusional depression. *Am J Psychiatry* 153: 1631–3.

Zanardi, R., Franchini, L., Gasperini, M., et al. 1997. Long-term treatment of psychotic (delusional) depression with fluvoxamine: An open pilot study. *Int Clin Psychopharmacol* 12: 195–7.

Zanardi, R., Franchini, L., Gasperini, M., et al. 1998. Faster onset of action of fluvoxamine in combination with pindolol in the treatment of delusional depression: A controlled study. *J Clin Psychopharmacol* 18: 441–6.

Zanardi, R., Franchini, L., Perez, J., et al. 1999. Dr. Zanardi and colleagues reply. *Am J Psychiatry* 156: 978.

Zanardi, R., Franchini, L., Serretti, A., et al. 2000. Venlafaxine versus fluvoxamine in the treatment of delusional depression: A pilot double-blind controlled study. *J Clin Psychiatry* 61: 26–9.

Zimmerman, M. and Spitzer, R. L. 1989. Melancholia: From DSM-III to DSM-III-R. *Am J Psychiatry* 146: 20–8.

Zimmerman, M., Chelminski, I., and McDermut, W. 2002. Major depressive disorder and axis I diagnostic comorbidity. *J Clin Psychiatry* 63: 187–93.

Zwanzger, P., Ella, R., Keck, M. E., Rupprecht, R., and Padberg, F. 2002. Occurrence of delusions during repetitive transcranial magnetic stimulation (rTMS) in major depression. *Biol Psychiatry* 51: 602–3.

Index

Printed in the United States
by Bookmasters

Printed in the United States
By Bookmasters